M I L E

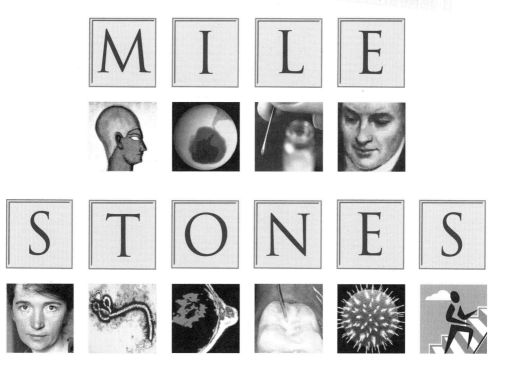

S T O N E S

IN PUBLIC HEALTH

ACCOMPLISHMENTS
IN PUBLIC HEALTH
OVER THE LAST
100 YEARS

Acknowledgments

Milestones in Public Health is a journey through the seminal accomplishments in the field of public health during the 20th century, as well as an inquisitive—and hopefully—inspirational look at the next set of challenges faced by our nation's public health system. It is not intended to be a textbook or research publication. Rather, it is a general-interest book about public health that should appeal to students in any health-related field, as well as public health professionals and others with a keen interest in this field. At the same time, I hope, in a very personal way, that this book will engage those with little knowledge of the field to learn more about it. I know that a book can change a life's direction, as I myself entered public health after a book awakened my curiosity about the prevention and control of infectious diseases.

Readers will note that we have listed all sources by chapter at the end of the book rather than annotating each fact as it appears in the body of the text. This conscious decision on our part should make the book more readable while allowing those who would like to pursue particular topics to find useful references.

Milestones in Public Health is the third in a series of books published by Pfizer Inc's Public Health Group. These books are a part of our ongoing commitment to public awareness and understanding of the field of public health. As with our previous publications – *Advancing Healthy Populations: The Pfizer Guide to Careers in Public Health* and *The Faces of Public Health* – this book represents the collective efforts of many individuals who have dedicated countless hours to its development and production. Our sincere thanks go to Dilia Santana and Oscar Perdomo, U.S. Public Health, Pfizer Inc; Ana Rita González, ScD, Sydney Ann Neuhaus, and Nadjha Acosta of Fleishman-Hillard International Communications; David L. Farren; and Matt Warhaftig of Warhaftig Associates.

Special thanks must also go to our expert reviewers: Myron Allukian, retired from the Boston Health Commission *(Oral Health)*; Susan Baker, Bloomberg School of Public Health, Johns Hopkins University *(Automotive Safety)*;

Joseph Califano, Executive Director, CASA, Columbia University *(Addiction)*; James Curran, Dean, Rollins School of Public Health, Emory University *(Infectious Disease Control)*; D.A. Henderson, Center for Biosecurity, University of Pittsburgh Medical Center and Dean Emeritus, Johns Hopkins University School of Hygiene and Public Health *(Vaccines)*; Richard Jackson, California Department of Health Services *(Environmental Health)*; William Keck, Northeastern Ohio Universities College of Medicine *(Public Health Infrastructure)*; Thomas Pearson, School of Medicine & Dentistry, University of Rochester *(Cardiovascular Disease)*; Allen Rosenfield, Dean, Mailman School of Public Health, Columbia University *(Maternal and Child Health)*; John A. Seffrin, Executive Director, American Cancer Society *(Cancer)*; and Ernest Julian, Director of Food Protection, Rhode Island Department of Health *(Food Safety)*. We appreciate as well the contributions of David Satcher, former Surgeon General and Interim President, Morehouse College of Medicine.

We are especially grateful to Hugh Tilson, School of Public Health, University of North Carolina at Chapel Hill. Deeply committed to raising the visibility of the public health community, Hugh provided important perspective and insights throughout the development of this book. His energy and enthusiasm for our entire series of books are invaluable and drive us toward continued partnership with this special community.

Barbara A. DeBuono, MD, MPH
November 2005

Contents

Prologue ———————————————————— *1*
>   With remarks by David Satcher, MD, PhD
>   Morehouse School of Medicine,
>   16th U.S. Surgeon General

1. Vaccines and the Eradication of Smallpox ——————— *5*
>   Expert Reviewer: D.A. Henderson, MD, MPH
>   Center for Biosecurity, University of Pittsburgh;
>   and Dean Emeritus, Bloomberg School of Public Health,
>   Johns Hopkins University
>
>   *Looking Back* ————————————————— *5*
>   *Case Study:* Eradication of Smallpox ——————— *9*
>   *Vignette:* Hib Vaccine ————————————— *15*
>   *Looking Ahead:* Advances in Vaccine Research ——— *16*

2. Automotive Safety ——————————————————— *21*
>   Expert Reviewer: Susan Baker, MPH
>   Bloomberg School of Public Health,
>   Johns Hopkins University
>
>   *Looking Back* ————————————————— *21*
>   *Case Study:* Development of Seat Belts ——————— *28*
>   *Vignette:* Air Bags ————————————————— *31*
>   *Looking Ahead:* Advances in Automobile
>   Manufacturing ————————— *33*

3. Environmental Health ——————————————————— *37*
>   Expert Reviewer: Richard Jackson, MD, MPH
>   Division of Environmental Health Sciences
>   University of California, School of Public Health
>
>   *Looking Back* ————————————————— *37*
>   *Case Study:* Lead Poisoning ————————————— *41*
>   *Vignette:* Asbestos ————————————————— *49*
>   *Looking Ahead:* Asthma ———————————————— *51*

4. Infectious Disease Control —————————————— *59*
>   Expert Reviewer: James Curran, MD, MPH
>   Rollins School of Public Health, Emory University
>
>   *Looking Back* ————————————————— *59*
>   *Case Study:* HIV/AIDS ——————————————— *65*
>   *Vignette:* Development of Penicillin ——————— *73*
>   *Looking Ahead:* Antibiotic Resistance ——————— *76*

5. *Cancer* _____ *83*

    Expert Reviewer: John Seffrin, PhD
    American Cancer Society

    Looking Back _____ *83*
    Case Study: Screening Tools for Cancer Detection __ *90*
    Vignette: Skin Cancer and Sunblock/SPF Products __ *100*
    Looking Ahead: Genomic Research and Medicine ___ *101*

6. *Cardiovascular Disease* _____ *107*

    Expert Reviewer: Thomas A. Pearson, MD, MPH, PhD
    University of Rochester School of Medicine

    Looking Back _____ *108*
    Case Study: Risk Assessment _____ *111*
    Vignette: Statins _____ *114*
    Looking Ahead: Obesity in Young Populations _____ *116*

7. *Safer and Healthier Foods* _____ *123*

    Expert Reviewer: Ernest Julian, PhD
    Rhode Island Department of Health

    Looking Back _____ *123*
    Case Study: Jack in the Box *E. coli* Outbreak _____ *132*
    Vignette: Nutrition Labeling on Food Packaging ___ *138*
    Looking Ahead: How to Ensure a Safe Food Supply_ *142*

8. *Advances in Maternal and Child Health* _____ *147*

    Expert Reviewer: Allen Rosenfield, MD
    Mailman School of Public Health, Columbia University

    Looking Back _____ *147*
    Case Study: Folic Acid _____ *158*
    Vignette: Amniocentesis _____ *161*
    Looking Ahead: Genetic Screening _____ *163*

9. *Oral Health* _____ *167*

    Expert Reviewer: Myron Allukian, DDS, MPH
    Former Director of Oral Health,
    Boston Public Health Commission

    Looking Back _____ *167*
    Case Study: Fluoridation _____ *176*
    Vignette: Dental Sealants _____ *182*
    Looking Ahead: Oral Diseases, Still
                 a Neglected Epidemic _____ *183*

Contents

10. Addiction ———————————————————————— *191*
        Expert Reviewer: Joseph A. Califano, Jr.
        National Center on Addiction and
        Substance Abuse, Columbia University

        Looking Back ———————————————————— *191*
        Case Study: Tobacco ——————————————— *199*
        Vignette: Mothers Against Drunk Driving (MADD) *204*
        Looking Ahead: Fighting Addiction
                in Young Women ——————————— *207*

11. U.S. Public Health Infrastructure ——————————— *213*
        Expert Reviewer: C. William Keck, MD, MPH
        Northeastern Ohio Universities College of Medicine

        Looking Back ———————————————————— *213*
        Case Study: The Creation of CDC ——————— *222*
        Vignette: Surgeon General's Report of 1964 ——— *225*
        Looking Ahead: Public Health –
                A 21st Century Perspective ——— *227*

Epilogue ———————————————————————————— *233*
        Barbara A. DeBuono, MD, MPH
        Pfizer Inc.

References ———————————————————————————— *238*

Prologue

Public health is the art and science of protecting and improving the health of a community through an organized and systematic effort that includes education, assurance of the provision of health services and protection of the public from exposures that will cause harm. In other words, public health is what we as a society do collectively to assure the conditions in which people can be healthy. In order to effectively address challenges to people's health, public health practice requires an organized and sustained population-based approach.

Milestones in Public Health portrays public health as the vital, critical field it is today in the United States. Each chapter in the book celebrates an acknowledged milestone of public health, exploring first its historical developments, followed by an in-depth case study of the milestone and a vignette that illustrates another facet of the milestone, and concluding with a look ahead. The "Looking Ahead" section predicts advances yet to come in each of the broad areas of public health where milestones occurred, and acknowledges the paramount issue of preparedness now facing the public health community. The "Looking Ahead" sections may also explore issues of particular concern to the public health community – such as asthma or obesity in young people – that have yet to be fully resolved or eradicated.

What are these milestones? In keeping with the list of ten acknowledged milestones in public health that have been identified by the Centers for Disease Control and Prevention, they are advances in addiction, automotive safety, cancer, cardiovascular disease, environmental and occupational health, food safety, infectious disease control, maternal and child health, oral health, and vaccines. To bring it all together, the concluding chapter explores how the development of the public health infrastructure in the United States has contributed greatly to advances in public health, serving as a model for the world.

The milestones identified in this book signify the most significant achievements in public health from the last century. As you read the chapters, the long, rich history of public health should come to life. Through the historical developments, case studies and vignettes, your insights into the many successes of public health and the challenges that were overcome should deepen. Too often we fail to appreciate the way public health, so basic to the overall health of Americans, improves our daily lives. Public health works best when its successes are hidden, forestalling crises before the public grows alarmed. This book seeks to shed light on the underappreciated achievements of public health and to lay claim, in the open, to its vital work. It is time to celebrate public health.

Milestones in Public Health also seeks to reinforce a core trait of public health, namely that success redefines the challenge. Whether with cancer, infectious diseases, oral health, vaccines, or a host of other areas, advances yet to come owe their possibility to the hard, focused work of public health professionals today and in preceding decades. For example, in the chapter on vaccines, we learn that global eradication of smallpox finally succeeded in 1977 only after an intense, years-long effort led by the World Health Organization in sub-Saharan Africa and South Asia. Currently, public health professionals are overseeing an intense worldwide effort to eradicate polio. Once they succeed, other debilitating diseases will become targets, and the hard work of global eradication will continue. With each succeeding battle, refinements in the particular skills and techniques of public health will allow millions more of the world's people to benefit from advances that have benefited the people of the United States.

Another example of how success redefines the challenge comes from the chapter on oral health. Each community in the United States that has fluoridated its water supply demonstrates a reduction in the rate of dental caries in its young population. Yet, despite compelling evidence, the process of fluoridating the nation's water supply is far from complete. Even as public health experts gather and share statistics that demonstrate the good of a particular milestone, the challenge never dissipates.

Each case study and vignette in this book examines in depth the complexities of public health, highlighting how each milestone contributed so remarkably to the health of the American public. Furthermore, the lessons learned from these contributions promise to benefit the world's population. For example, in the chapter on infectious disease control, the public health response to the AIDS pandemic, which was first identified in 1981, demonstrates truly astounding progress against a disease that was at first always fatal and is now often a treatable, chronic condition. Despite this progress, however, the public health community still confronts the threat of a continuing AIDS pandemic, especially in sub-Saharan Africa, and the cold truths of no vaccine, no cure, and no inexpensive treatment therapies. As with the global eradication of smallpox, progress in fighting an epidemic – whether it is AIDS, dental caries, or polio, in one country or in one county – redefines the challenge. Always, new aspects of epidemics and new populations around the world await the vital work of the public health community.

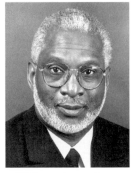

David Satcher, MD, PhD, former U.S. Surgeon General and current Interim President of the Morehouse School of Medicine in Atlanta, observes, "It is certainly true that public health always faces new challenges. However, embedded within these challenges are also new opportunities. It is clear that the focus of *Healthy People 2010* on the quality of life and on the targeting of disparities in health among different racial, ethnic and socioeconomic groups, represents both new challenges and new opportunities for public health. Public health is challenged to improve communication and to become more visible while developing new partnerships with and in the communities. Through these partnerships, the opportunity to better impact the all-important social determinants of health is real and tremendous."

The fact that public health is often invisible to the society it serves does not mean that its successes need to be hidden. *Milestones in Public Health* seeks to highlight how public health is at the core of our nation's progress and development and, at the same time, at the center of every family and community. *Milestones in Public Health* celebrates innovative solutions to public health challenges and the people and institutions that have implemented them. We hope this book will inspire new generations to become public health professionals and to hold in their hands the privilege and responsibility of building new milestones in public health. ◘

Chapter 1

Vaccines and the Eradication of Smallpox

Looking Back

"Ring around the rosy / A pocket full of posies / Ashes, ashes / We all fall down!"

Who isn't familiar with this childhood song? Many people might be surprised that this verse from the 1600s refers to an outbreak of the plague that devastated much of western Europe. Humans are still vulnerable to infectious diseases that through history have run rampant and killed vast numbers of people. The plague and smallpox did just that through much of the Dark and Middle Ages. New viruses such as HIV and SARS threaten humans in this century. The development of vaccines, therefore, is one of man's

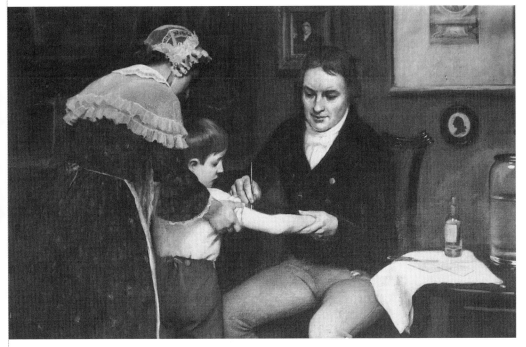

Dr. Edward Jenner inoculating a child with vaccinia virus taken from a cow.

greatest achievements. Vaccines protect people from fatal diseases, increase life expectancy and spare countless millions from pain and suffering.

The word *vaccine* comes from "vaca," Latin for cow. In 1796 in Gloucestershire, England, Dr. Edward Jenner discovered the first vaccine for smallpox. Jenner used material from a skin pustule which contained live *vaccinia virus*, a virus believed to be spread by cows to milkmaids, causing cowpox. Milkmaids who contracted cowpox, a mild disease in humans, seemed to be immune to smallpox, a virulent disease in humans. Jenner inoculated 24 children with the *vaccinia virus* and, like the milkmaids, they became immune to smallpox. Despite its success, the smallpox vaccine never became widespread enough to fully control the disease until late in the 20th century. It was especially problematic in the tropics, where suspensions could not be kept cool enough to be effective.

In 1895, Louis Pasteur developed the second vaccine, this one for rabies, a groundbreaking achievement. As the first example of a pathogen being altered for a therapeutic purpose, Pasteur's success opened the door to the field of immunobiology. That same year, Emil von Behring of Marburg University in Germany introduced the diphtheria vaccine. Three other vaccines – for typhoid, cholera and plague – were also developed late in the 19th century, but their use was not widespread at the beginning of the 20th century. Too many impoverished countries had no public health infrastructure, and the costs of vaccine distribution were prohibitive.

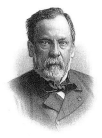

Louis Pasteur

Although smallpox was still widely prevalent in the United States at the beginning of the 20th century, it was by no means the only infectious disease to affect the American population. In 1920, for example, 469,924 cases of measles resulted in 7,575 deaths. That same year, nearly 148,000 diphtheria cases resulted in more than 13,000 deaths and 107,473 pertussis cases resulted in more than 5,000 deaths.

The development of the polio vaccine in 1955 had a radical impact on the use of vaccines in the United States. Parents were eager to protect their children from the "iron lung" disease, and Congress appropriated funds to inoculate school children with the polio vaccine. The U.S. government then began a major push to promote the use of vaccines. Today, most Americans don't think twice about vaccination. Children routinely undergo a series of vaccinations from birth through early childhood. These include vaccinations against diphtheria, pertussis, tetanus, poliomyelitis, measles, mumps, rubella, chicken pox and *Haemophilus influenzae*

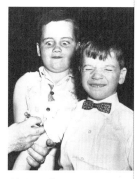

1955 polio vaccination.

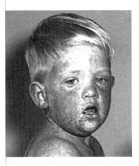

Child with the red blotchy pattern of measles.

type b (Hib). Some of these vaccines – measles, mumps and rubella (MMR), for example – have been combined and can be administered in one dose.

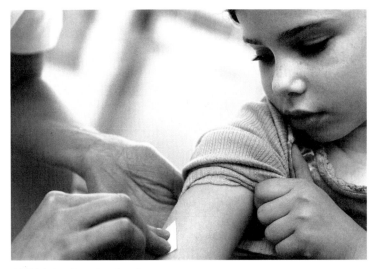

Child being inoculated today.

What exactly is a vaccine, and how is it made?

A vaccine is formally defined as "a preparation of killed, weakened, or fully infectious microbes that is given to produce or increase immunity to a particular disease." It can be given as an injection or in a form that can be swallowed (such as the polio vaccine). Vaccine researchers are inventing other means of safely and effectively delivering vaccines, such as nasal sprays.

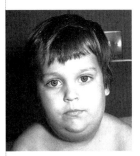

Child with mumps before vaccine was introduced in 1967.

Vaccines fall into three broad categories:

- ◆ Live (Attenuated) Vaccine. This type of vaccine uses a live, although weakened, version of the virus; it usually provides lifelong immunity to the recipient. Measles, mumps and rubella vaccines are examples of the live vaccine type.

- ◆ Killed (Inactivated) Vaccine. This vaccine uses a pathogen exposed to Formalin, a chemical that kills its genetic material, leaving just its shell. This form of vaccination usually requires several injections. The typhoid and Hib vaccines are examples.

- Toxoid Vaccine. This type of vaccine uses protein toxins that have been secreted by pathogenic bacteria but are inactivated. These vaccines also require several injections; diphtheria and tetanus vaccines are examples.

Since 1900, vaccines have been developed and licensed against 21 other diseases, with ten limited to selected populations at high risk according to residence, age, medical condition or risk behaviors. At the start of the 21st century, the vaccine-delivery system in the United States has evolved into a collaboration of all levels of government (federal, state, local) and public and private health care providers. The system continues to harness the latest technological advances. ◻

Case Study

Eradication of Smallpox

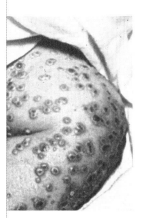

Smallpox

The story of vaccines begins with smallpox. Over thousands of years, hundreds of millions of people contracted the disease. The mummified body of Pharaoh Ramesses V of Egypt, who died in 1157 BC, shows a pustular rash, the earliest physical evidence of smallpox. During the next thousand years, traders carried the disease from Egypt to India, and from there it swept into China. It reached Japan by the 6th century and Europe by the 11th century, spread by returning crusaders. In the 20th century alone, an estimated 300 million people are believed to have died from it. Although smallpox was declared eradicated in 1980, the threat that it might be distributed by a terrorist has created fear.

Smallpox was particularly contagious and deadly in populations exposed for the first time to explorers from Europe. It paved the way for Spanish conquests in Latin America. ► Historians say that smallpox made the Spanish conquest of Mexico possible when Cortés and his *conquistadors* unintentionally introduced it to the Aztec population in Techotitlan in 1520. Smallpox ravaged the Aztecs, who had no natural immunity. Cortés and his men then proceeded to conquer a vastly weakened Aztec empire. During the French and Indian War, Lord Jeffrey Amherst deliberately infected blankets with smallpox and distributed them to Indians outside Fort Ticonderoga, the first known example of germ warfare.

Smallpox affects only humans. Transmission occurs when the *variola virus* (an *orthopoxvirus*) is inhaled in droplets or aerosols from the respiratory tract. Transmission also occurs through contact with skin lesions of infected patients or their bedding or clothing. The incubation period lasts seven to 17 days, with an average of 12 days. The disease presents first with fever for two to four days, followed by a rash lasting for weeks. The rash evolves slowly from papules to vesicles, then pustules and finally scabs, all at the same stage in any one area. Transmission

▼

Historians say that smallpox made the Spanish conquest of Mexico possible when Cortés and his *conquistadors* introduced it to the Aztec population in Techotitlan in 1520.

occurs mainly during the rash phase and diminishes as the lesions scab. Historically, about 50 percent of unvaccinated family members became infected. The mortality rate was 20 percent to 30 percent in unvaccinated populations, but many survivors were left with severe scarring and some with blindness.

Noting that survivors enjoyed lifelong immunity from any recurrence of the disease, physicians in China and India in the 10th century began to experiment with inoculation. In a process called *variolation*, these physicians introduced pus from smallpox pustules on infected people into non-infected people. Usually, the person who was inoculated would develop only a few pustules and a fever. However, in up to two percent of the cases, a virulent or aggressive form of the disease developed, causing death. Nonetheless, the odds were great that an inoculated person would sur-vive and, thereafter, enjoy lifelong immunity. The idea of *variolation* spread to Europe.   ►   In a famous case in 1721, Lady Mary Wortley Montagu, a smallpox survivor left with unsightly pockmarks, learned of *variolation* while her husband was posted to Constantinople as the British ambassador. She inoculated her children and persuaded the Princess of Wales to do the same. In fact, Edward Jenner, the discoverer of the smallpox vaccine, had been so inoculated.

In 1796, Dr. Jenner vaccinated 24 children with pus he had extracted from a milkmaid's cowpox pustule. First, he experimented with James Phipps, an eight-year-old boy, by introducing the cowpox strain through a cut in the arm. After purposely exposing the young boy to smallpox, Jenner followed the boy's status closely and concluded that the introduced *vaccinia virus* conferred immunity from smallpox. Next, Jenner inoculated his own 11-month-old son with the same result. The cowpox vaccine proved effective with all 24 children, conferring lifelong immunity from smallpox. By today's standards, Jenner's experiments on human subjects would not be considered ethical. Fortunately, the fact that his cowpox vaccine worked is not in dispute, and his discovery would protect millions of lives in the future.

▼

In 1721, smallpox survivor, Lady Montagu, learned of variolation while in Constantinople. She inoculated her children and persuaded the Princess of Wales to do the same.

Smallpox continued to appear in outbreaks throughout the world into the 20th century. In fact, a deadly smallpox outbreak in the United States between 1900 and 1904 caused an average of 48,164 cases in each of those years and resulted in an average of 1,528 deaths annually. Due to improved tracking and containment, outbreaks of the severe form of the disease *(variola major)* ended abruptly in 1929 in the U.S.; outbreaks of *variola minor*, the milder form, declined in the 1940s with the last U.S. case reported in 1949.

One scare in New York City in 1947 resulted in the city vaccinating more than six million residents. A Mexican businessman who traveled by bus to the city, unaware that he was incubating smallpox, spread the disease to 12 people, two of whom died, including him.

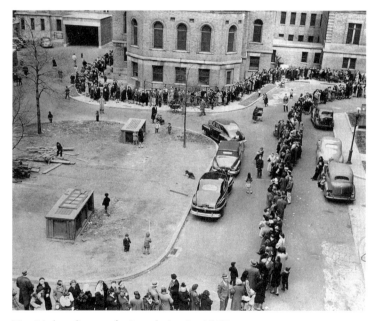

New Yorkers line up for inoculation in 1947.

Fearing the worst in the densely populated city, health authorities took no chances and ordered the mass vaccination, which took place within one month at hundreds of stations in hospitals, police stations and firehouses.

A resolution proposed by a delegate from the former USSR at the 11th World Health Assembly in 1958 and passed by the assembly in 1959 paved the way for a worldwide effort to eradicate smallpox. In 1966 at the 19th World Health Assembly, the World Health Organization (WHO) called upon all the world's governments to support and give financial backing to a newly created Global Smallpox Eradication Campaign.

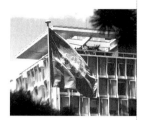

World Health Organization in Geneva.

Why did smallpox, of all diseases, become a candidate for worldwide eradication? An important reason was that it remained a powerful killer throughout the world. In the year prior to the start of the WHO eradication program, an estimated 15 million people contracted the disease and an estimated two million people died from it. Smallpox lent itself to the possibility of complete eradication for other reasons as well.

♦ Only humans are hosts; no animal reservoir exists, so smallpox cannot jump from animals to humans.

♦ A prompt antibody response allows exposed people to be protected.

♦ The vaccine is very inexpensive, easy to administer, does not require refrigeration, and provides long-term protection.

♦ Smallpox has no subclinical infection, or hidden carrier state, to contend with. The disease is always overt and can, therefore, be traced and contained.

The Global Smallpox Eradication Campaign became a worldwide public health program like no other. The WHO chose Donald Ainslie (D.A.) Henderson to head the campaign. He moved to Geneva, Switzerland, from Atlanta, where he had headed the CDC's Infectious Diseases Surveillance Unit.

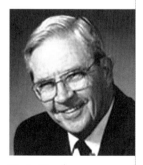

D.A. Henderson

D.A. Henderson was born in 1928 in Ohio, attended Oberlin College, and graduated from the University of Rochester's medical school. Immediately after, he joined the Epidemic Intelligence Service (EIS) at CDC and continued his career there. His work in containing various infectious diseases in the United States and in hot spots throughout the world had earned him international acclaim. He pioneered improved methods for disease control that emphasized better reporting of infectious diseases so that control measures could begin sooner to control the diseases. This became the most important strategy in smallpox eradication – surveillance to detect cases as early as possible and vaccination of all contacts of patients by specialized teams so that the outbreak would not spread.

In 1967, the campaign got under way using D.A. Henderson's methods. The WHO worked with health workers in all the infected countries to form surveillance teams ready to track down smallpox outbreaks and armed with "recognition cards" that explained the disease simply. As the number of smallpox cases decreased, the teams offered rewards to encourage reporting. The earliest successes came in western and central Africa. Smallpox turned out to spread less readily than had previously been thought, ► and the world began to understand that prompt detection and containment could lead to the eradication of the disease. Although the western African countries reporting endemic cases at the beginning of the campaign were among the poorest in the world and had heavy infection rates, all but one of them became free of smallpox within three years. Brazil recorded the last case in the Western Hemisphere in April 1971. Well-executed eradication programs eliminated smallpox transmission in East Pakistan (now Bangladesh) in 1970 and in Indonesia and Afghanistan in 1972. In eastern and southern Africa, smallpox had been eliminated in all but three countries by the end of 1971.

The introduction of potent, freeze-dried vaccine and the bifurcated needle had remarkable effects on smallpox prevalence, even in countries where eradication programs stalled. The freeze-dried version solved the problem of the vaccine losing potency in the heat of the tropics. The bifurcated needle, which was easy to transport, simplified administering the vaccine.

Unfortunately, setbacks did occur. In 1972, refugees returning to Bangladesh after its war for independence reintroduced the disease. In Botswana, introduction of the disease from South Africa created an epidemic, and

▼

...and the world began to understand that prompt detection and containment could lead to the eradication of the disease.

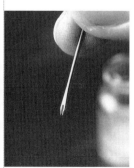

The bifurcated needle, which simplified administration of the vaccine.

in Iran, Iraq and Syria, cases were imported, and epidemics occurred. However, by late 1973 outbreaks had been contained except in Bangladesh. That year, intensified campaigns began in the five countries with remaining endemic cases – Bangladesh, India, Nepal, Pakistan and Ethiopia. India alone reported 64 percent of the cases worldwide.

By 1976, only Ethiopia remained with smallpox, and all attention turned to it. The milder strain, *variola minor*, spread tenaciously across a vast, sparsely settled region made destitute by civil war. The last outbreak was finally contained in the Ogaden Desert in August 1976.
►   However, an affected nomad population had already migrated into Somalia, and it was there that the last known outbreak occurred on October 26, 1977.

In 1980, the WHO declared smallpox eradicated. The steps taken to get to that point illustrated how the surveillance and containment programs could be adapted to individual countries to allow teams to succeed in very different populations. The combination of a persistent, coordinated international effort, spearheaded by the WHO, and innovative approaches at local levels led to success. Lessons learned from the eradication campaign are relevant in the 21st century as the threat of weaponized smallpox forces the public health community to confront a scourge it hoped had been conquered. ▫

▼

However, an affected nomad population had already migrated into Somalia, and it was there that the last known outbreak occurred on October 26, 1977.

Vignette
Hib Vaccine

The story of the Hib vaccine demonstrates how the painstaking work of research scientists in their laboratories can have immediate and profound impact on serious bacterial diseases in very young children. For years, serious infection with the bacteria *Haemophilus influenzae* type b (Hib) had led to complications in infants and young children under the age of five. Invasive Hib disease was the leading cause of epiglotitis and bacterial meningitis in very young children. About five percent of children who developed Hib meningitis died; and in 35 percent of the children who survived, serious complications occurred. These included neurological problems, such as seizures, deafness and mental retardation. A special vaccine would be needed to produce antibodies in very young, vulnerable children under the age of five, thereby immunizing them against the disease. An estimated 20,000 cases of Hib disease occurred annually in the United States before the vaccine appeared.

The Hib vaccine emerged from groundbreaking research in the 1960s by Porter Anderson, David Smith and Richard Insel at Strong Memorial Hospital of the University of Rochester. The first study took place in Finland in 1975 with more than 100,000 infants and children vaccinated with a polysaccharide product, with mixed results. While the trial vaccine worked in older children, it did not work in infants, whose immune systems failed to produce protective antibodies.

In 1985, after further trial and error, the vaccine was made available as a polysaccharide–protein conjugate product for use in children aged 18-24 months. In 1987 after further development, the vaccine was licensed for children aged 18 months, and in 1990 was finally licensed for children aged two months. By 1993, the Centers for Disease Control and Prevention reported a remarkable 95 percent reduction in invasive Hib disease in the United States. In 1997, Merck & Co. introduced a combination vaccine – Hib and Hepatitis B – that reduces the number of injections required in the first 18 months of life from 15 to as few as 11. In 1998, only 125 cases of Hib disease among children less than five years of age were reported. In less than a decade, the Hib vaccine had nearly eliminated invasive Hib disease among very young children. ◻

Looking Ahead

Advances in Vaccine Research

The need for new vaccines and new vaccine technologies has never been greater in light of the events of September 11, 2001. Vaccines are likely to be the only practical means of protection in the event that biological weapons of mass destruction are unleashed on an unsuspecting population. Weapons that use diseases to kill large numbers of people, that can be readily transmitted person to person – anthrax, smallpox, and plague being the foremost threats – call for new types of second-generation vaccines to be developed and stockpiled.

Currently, only small amounts of anthrax vaccine are produced in the United States with use limited to those in the military. Planning is in progress, however, to produce large quantities of a more modern vaccine that could be used in the general population in case of a serious threat or attack.

In August 2003, D.A. Henderson, who now serves as a senior adviser at the Center for Biosecurity, University of Pittsburgh Medical Center, and Dean Emeritus at the Bloomberg School of Public Health at Johns Hopkins University, addressed the issue of preparedness to deal with a possible smallpox release. "Preparedness is much better than it was at 9/11," he said. "We have ample vaccine and needles, a better-educated public health and medical community, most hospitals have negative pressure examination rooms and some areas are prepared for large-scale vaccination should that be necessary. In all, 700,000 in the military and some 40,000 civilian health workers have now been vaccinated, far fewer in the civilian sector than we believe desirable. Work remains to done, but progress in moving toward a full preparedness has been gratifying."

In the United States, ▶   an estimated 11,000 births each day place stress on the vaccine-delivery system. Each newborn currently requires a series of between 15 and 19 vaccine doses in the first 18 months of life. New combination vaccines may reduce that number to 11, but as additional vaccines are developed, the number of doses may well rise again. Parents tend to value immunization, a sign of public trust that all successful vaccine programs count

▼

...an estimated 11,000 births each day place stress on the vaccine-delivery system.

on. Adverse results, although rare, still occur, however, and surveillance to detect these events must continue, along with research into possible risk factors and their management. For each new vaccine program, an accompanying public-information campaign is essential. Professional and advocacy groups must be kept informed every step of the way, as must legislators, educators and the media.

In 1998, an article in *The Lancet* suggested that the MMR (measles, mumps, rubella) vaccine might be linked to increases in autism. As D.A. Henderson points out, however, "I, for one, am fully persuaded by several studies that demonstrate conclusively there is no relationship between MMR and autism. The problem: poor science in the first place and a press eager to publicize the spectacular. Regrettable." After the *Lancet* article, some parents refused the MMR vaccine for their children, and this eventually resulted in measles outbreaks that would have been prevented. Concerns over adverse events must be balanced with the knowledge that vaccines avert misery. Many a grandparent owes a long life not just to clean water, but also to remarkable advances in vaccines. ► Vaccines have saved more lives than any surgical technique or any medication, including antibiotics.

▼

Vaccines have saved more lives than any surgical technique or any medication, including antibiotics.

Despite the success of smallpox eradication, many diseases that vaccines prevent still persist, especially in developing countries. Polio, measles and rubella are still threats to millions of children and adults worldwide. According to the WHO, infectious diseases were the leading causes of death worldwide in 1996, with 17 million deaths annually compared to ten million from heart disease and seven million from cancer. Even in the United States and other industrialized countries, infectious diseases caused 18 percent of deaths.

The world has seen infectious diseases both old and new continue to emerge rather than decline as it enters the 21st century. Malaria has risen dramatically, thanks in part to resistant strains, as has gonorrhea, tuberculosis and typhoid – diseases that had been previously controlled with standard antimicrobial therapy. Devastating diseases such as Ebola haemorrhagic fever, hepatitis C, HIV/AIDS, Lyme, monkeypox, SARS and West Nile virus, have appeared suddenly. Until there are effective vaccines, these unexpected diseases will continue to affect various populations around the world.

Vaccines now in development to fight infectious diseases include vaccines against additional serotypes of pneumo-coccal and meningococcal infections, influenza, parain-fluenza and respiratory syncytial virus (RSV). Another exciting area of research is therapeutic vaccines against noninfectious diseases, such as cancer. Experimental vac-cines to fight cervical cancer caused by human papilloma virus and other cancers are currently being researched in clinical trials. Other promising vaccines in development include those to fight autoimmune diseases, gastric ulcers, and rheumatic heart disease as a result of Group A strepto-coccal infection. Trials are also under way for vaccines to prevent HIV infection, the cause of acquired immunodefi-ciency syndrome (AIDS). ▶   Hopeful developments may soon make trials possible for vaccines to fight Alzheimer's and breast cancer, two devastating diseases that affect large numbers of people.

The recent declaration by the WHO to eradicate polio globally by 2005 promises relief for a large part of the world's population. While polio was eliminated from the Western Hemisphere through vaccination in 1991, the disease is still endemic in three countries of Asia and four others in Africa, but all have mounted vaccination campaigns to stop the disease. By 2010, vaccines against several types of meningitis, pneumonia, as well as rotavirus-caused diarrhea and human papilloma virus (the cause of cervical cancer) should be introduced. In the future, vac-cines against AIDS, malaria and pulmonary tuberculosis may begin saving lives, and measles should be controlled throughout the globe as well. Thanks to advances in vac-cine technology, infants may well be protected throughout their lives against many of the pathogens that threaten their health today. Developments under way promise one day to provide immunologic protection against conditions such as asthma, multiple sclerosis and diabetes.

In the last quarter of the 20th century alone, new vaccine-delivery technology made rapid strides. Modern biotechnol-ogy gave rise to conjugate vaccines, live vector vaccines, new

▼

Hopeful develop-ments may soon make trials possi-ble for vaccines to fight Alzheimer's and breast cancer, two devastating diseases that affect large numbers of people.

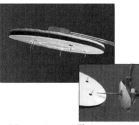

New microneedle developed to improve vaccine delivery.

adjuvants, genome-based proteomic vaccines, DNA vaccines and recombinant strains. New delivery approaches have included transgenic plants and transcutaneous immunization.

As vaccines prevent diseases, it follows that the more people are vaccinated against preventable diseases, the more health systems can marshal resources to fight diseases that are not preventable. This is why the invention of new vaccines and new technologies for vaccine delivery are so vital. Not only will health care systems be more successful at fighting disease, the world's population will enjoy marked improvements in overall health.

Chapter 2

Automotive Safety

Looking Back

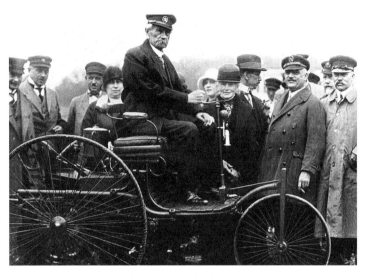

The first gasoline-powered automobile, built by Karl Benz in 1885.

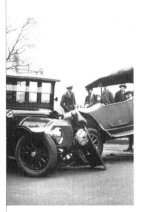

A 1924 pileup.

The United States became a motorized society during the 20th century, as did much of the rest of the world. The first recorded fatal traffic accident occurred in London in 1896 when an automobile struck an onlooker during a demonstration drive. The onlooker later died of head injuries caused by the collision. Today, people in the developing world drive only 20 percent of the world's cars but suffer nearly 90 percent of the world's traffic deaths. The World Health Organization, recognizing a growing global health issue, predicts that by the year 2020 traffic accidents will be the third leading cause of death and disability.

Despite this looming threat, improvements in automotive safety have occurred throughout the 20th century and into the 21st century. In 1901, Oldsmobile introduced the first speedometer, and in 1908, General Motors introduced the first electric headlamp. In 1924, GM opened the automobile industry's first proving-ground facility in Milford, Michigan and, over the years, improved dummies in crash testing that helped narrow injury tolerances for humans.

In 1928, shatterproof glass on all vehicle windows was introduced; and two years later, tinted windshields to help eliminate nighttime glare from oncoming headlamps went into volume production. Rear-turn signals became standard equipment on GM cars in 1939. ► Over the decades, these improvements and many more – such as seat belts and air bags – have saved countless lives.

In 1966, Congress passed the Highway Safety Act and the National Traffic and Motor Vehicle Safety Act, authorizing the federal government to set and regulate standards for motor vehicles and highways. Under the leadership of Dr. William Haddon, Jr., the first administrator of the National Highway Traffic Safety Administration (NHTSA), these landmark acts introduced many changes in both vehicle and highway design. Car manufacturers were required to incorporate new safety features – headrests, energy-absorbing steering columns, shatter-resistant wind-shields and safety belts – and highway construction stan-dards were improved. Highways began to be built with better alerts to curves (reflectors and line stripes in the center and at the edge), improved lighting, barriers separat-ing oncoming traffic lanes and guardrails. The design of traffic signs also improved, with breakaway features added to roadside signs and utility poles, especially on interstate highways. By 1970, deaths caused by motor vehicles began to decline both by the public health measure (deaths per 100,000 population) and the traffic safety indicator (deaths per vehicle mile traveled, or VMT).

Since the 1960s, NHTSA and the Federal Highway Administration within the U.S. Department of Trans-portation have provided national leadership to the auto-motive safety movement. Dr. Jeffrey Runge, an emergency room physician, currently heads NHTSA. A month before he took his post, Runge witnessed the aftereffects of a horrific car crash involving teenagers. Sarah Longstreet, known in her high school for her friendliness and church activities, had been belted in when a sport utility vehicle (or SUV) veered across the centerline and plowed over the hood of her smaller car. Although her air bag inflated just as it was meant to, the incompatibility in the design of the two cars caused her to die instantly, an unnecessary fatality. Sarah's death became a motivator for Runge in his new job as he seeks ways to improve the design of SUVs and pickup

▼

Over the decades, these improve-ments and many more – such as seat belts and air bags – have saved countless lives.

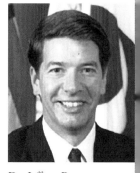

Dr. Jeffrey Runge, NHTSA administrator from 2001 to 2005.

trucks to eliminate design incompatibilities as a cause for traffic accidents.

Breath analyzer

Since 1986, the Centers for Disease Control and Prevention (CDC) has funded university-based centers for injury control which have pursued research on injury biomechanics, epidemiology, prevention, acute care and rehabilitation. In 1992, CDC established the National Center for Injury Prevention and Control (NCIPC) to contribute a public health direction to automotive safety as well as other injury areas. NCIPC targets the high-risk populations of alcohol-impaired drivers, young drivers, and passengers and pedestrians in an effort to reduce fatalities in motor vehicle accidents. NCIPC advocates the use of occupant-protection systems including safety belts, child-safety seats and booster seats.

NCIPC recognizes the role state and local governments play in enacting and enforcing laws that affect motor vehicle and highway safety, driver licensing and testing, vehicle inspections and traffic regulations. Nonetheless, federal guidelines influence these state and local decisions. The awarding of federal highway construction funds, for example, allows the federal government to exert some control over the way localities enforce rules that are meant to improve highway safety.

▼

...nearly 43,000 people still die annually on U.S. highways.

► Although automotive safety in the United States is light-years ahead of the developing world, nearly 43,000 people still die annually on U.S. highways. Since the early 1990s, this number has gradually increased as the population has increased − i.e., the death rate has changed very little. Factors contributing to the toll include poor design of secondary roads, high speeds, drunken drivers, and too few drivers and passengers wearing seat belts. The highest rates of traffic deaths are at ages 16-24 and 75 and older. Deaths linked to drinking have increased steadily since 1999 despite social marketing campaigns and tougher enforcement designed to curb drinking and driving. Furthermore, some 19,000 individuals killed in crashes in 2002 were not wearing seat belts, with young men between the ages of 18 and 34 most at risk.

The number of deaths from rollovers, which are caused in part by design flaws in SUVs, is an increasing concern. In fact, 59 percent of the overall increase in fatalities of motor-vehicle occupants came among passengers in pickups, vans and SUVs. Other risks for motor vehicle crashes are driving while drowsy, especially among college students and the elderly, and excessive speed. Much more attention is now being paid to the dangers of sleep-deprived drivers on the nation's roadways. Two examples are the increased efforts to educate drivers about the need to stop and rest, often through roadside billboards, and the placement of "wake-up" bumps along road shoulders to minimize crashes.

Mothers Against Drunk Driving (MADD), an advocacy organization formed in 1980 that now has 600 chapters, seeks to stop drunk driving by advocating for tough laws and appropriate sentences. MADD seeks especially to educate young people about the dangers and consequences of underage drinking, alcohol-related traffic crashes, alcohol

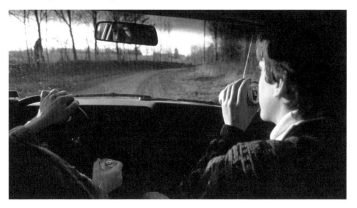

poisoning, and other harms resulting from illegal drinking under the age of 21. MADD's message for teens is not to use alcohol. In addition to stopping drunk driving and underage drinking, MADD supports the victims of the violent crime of drunk driving. A group of outraged women in California formed the organization after a repeat-offender drunk driver killed a teenage girl.
▶   Thanks, in part, to the efforts of MADD since its founding, more than 2,300 drunk-driving laws have been enacted by state legislatures. These laws range from permissible levels of alcohol in drivers to sanctions against tavern owners who serve drivers who then cause traffic accidents. In 2004, more than 16,500 people died in alcohol-related traffic crashes. In 2002, approximately 1.45 million drivers were arrested for driving under the influence of alcohol or narcotics. The blood alcohol concentration (BAC) of 0.08 percent, more stringent than before and now in effect in

▼

Thanks, in part, to the efforts of MADD...more than 2,300 drunk-driving laws have been enacted....

all 50 states and Washington, D.C., accounts for some of this increase.

In addition to the need to prevent drunk driving, another focus of automotive safety is immigrants who learn to their surprise that every state requires infants to be placed in child seats. Often, they choose to do without seats because they think they are unaffordable, although a good safety seat costs as little as $40 and some organizations have car seat loaner programs. A 1998 study done by the Johns Hopkins School of Public Health and the Insurance Institute for Highway Safety showed that Hispanic children between the ages of five and 12 are 72 percent more likely to die in a traffic accident than non-Hispanic whites of the same age.

► In 2000, CDC found that the leading cause of death for Hispanics between the ages of one and 44 was motor vehicle accidents. The number of Hispanic children from newborn to age 19 killed in vehicle accidents in 2000 jumped nearly 11 percent from the year before, to 1,115. Meanwhile, deaths among non-Hispanic white children actually fell by one percent during the same year.

An important trend in recent years comes from the enactment of Graduated Driver Licensure (GDL) programs to help reduce novice drivers' extremely high crash rates. GDL allows new drivers to face increasing challenges as they become more experienced. Between 1996 and 2004, 40 states and Washington, D.C., enacted three-stage GDL programs. The initial stage, requiring supervision by an older driver, is followed by an intermediate stage that permits some unsupervised driving while continuing to restrict nighttime driving and carrying passengers. The third stage is full licensure. These programs, especially those with more stringent requirements, have been associated with significant reductions in crashes of teenage drivers.

Among the many advances in traffic enforcement that have improved motor vehicle safety are radar detectors, speed cameras, red-light cameras and aerial surveillance. Traditional patrol car enforcement has its limits. About a third of motor vehicle deaths involve a single vehicle leaving the roadway and hitting a fixed object such as a tree or utility pole. Primarily a rural problem, an increasing number of deaths are caused by roadside hazards.

▼

In 2000, CDC found that the leading cause of death for Hispanics between the ages of 1 and 44 was motor vehicle accidents.

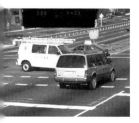

A red-light camera photograph of a violator.

Related to improvements in traffic enforcement are traffic courts. In 1943, when the United States lost more soldiers in traffic accidents than in combat, James Economos began the ABA Traffic Court Program. He established the first continuing education program for judges and the first application of computers to court administration. He also proposed the first anti-drunk driving law based on percentages of alcohol in the driver's blood and popularized the Model Rules Governing Procedure in Traffic Cases, which helped eliminate ticket-fixing.

Ongoing improvements in automobile design also contribute to driver and passenger safety. Engines in some

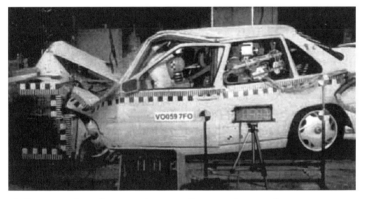

A demonstration of automotive crumple zones in a crash test.

vehicles are mounted to drop down immediately upon impact, saving front seat passengers from having an engine driven directly into them. Tires have been designed with interior walls that absorb the worst effects of blowouts and allow a car to be pulled over safely to the side of the road. Daytime running lights, long required in Scandinavia with its limited daylight during winter months, have become more prevalent in the U.S. and have been shown to help reduce traffic accidents, specifically when visibility is impaired by fog or smoke.

► Highway construction improvements have also been key to improving automotive safety. Evidence-based traffic engineering measures are designed to reduce pedestrian injury and death by managing vehicle speed, separating pedestrians from vehicles and increasing pedestrian visibility. Pedestrian deaths are primarily an urban problem and significant among the elderly; even with improving numbers – pedestrian deaths per 100,000 decreased 51 percent

▼

Highway construction improvements have also been key to improving automotive safety.

between 1975 and 2002 – they still account for 11 percent of motor vehicle deaths. Among the construction improvements that have led to safer highways are rumble strips that alert drowsy drivers they are leaving the roadway and reflective road markers that enhance visibility. Increased use of roundabouts in local road design has proved to reduce traffic accidents, as has the installation of more prominent traffic signals and a greater number of streetlights.

In summary, the strides made in automotive safety in the United States during the last century and the early years of the current century have significantly reduced deaths from traffic accidents. ► Much progress in further reducing risks remains to be realized, however. The challenge for car manufacturers, traffic safety engineers, ergonomists and legislators is to work together to develop and implement new improvements that will help the U.S. break through the current plateau in the number of traffic fatalities. ◻

▼

Much progress in further reducing risks remains to be realized, however.

Case Study

Development of Seat Belts

Volvo, a Swedish car manufacturer recognized by the industry for its innovations in automotive safety, led the way in the development of seat belts. Based on the wartime experience of airplane pilots, Volvo installed seat belts in cars it manufactured in Sweden starting in 1956, first just as an accessory but soon as a required feature because the evidence proved that seat belts saved lives. Car manufacturers in the United States, impressed by the evidence, soon followed Volvo and offered seat belts as an option.

After several decades during which physicians urged car manufacturers to provide lap belts in new cars, the Colorado State Medical Society led the way in 1953 by publishing a policy supporting installation of lap belts in all automobiles. In 1954, the Sports Car Club of America required compet-ing drivers to wear lap belts, and the American Medical Association House of Delegates voted to support their installation in all automobiles. In 1955, the California Vehicle Code was amended to require state approval of seat belts before their sale or use, and the Society of Automotive Engineers (SAE) appointed a Motor Vehicle Seat Belt Committee. In addition, the National Safety Council, American College of Surgeons and the International Association of Chiefs of Police all voted to support installation of seat belts in all automobiles.

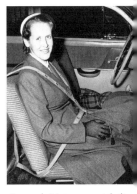

An early Y-type seat belt design.

In 1956, Volvo introduced the two-point, cross-chest diagonal belt as an accessory, while Ford began a two-year campaign emphasizing safety with a heavy focus on seat belts. Ford and Chrysler offered lap belts in front as an option on some models. In 1957, the U.S. House of Representatives Special Subcommittee on Traffic Safety opened hearings on the effectiveness of seat belts in auto-mobiles, while Volvo refined its belt by providing anchors in front for their two-point diagonal belts.

In 1958, Nils Bohlin of Volvo patented a three-point safety belt, replacing the single lap belt that risked injury to abdominal organs in high-speed crashes. Volvo also provided anchors for two-point diagonal belts in the rear. Bohlin, who died in 2002, may have saved as many as one million lives with his invention. Before joining Volvo in 1958,

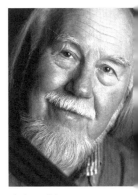

Nils Bohlin

Bohlin designed ejection seats and pilot rescue systems for the Saab Aircraft Company. His three-point solution for automobiles allowed occupants to buckle up with one hand, using one strap across the chest and another across the lap, with the buckle placed next to the hip.

In 1959, Volvo introduced three-point belts in front as a standard in Sweden. The New York State legislature considered, but rejected, legislation requiring seat belts, as it did again the next year. In 1961, however, New York finally enacted a law requiring that seat belt anchors be placed in the front outboard seat positions, effective January 1, 1962. In the same year, the SAE issued standards for U.S. seat belts and Wisconsin also required seat belt anchors.

In 1962, Virginia Trailways became the first U.S. bus company to install passenger safety belts. U.S. automobile manufacturers began to provide seat belt anchors in the front outboard positions as standard equipment, and the ripple effect of U.S. states requiring them began, with six states enacting legislation. Meanwhile, the Association for Aid to Crippled Children and the Consumers Union sponsored a landmark conference on "Passenger Car Design and Highway Safety" with occupant protection the sole theme.

In vehicles sold in the U.S. in 1963, Volvo introduced its three-point belt in front as standard. As well, several U.S. car manufacturers began to provide lap belts in front outboard positions. Meanwhile, 23 states now required seat belts in front, most enacting their laws to become effective on January 1, 1964. Recognizing this trend toward seat belts, the U.S. Congress passed a law to encourage the Commerce Department to issue mandatory standards for seat belts sold in interstate commerce, which the Department accomplished in 1965. Some U.S. manufacturers began to provide automatic-locking retractors (ALRs) in front seat belts.

In 1966, the Sports Car Club of America required drivers in competitions to wear a shoulder harness as well as a lap belt. Meanwhile, in an effort to improve the safety features of seat belts, Swedish regulators prohibited two-point cross-chest diagonal seat belts at seats next to a door and the Y-type of three-point belt altogether.

Laws requiring drivers and passengers to wear seat belts, first enacted in Victoria, Australia, in 1971, were not enacted in

the United States until 1984, when New York became the
first state with a seat belt use law. As Susan P. Baker, MPH,
professor and head of the Center for Injury Research and
Policy at Johns Hopkins School of Public Health, points
out, "Resistance to the use of seat belts endured for several
decades, often based upon such misconceptions as 'being
thrown clear is better' (not realizing this could mean clear
to eternity) and fear of being trapped by fire (even though
being trapped by one's injuries was a far greater risk). In
addition, as seat belt laws were considered, issues of personal
freedom inevitably entered the debate." Since 1984, however,
all states except New Hampshire have passed such laws.

In 1987, New York State once again led the way in requiring
large school buses to install two-point seat belts, although
compliance was left to individual school districts. Since then,
most new seat belt laws in state legislatures concern restraint
use in school buses. In 1998 and 1999, NHTSA conducted
a research project to develop the next generation of occupant protection systems for school buses. At present, most
school bus seats are padded to reduce crash forces and do
not have lap belts, which can contribute to head injuries if
a lap belt restrains the pelvis while the head impacts the seat
in front.

According to a 2003 NHTSA survey, compliance in wearing
seat belts has reached 79 percent, the highest level in the
nation's history. In most states the laws cover front-seat
occupants only, but the laws in 18 states also cover passengers in rear seats. In some jurisdictions, however, occupants
in some vehicle classifications, usually pickups, are exempt
from the law. Of the 49 states, only 21 allow law enforcement officers to stop drivers for failure to comply with the
mandatory seat belt laws; this "primary enforcement" has
been associated with greater seat belt use. The other states
require that officers first stop a vehicle for another reason
before citing noncompliance with the mandatory seat belt
law. However, all 50 states and the District of Columbia have
child restraint laws. These laws require that children travel in
approved child restraint devices, either car seats for young
children or booster seats or seat belts for older children. If
seat belt use continues at 79 percent or higher, it is estimated
that at least 15,000 lives will be saved in each future year. ◻

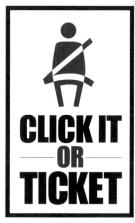

*One of several
seat belt promotion
logos published by
the NHTSA.*

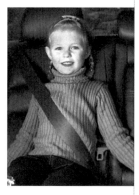

*NHTSA-
recommended
child safety seat.*

Vignette

Air Bags

Seat belts by themselves are active restraint systems, meaning that motor vehicle occupants must consciously belt themselves in. Belts therefore can save lives only when drivers and passengers use them. Air bags, on the other hand, are passive restraint systems, requiring no conscious decision on the part of a motor vehicle occupant. Assuming universal implementation of effective passive restraint systems, air bags could save even more lives than active restraint systems.

The first patent on air bag restraint systems was issued to John W. Hetrick in 1952, covering designs for safety cushions that would inflate automatically when a vehicle suddenly slowed. In 1964, Carl C. Clark reported on his work at the Martin Company on experiments that verified various air bag restraint designs and described their advantages and limitations. Some of the experiments involved him as the subject. Using pre-inflated designs, Clark's research was the first to demonstrate the potential benefits of air bag restraints.

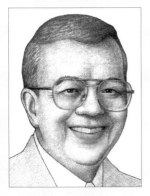

Allen K. Breed

To actually inflate air bags prior to a crash requires a sensing device. Allen K. Breed founded Breed Corp. in 1961 and secured a contract with the U.S. military to develop safety and arming devices. Seven years later, in 1968, he and his brother David invented an electromechanical sensor (a moving weight triggering a switch after the acceleration threshold is reached). The Breed sensor was a simple design, with reproducible results, and was widely used as air bags began to be produced commercially.

The key to the success of air bags is a reliable crash sensor so that an air bag will inflate the instant a serious crash occurs. Since the 1999 model year, the federal government has required automobile manufacturers to install driver and passenger air bags for frontal impact protection in all cars, light trucks and vans.

It became apparent that air bags inflating instantly with great force must vent some air to prevent trauma to the head and upper torso. Aside from routine injuries caused when air bags inflated with too much force – usually minor abrasions to people's hands, arms and

faces – air bags caused fatal head injuries in young children. The force
of the air bag smashing either directly into young children or into
rear-facing child safety seats, sometimes when vehicles collided at
relatively low speeds, caused these head injuries. The fear of air bags,
plus information about the importance of keeping children out of
the front seat, has led parents to banish children to the rear seats of
cars, vans and SUVs, a step that has helped reduce the number of
child traffic fatalities. Automobile manufacturers also allow the
passenger-side air bag to be disabled for adults and children.

GM tested air bags on the 1973 model Chevrolet sold only for
government use. In 1975 and 1976, GM offered buyers of full-sized
Oldsmobiles and Buicks driver-side air bags, and both driver and
passenger-side air bags to buyers of Cadillacs during those same years.
Today, dual front air bags are standard in all automobiles sold in the
United States. In addition, side air bags are options offered by many
manufacturers and are standard in many models. In second-generation
air bags, the force used to inflate the air bag has been further reduced,
an important modification that helps cut down on the number of
injuries to the head and upper torso caused by air bags during motor
vehicle crashes. As of late 2003, NHTSA estimates that more than
13,000 lives have been saved by air bags, mostly drivers but with a
significant number of front-right passengers. ◻

Looking Ahead

Advances in Automobile Manufacturing

The next frontier in automotive safety is saving bad drivers from mistakes that contribute to most crashes.   ►   To prevent drivers from making life-threatening mistakes, automobile manufacturers have begun to provide linked systems of safety features that they are either improving or designing from scratch.

The anti-lock brake system is the foundation of these linked safety systems. Anti-lock brakes, controlled by a computer, pump themselves automatically to avoid locking the wheels and sending the vehicle into a skid. This same basic hardware also applies braking force when sensors detect a vehicle skidding sideways or rocking violently side to side. When they do so, the anti-lock brakes become an electronic stability control system.

Since every vehicle has a mechanical suspension system, with shock absorbers and (preferably) stabilizer bars that are designed to control the vehicle's side-to-side motion, engineers can make these suspensions smarter using electronics and software. For instance, one manufacturer has devised a system called Active Stabilizer Bar in which the electronics push back against the forces that cause the vehicle to sway from side to side and go out of control in a violent turn. Another system uses shock absorbers filled with a magnetic fluid. Sensors read the road and send an electric current through the magnetic fluid, and depending on conditions, the shock absorbers will get either stiffer or softer to keep the car level even on rough roads.

These advances in safety systems, employing software and electronic control technology, could mean that showrooms will soon feature cars that weave a safety net around drivers. The safety net will integrate skid controls, stability sensors, steering, brakes and the throttle in a system that rectifies driver error automatically the instant it occurs. The challenge for automotive technology manufacturers is to persuade car manufacturers to spend the extra money to make their advances more widely available and bring automotive safety to the next level. The challenge for car manufacturers is

▼

To prevent drivers from making life-threatening mistakes, automobile manufacturers have begun to provide linked systems of safety features....

to persuade car buyers that these technologies are worth paying for.

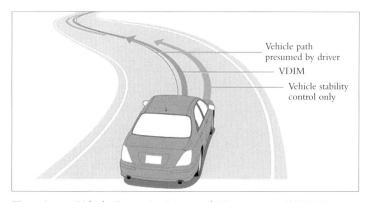

Toyota's new Vehicle Dynamics Integrated Management (VDIM) enhances handling and traction control systems, thus, improving preventive safety.

In late September 2004, NHTSA released a preliminary study that showed SUVs equipped with stability-control systems had 63 percent fewer fatal crashes. Cars equipped with stability controls had 30 percent fewer fatal crashes. However, the sample size was small – only 7.4 percent of light vehicles sold in 2003 had some kind of electronic stability control. Meanwhile, as pickups and SUVs with high centers of gravity grow increasingly popular with consumers, the problem of rollovers persists. Rollovers represent two percent of all crashes, but 33 percent of fatal crashes. Studies show that an SUV that skids into a curb at speeds as low as nine to 13 miles per hour is at high risk of flipping over. Cars will also flip over if they trip on a curb, but not until they attain speeds of 11-18 miles per hour. If electronic stability control (ESC) is to catch hold, the makers must advertise the benefits of their systems and stage demonstrations for the automotive press who, in turn, would spread word to consumers.

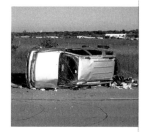

...an SUV that skids into a curb at nine to 13 miles per hour is at high risk of flipping over.

The challenge for automotive safety in the 21st century is to sustain and improve manufacturing and highway safety innovations. The role of public health in future successes, as measured by decreasing traffic fatalities and injuries, will come through the following approaches:

◆ Continue efforts to reduce alcohol-impaired driving and related fatalities and injuries.

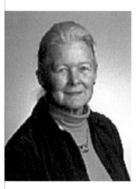

*Susan Baker,
Bloomberg School of
Public Health, Johns
Hopkins University.*

▼

By far the
greatest challenge
for public health
is extending
to developing
countries the
knowledge and
technology that
have enabled the
United States to
better protect its
road users.

◆ Promote strategies such as graduated licensing that discourage teenage drinking and speeding.

◆ Enhance pedestrian safety, especially for children and the elderly, through engineering solutions that reduce exposure to traffic and permit crossing streets safely and by encouraging safer pedestrian behaviors.

◆ Accommodate the mobility needs of persons aged 65 years and older – a population estimated to double to 65 million by 2030 – through a combination of alternative modes of transport.

◆ Encourage routine seat belt use by drivers and passengers.

◆ Encourage proper use of child safety seats.

◆ Conduct biomechanics research to better understand the causes of nonfatal disabling injuries, particularly brain and spinal cord injuries.

► By far the greatest challenge for public health is extending to developing countries the knowledge and technology that have enabled the United States to better protect its road users. This will require surmounting economic and cultural barriers. Susan Baker of Johns Hopkins School of Public Health says, "Advances in automotive safety in this country can point the way to improved safety in the developing world. Hopefully, those countries and that vast population will not have to learn from hard experience, as we did, that government regulations, wisely implemented, are the best way to protect public health." ◻

Photo credits

Chapter 3

Environmental Health

Looking Back

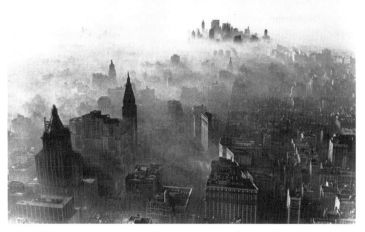

Air pollution over Lower Manhattan in November 1953.

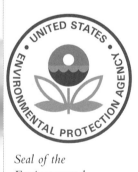

Seal of the Environmental Protection Agency.

Historians will likely regard Earth Day in April 1970 as a signal achievement in awakening the American public to environmental issues. Several months later, Congress passed significant amendments to the Clean Air Act of 1967, imposing statutory deadlines for states to comply with federal emission standards. The previous approach, allowing regions to set their own air quality standards, had produced little headway against air pollution. Earth Day provided the impetus to enact the amendments. These amendments were strengthened further in 1977, and Congress has continued to keep environmental protection at the forefront of its concerns. The year 1970 also saw the creation of the Environmental Protection Agency (EPA), consolidating under one roof a host of federal bureaus and

The Environmental Protection Agency	Previous Cabinet Department
National Air Pollution Control Admin.	Health, Education and Welfare (HEW)
Environmental Health Service	HEW
Environmental Control Admin.	HEW
Bureau of Solid Waste Management	HEW
Bureau of Water Hygiene	HEW
Bureau of Radiological Health	HEW
Federal Water Quality Admin.	Interior
Bureau of Commercial Fisheries	Interior
Agricultural Research Service	Agriculture

agencies to deal with pollution and environmental health issues. Previously, these bureaus and agencies had been housed in different cabinet departments, only loosely coordinated.

The creation of EPA gave the public health community regulatory power to fight manufacturing and industry pollution. Prior to EPA, the public health community had played David to the Goliath of industry, the source of most environmental pollution. The public health focus on environmental health became much sharper once EPA began to systematically address the effects that air, water and soil pollution have on the environment and on people's health.

EPA's mission is to protect human health and to safeguard the natural environment – air, water and land – upon which life depends. EPA accomplishes this mission by establishing and enforcing environmental protection standards consistent with national environmental goals. At the same time, EPA conducts research on the adverse effects of pollution. ► Because legislation to address pollution was urgently needed, the field of environmental health law rose to prominence with the creation of EPA.

▼

...legislation to address pollution was urgently needed, the field of environmental health law rose to prominence with the creation of EPA.

Knowing that businesses would be reluctant to transform their operations in a vacuum, EPA held all competitors to the same strict standards, and this helped prompt industry to act. International trade complicates the level playing field, however, sometimes leading multinational corporations into a "race to the bottom." If multinational corporations can freely transfer a polluting industry to another country with more lenient pollution standards, nations may resist restricting their own industry through legislation. To a greater extent than perhaps any other area of public health, environmental health must regulate the global marketplace. Environmental health officials, key sources of information on pollution, have become catalysts for policy change to protect the environment and advocate for environmental health precautions across national boundaries.

How pervasive was environmental pollution in the United States before EPA stepped in to regulate the worst offenders? Rachel Carson's *Silent Spring*, published in 1962, became a landmark work in the environmental movement. Through the lens of Carson's fervent appeal to regulate the pesticide DDT, the benevolent environment most Americans perceived became menacing. The chemical

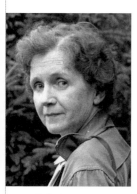

Rachel Carson, 1962, in Maine.

▼

Unlike other insecticides that were narrow in their targets, DDT killed hundreds of species at once.

industry, led by Monsanto, characterized Carson's findings as one-sided for failing to point out how pesticides had eliminated malaria, typhus and other human scourges. In mounting a public relations campaign to alleviate the public anxiety caused by *Silent Spring*, however, the chemical industry suffered a backlash when the public implicitly recognized Carson's solid research and the interconnectedness of the natural environment.

Rachel Carson, a trained marine biologist, worked for the U.S. Fish and Wildlife Service writing educational brochures. She earned a reputation as a meticulous researcher and evocative writer able to make science seem poetic. In the 1950s, she wrote two popular nature books, *The Sea Around Us* and *The Edge of the Sea*, which sold well enough to give her financial independence. The books also introduced her readers to ecology. Carson next turned her attention to the effects DDT had on the environment. A miracle insecticide that saved American servicemen from malaria in the Pacific islands during World War II, DDT found immediate and widespread use in agriculture in the years following the war. ► Unlike other insecticides that were narrow in their targets, DDT killed hundreds of species at once. Carson observed the effects of DDT on wildlife, specifically how it thinned the eggshells of raptors – eagles, falcons and hawks – leading to a decline in their populations, which, in turn, threw the ecosystem out of balance.

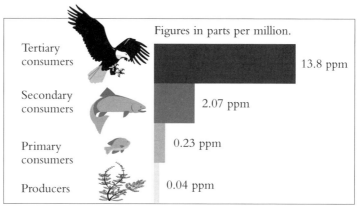

DDT becomes increasingly concentrated as animals prey on those lower in the food chain.

"For each of us, as for the robin in Michigan, or the salmon in the Miramichi, this is a problem of ecology, of interrelationships, of interdependence. We poison the caddis flies in the stream and the salmon runs dwindle and dwindle. We spray our elms and following springs are silent of robin song, not because we sprayed the robins directly but because the poison traveled, step by step, through the now familiar elm leaf-earthworm-robin cycle. These are matters of record, observable, part of the visible world around us.   ▶   They reflect the web of life-or-death that scientists know as ecology."

The publication of *Silent Spring* led to public clamor for a ban of DDT. The government's initial response, at the behest of the Kennedy administration, was to increase oversight of DDT's use. Not until 1972, however, did EPA implement a total ban. Banning DDT was the first major victory of the environmental movement. ◻

▼

"They reflect the web of life-or-death that scientists know as ecology."

Case Study

Lead Poisoning

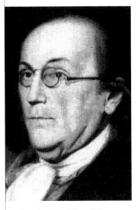

Benjamin Franklin

"The history of child lead poisoning in the past century in this country is a good example of how powerful economic interests can prevent the implementation of a 'useful Truth.'"
— Benjamin Franklin

In 1786, Benjamin Franklin listed in a letter to a friend every profession for which lead posed a health hazard. He then predicted that years would pass before the truth of a public health tragedy would be confronted. In fact, long after the lead and lead-paint industries became aware of the hazards posed by lead, particularly in young children, they continued to market their products aggressively. They lobbied legislatures to forestall regulation, suppressed research findings and advertised falsely and, in doing so, created a public health problem that grew to major proportions over decades. Benjamin Franklin's prediction proved correct.

Lead-poisoning, one of the most common environmental health problems affecting young children, is a preventable disease. Normal hand-to-mouth behavior makes children under six particularly at risk for ingesting lead from the environment. Exposure to even small amounts of lead can adversely affect children's growth and development.

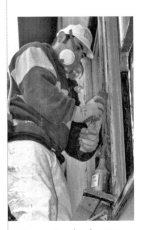

Removing lead paint.

Lead-poisoning symptoms include severe stomach cramps, joint and muscle pain, extreme weakness in the ankles and the wrists, blindness, convulsions, coma and death. These symptoms have all been well-documented in lead-poisoned children. Although lead poisoning affects virtually every system in the body, it can occur without distinctive symptoms. If lead poisoning goes unnoticed, it can damage a child's central nervous system, kidneys and reproductive system. It can also result in lower intelligence, hyperactivity, impaired hearing, decreased stature and growth, learning difficulties and behavioral problems that may persist into adulthood.

Exposure to lead has been a known risk factor to the public's health and well-being for the past two centuries. As Benjamin Franklin pointed out in his letter, he could list every profession for which lead posed a hazard and every health condition caused by exposure to lead.

▶   Still, as Franklin predicted, the remedies were years in the future – nearly 200 years, in fact.

Throughout the 1920s and 1930s, public health took a back seat to the belief that health care should focus on the individual. Charles Chapin, the health commissioner of Providence, Rhode Island, expressed this viewpoint in the late 1920s as follows:

"With minor exception, municipal cleanliness does little to prevent infection or decrease the death rate. Municipal cleanliness is no panacea. It will make no demonstrable difference in a city's mortality whether its streets are clean or not, whether the garbage is removed promptly or allowed to accumulate, or whether it has a plumbing law."

As shocking as this statement seems today, it reflects the prevailing view of health care professionals of the time. The public health community's lack of success in addressing a population-based tragedy can readily be seen. In addition, doctors often failed to diagnose childhood lead poisoning, compounding the problem.

The tragic case of the gasoline additive tetraethyl lead (TEL), closely related to white lead, illustrates how industry controlled the terms of debate and determined the outcome of a controversy. General Motors, under the substantial control of DuPont, joined with Standard Oil of New Jersey (now known as Exxon Mobil) to form the Ethyl Corporation. The company's main focus was to produce TEL to reduce engine "knock" while boosting engine power. Ethanol, produced from corn, could have reduced engine knock equally, but royalties from such a common product would not have been as lucrative to the corporations. When several TEL production workers died and New York City subsequently banned the lead additive, the Ethyl Corporation sought ways to calm the public.

With the full knowledge of GM, DuPont and Standard Oil, the Ethyl Corporation engineered a fraudulent research agenda that produced the desired result – proof that TEL was a safe product. In 1924, with the public increasingly worried by worker deaths, Ethyl contracted with the U.S. Bureau of Mines to conduct animal studies of TEL. Ethyl controlled both the content and the release of results, and

▼

Still, as Franklin predicted, the remedies were years in the future – nearly 200 years, in fact.

not surprisingly, the animal studies gave Ethyl a clean bill of health. Workers continued to die, however, and in the face of public panic, the U.S. Public Health Service held public hearings. Predictably, industry representatives dominated these hearings and no actions were taken. Worker deaths did not abate, however, and the public became increasingly agitated. To put the controversy to rest, the Surgeon General appointed an advisory committee to conduct a definitive study and make recommendations regarding the production and sale of tetraethyl (TEL) lead. The study lasted several months, not long enough to properly gauge the effects of TEL on workers. In the end, TEL was approved for unrestricted use.

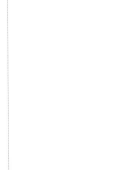

Dr. Herbert Needleman

Almost 50 years later, in the 1970s, a study by Dr. Herbert Needleman at Harvard Medical School provided the first clear evidence that lead, even at very low levels, could affect a child's IQ. In a series of follow-up studies, he determined that lead poisoning affected a child's attentiveness, behavior and school success with long-term implications. The lead industry attacked Dr. Needleman's findings, accusing him of scientific fraud and misconduct. He fought back successfully, however, winning exoneration and the right for all scientists accused in this way to have an open hearing with legal representation. Dr. Needleman's findings prompted CDC to issue guidelines for the diagnosis and management of lead poisoning in children. EPA took note, and Dr. Needleman's studies became the basis for the mandate to remove lead from gasoline. The Consumer Product Safety Commission also took note and called for a ban on lead in interior paints, while the Department of Housing and Urban Development (HUD) began to remove lead from thousands of housing units across the country.

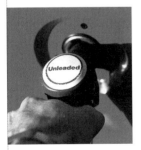

By 1976, auto and fuel manufacturers had made the changes necessary to begin to eliminate lead from gasoline. The U.S. phaseout of lead began that year when the first catalytic converters in automobiles were introduced to the market. In 1986, a complete ban finally took effect, and all gasoline was unleaded. This phaseout was strikingly successful in reducing child blood lead levels. Before the ban was implemented, 88 percent of children in the United States had blood lead levels (BLL) higher than 10 µg/dL. Afterwards, only nine percent had elevated blood lead levels.

The blood lead levels of all Americans declined 78 percent between 1978 and 1991, falling in exact proportion to the declining levels of lead in the overall gasoline supply. As a result of EPA's regulatory efforts to remove lead from gasoline, between 1980 and 1999 emissions of lead from the transportation sector declined by 95 percent, and levels of lead in the air decreased by 94 percent.

Following years of heated debate, Congress banned lead-based paints for use in housing in 1978. By the time the ban went into effect, the industry no longer opposed the ban, reeling from negative publicity and a precipitous decline in sales of lead-based paint. ► However, approximately 24 million housing units in the United States still have deteriorated leaded paint and elevated levels of lead-contaminated house dust. Young children live in more than four million of these homes. Roughly two-thirds of homes built before 1940 and one-half of homes built from 1940 to 1960 contain lead-based paint. Responding to this continuing threat, Congress passed the Residential Lead-Based Paint Hazard Reduction Act, known as Title X, in 1992. The law requires that home sellers and landlords provide known information on lead-based paint hazards during sales and rentals of housing built before 1978.

In 2001, the U.S. government settled cases against land-lords in Chicago, Los Angeles and New York that resulted in 16,000 apartments across the country being made lead-safe. The Department of Justice (DOJ), HUD and EPA collaborated in pressing the cases, basing them on Title X and the obligation of landlords to divulge hazardous conditions. Also in 2001, HUD and DOJ brought the first-ever criminal case based on Title X. A landlord in the Washington, D.C., area who had failed to notify tenants of lead-based paint hazards pleaded guilty to obstructing a HUD investigation and falsifying documents. The land-lord agreed to serve two years in prison and pay more than one million dollars in fines for six felony counts.

Prior to the 1950s, only Baltimore, Maryland, had a program to reduce blood lead levels in children. In the 1940s, a half-hearted effort by the federal government through the Children's Bureau to alert the public to the dangers of lead paint dissipated in the face of industry opposition. Although medical journals addressed the issue periodically,

▼

....approximately 24 million housing units in the United States still have deteriorated leaded paint and elevated levels of lead-contaminated house dust.

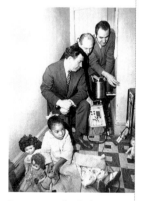

Inspectors check for lead in paint in a Manhattan apartment.

the record shows that public health journals virtually ignored the subject. The American Public Health Association did not take a public stand on childhood lead poisoning until 1969.

► Today, Rhode Island leads the way in reducing the incidence of childhood lead poisoning, pushed to do so because a disproportionate number of the state's families still live in older homes. Rhode Island owes its success, in large part, to the nonprofit Childhood Lead Action Project, founded in 1992, which serves as a catalyst for lead poisoning prevention. The project provides leadership to the Get-the-Lead-Out Coalition, a statewide network of environmental, housing, health, social service and church groups, and other advocates promoting public policy changes.

Community-based approaches to prevent childhood lead poisoning, as in Rhode Island, have proven highly effective. In 1995 in North Carolina, Edgecombe and Nash counties and the city of Rocky Mount initiated a comprehensive, communitywide program to prevent childhood lead poisoning. In a population of 143,000 in the combined counties at that time, 17 percent of families lived in poverty, and roughly 90 percent of children with lead poisoning lived in Rocky Mount. This community-based approach provides a model that can be emulated anywhere children are at risk of lead poisoning.

1. *Create a broad-based community coalition or advisory group.*

   A task force of 50 members meets quarterly to mobilize the entire community to eliminate the environmental sources that cause lead poisoning in children.

2. *Involve community members most at risk in all stages of the program.*

   In a 16-block area in the center of Rocky Mount, education and cleanup activities became watchwords, spearheaded by a local chapter of United Parents Against Lead (UPAL).

3. *Secure diverse and dedicated sources of funding.*

   Funding came from county and state health departments, the city of Rocky Mount, HUD and, indirectly, CDC through the North Carolina Division of Environmental Health. Most importantly, a regional

Smart Start Agency, the Down East Partnership for Children, allowed for program planning and the hiring of a community development specialist.

4. *Designate outreach and education staff.*

The leader of the Edgecombe and Nash counties program has a background in environmental health and has also worked in real estate. She educates land-lords and mortgage officers, an important constituency.

5. *Develop culturally appropriate educational materials and dissemination strategies.*

Communitywide education in libraries, schools and businesses, as well as through the local media, targets the problem of childhood lead poisoning.

6. *Coordinate among local social service agencies.*

A million-dollar grant awarded by HUD helped align local health providers, local and state environmental specialists, a community development specialist and a state nursing consultant to provide early screening, medical management, and nutritional and educational counseling for children with elevated blood lead and those who are at high risk of lead exposure.

7. *Implement a variety of cleanup and repair strategies.*

Education, interim control counseling, abatement enforcement and contractor consultation have become routine activities.

8. *Conduct a targeted screening program.*

Screening has seen steady increases, conducted by health departments, doctor's offices, and at local festivals, fairs and expositions. A Mobile Area Health Clinic (MAHC) screens in high-risk neighborhoods, helping elevate awareness and finding actual cases to mediate.

9. *Implement policy changes.*

Lead-based paint hazards in homes, the leading cause of lead poisoning in children, have been addressed through a proposed local ordinance that, if adopted and enforced, should reduce cases by 80 percent.

In 1997, the Edgecombe and Nash counties project received the GlaxoWellcome Child Health Recognition Award, a well-deserved recognition for an exemplary community-based program to reduce childhood lead poisoning.

Data from the National Health and Nutrition Examination Survey (NHANES) and national childhood blood lead surveillance data from 19 states indicates that average blood lead levels in young children decreased during the late 1990s (see table below). This dramatic decline, owing much to community-based approaches to eliminate childhood lead poisoning, should encourage more communities across the country to implement similar strategies. Meanwhile, HUD has distributed federal funds to 250 localities identified as still being at risk, a key factor in helping communities reduce BLLs in children. In 2003, HUD released $6.5 million through Operation LEAP (Lead Elimination Action Program) to seven organizations across the country to help prevent childhood lead poisoning in the home.

NHANES* Blood Lead Level (BLL) Measurements for Children Aged 1-5 Years

Year	Geometric Mean[1] BLLs (95% CI[2])	Prevalence[3] BLLs ≥10μg/dL[4] (95% CI)	Estimated No. of Children With BLLs ≥10μg/dL (95% CI)
1976–1980	14.9 (14.1–15.8)	88.2% (83.8–92.6)	13,500,000 (12,800,000–14,000,000)
1988–1991	3.6 (3.3–4.0)	8.6%[5] (4.8–12.4)	1,700,000 (960,000–2,477,000)
1991–1994	2.7 (2.5–3.0)	4.4% (2.9–6.6)	890,000 (590,000–1,330,000)
1999–2000	2.2 (2.0–2.5)	2.2% (1.0–4.3)	434,000[6] (189,000–846,000)

* National Health and Nutrition Examination Surveys.

[1] A measure of central tendency that differs from an arithmetic mean because it uses multiplication rather than addition to summarize the data values.

[2] This confidence interval (CI) means that there is a 95% probability that the true number is within that range.

[3] The number of children with BLLs ≥10 μg/dL over the whole population at a given point in time.

[4] The CDC has determined a BLL of 10 micrograms per deciliter (μg/dL) to be a level of concern.

[5] This estimate differs slightly from values published previously due to updates in coding and weighting of the survey data.

[6] This estimate differs slightly from values published previously due to weighting of the survey data.

Lead encephalopathy (a metabolic disorder caused by the ingestion of lead compounds) and death from lead poisoning have been virtually eliminated in the United States over the past 20 years. ► A combination of preventive approaches – screening high-risk children, medically treating children with elevated blood lead levels and intervening to reduce environmental lead exposure – contributed to this success story. Most important, the removal of lead from gasoline and paint manufactured for residential use has dramatically reduced childhood lead exposure. At the start of a new century, public health should continue building a winning coalition – government, community-based organizations, city planners, developers and private medicine – to prevent disease and deaths caused by unnecessary lead exposure. ▫

▼

A combination of preventive approaches contributed to this success story – screening high-risk children, medically treating children with elevated blood lead levels and intervening to reduce environmental lead exposure.

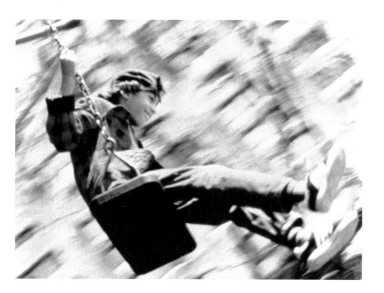

Vignette

Asbestos

Asbestos can be found in nearly every commercial and residential structure built in the United States from the early to mid-1900s. Prized for its insulating and fire-retardant characteristics, asbestos was added to concrete blocks, wallboard, insulation, gaskets and flooring materials, to name only a few building materials. Not until the 1960s did asbestos become a public health concern, too late for thousands of people who had either died or suffered from lung disease and other fatal illnesses caused by asbestos exposure. In 1964, an authoritative report presented by Dr. Irving J. Selikoff at the New York Academy of Medicine underscored what had become common knowledge – with asbestos, the magical properties to retard fire and insulate from heat came with a grave human cost.

Asbestos is a generic name for six naturally occurring minerals that have been mined since before recorded history. Ordinary silica boulders break apart first into rocks, then into stones, pebbles, grit and finally dust, always with a harmless quality of roundness. Asbestos, on the other hand, yields fibers when pulverized. These fibers, each composed of thousands of even smaller fibers woven tightly together, in turn, yield fibrils that are invisible to the human eye even under powerful microscopes. Asbestos causes harm only when it crumbles and releases submicroscopic fibrils into the air as a cloud of dust that is then breathed in or swallowed.

Lung disease can begin by chance when a single fibril embeds in a lung cell, something akin to a javelin thrown from one end of a football field landing in the exact center of a mattress at the other end. Since a single fibril can kill, there is no known safe level of exposure to asbestos. Unfortunately, asbestos is found everywhere in indoor environments, from acoustic ceiling tiles to ductwork insulation to taping compounds to vinyl floor tiles. Its use in exterior shingles and siding and in road-building materials is also pervasive. In the United States, laws did not curtail the use of asbestos as a fire-retardant and heat insulator in building materials until the late 1970s. Although asbestos remains harmless if left intact and undisturbed, once disturbed, its safe removal becomes a costly and laborious undertaking. Untold billions of dollars would need to be spent before all asbestos could be safely removed.

Meanwhile, the toll of fatal illnesses caused by submicroscopic asbestos fibrils continues to mount. Foremost in concern is mesothelioma, a rare form of lung cancer. Other debilitating lung illnesses caused by asbestos include asbestosis (a scarring of the lungs with fibrous tissue), pleural plaques, pleural thickening, asbestos pleurisy and lung cancer. Also, ingested fibrils can cause gastric tumors.

Mesothelioma causes particular pain to its victims and their families. Nearly always fatal unless it is discovered early, usually by chance, and treated aggressively, the usual course of the disease after diagnosis is an exceptionally painful two-year decline in lung function. The symptoms typically appear 20 to 30 years after the first exposure. Beyond construction workers, miners and shipyard workers who are known to be at risk, most people do not know whether they have been exposed. Consequently, the disease often takes people by surprise. Long-ago exposure to any material containing asbestos that crumbled or became a powder from sawing, scraping or sanding creates the condition for the disease.

While incidence of the disease in the United States remains relatively low, with 14 cases per million people per year, a threefold increase in mesothelioma in males between 1970 and 1984 caused alarm in public health circles. Health officials traced the increased incidence to workplace conditions, especially in shipyards, and the legal community responded by filing class action lawsuits against manufacturers and mine owners. Currently, asbestos litigation wends its way through courts across the country. In the case of Johns Manville, the world's largest asbestos company, bankruptcy proceedings further complicate pending legal remedies.

Tests in 2000 determined that even crayons contained unsafe levels of asbestos, a result of several leading crayon manufacturers using talc mined from one site in upstate New York. The mine's owner, backed by powerful members of Congress, had fought government regulators to a standstill for years. Meanwhile, workers in the crayon manufacturing plants continued to be exposed to fibrils made airborne in the talc. As public health authorities accumulated evidence of the health risks from crayon manufacturing and from crayons themselves, a battle with the mining industry and its powerful congressional supporters loomed. Only when evidence of the health risks became overwhelming were enforceable regulations enacted. Public health balances risk and precaution in addressing environmental public health issues, and the crayon issue illustrates how health threats often need to escalate before action is taken. ▫

Looking Ahead

Asthma

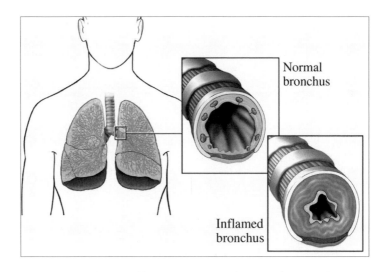

An estimated 31 million Americans have asthma today, more than triple the number in 1980, according to the U.S. Centers for Disease Control and Prevention (CDC). Characterized by a chronic inflammation and swelling of the airways that restrict breathing, asthma threatens the lives of people who have it and creates uncertainty in their daily lives. During a serious asthma attack, breathing becomes so constricted that the feeling is similar to drowning. At this stage, an emergency room visit for life-saving treatment becomes essential.

Asthma is debilitating and costly to the health care system. Although anyone can have asthma, regardless of age, income or ethnicity, the disease is particularly prevalent among low-income children in the inner cities. ► *The New York Times* reported in 2003 that one in four children in New York City's Harlem section has asthma, double the rate expected by researchers and one of the highest rates in the nation. In the early 1970s, because few people died from asthma attacks, they were not even reported. Now, just 30 years later, the disease causes 5,000 deaths a year and disproportionately affects African-Americans.

▼
...one in four children in New York City's Harlem section has asthma....

Why does the United States face this frightening public
health epidemic, and what should be done to address it?
Asthma can be characterized as a disease of industrialization. Epidemiologists, physicians, social workers and medical researchers have been hard at work trying to uncover
the environmental causes and aggravators of asthma. In
Harlem, the surprisingly high incidence of the disease
among children may stem from chronic pollution caused
by truck and automobile traffic, second-hand tobacco
smoke, unhygienic living conditions or a combination
of these factors. The research is not yet conclusive. Other
asthma triggers include industrial air pollution, dust mites,
cockroach and mouse droppings in tightly insulated homes,
and severe allergic reactions to common substances, such
as animal dander and pollen.

The exact causes of asthma in any particular person are still
subject to speculation. Heredity is thought to be a factor,
as children of asthmatics are more likely to develop the
disease. Atopy is a proven factor – people susceptible to
allergies are more likely to suffer from asthma. Race and

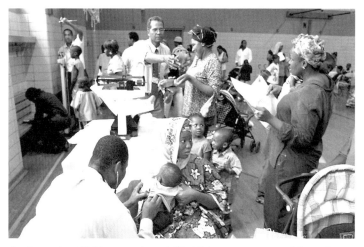

*In September 2002, more than 400 children were screened for asthma
at Public School 242 in Manhattan.*

ethnicity also appear to play a roll – African-Americans
suffer from the disease at an increased rate (5.8 percent
compared with 5.1 percent in whites) and are more likely
than whites to be hospitalized and die from asthma attacks.
In fact, the death rate from asthma in African-American
children is more than four times the rate in white children.

Epidemiological studies have yet to pinpoint the causes for this discrepancy, although for inner-city children, access to health care and the quality of residential environments are likely leading causes.

All asthma sufferers react in predictable fashion when they breathe airborne allergens, first with severe constriction of the trachea (windpipe), then with production of mucus that constricts the trachea further. Fortunately, asthma is a manageable disease. Patient and caregiver education is a key component of controlling asthma. The severity of the disease can be controlled by carefully monitoring exposures in the environment. For example, asthma sufferers should avoid tobacco smoke, stay away from pets, and abstain from foods that cause allergic reactions. ► Parents and caregivers must be exceptionally attentive to the triggers that cause asthma in the children in their care.

▼

Parents and caregivers must be exceptionally attentive to the triggers that cause asthma in the children in their care.

Given the enormous costs of asthma to society, significant medical research is dedicated to discovering new therapeutic approaches. Aside from the standard treatment of inhalers (anti-inflammatory drugs that prevent swelling in small airways branching off the trachea), some promising new approaches include antileukotrienes and bronchodilators. Leukotrienes are chemicals produced by cells that cause smooth muscles to constrict and fluid from blood vessels to collect in the lungs. Oral antileukotriene drugs developed by scientists prevent inflammation and constriction and show promise in treatment of asthma. Bronchodilators are medications that open constricted airways in the bronchial tubes and are available in tablet, capsule, liquid, inhaler or injectable forms. New approaches called tandem therapies combine approaches (i.e., bronchodilators work jointly with anti-inflammatory medications to control and prevent asthma symptoms). Recently, the National Heart, Lung and Blood Institute conducted research that shows that a long-acting beta-agonist (LAB), a bronchodilator, when taken with inhaled corticosteroids, helps improve asthma control.

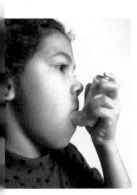

Girl using bronchial inhaler.

Other promising therapeutic approaches include monoclonal anti-immunoglobulin E (IgE) antibodies. Anti-IgE therapy is based on a "short circuit" approach to the allergic response, using the antibody to treat the first steps of the allergic response and thereby avoid symptoms caused by allergen exposure. Another new therapeutic approach, determining how to control lung acid levels in asthma patients, also promises to reduce symptoms. During an attack, asthma sufferers experience levels of lung acid up to 1,000 times higher than people without asthma. Researchers have discovered specific reasons for this imbalance and will soon make available therapeutics to prevent it and thus reduce symptoms.

Another promising avenue for therapeutics is genetic research. Although a single "asthma gene" has yet to be discovered, genetic studies have yielded significant advances in pinpointing the many genes thought to be involved in allergies and asthma. Understanding how these genes are inherited in families will enable researchers and physicians to better predict who is at risk for the disease and initiate therapies to control the symptoms. ▶ Many asthma researchers believe it is only a matter of time before advances in DNA technology and knowledge of the human genome will uncover the roots of asthma. Effective new treatment options will surely follow.

▼

Many asthma researchers believe it is only a matter of time before advances in DNA technology and knowledge of the human genome will uncover the roots of asthma.

The public health community views asthma and related breathing disorders as a key challenge in the new century. Moreover, asthma is a complex disease that requires a co-ordinated and multifaceted response from many organizations including those involved with transportation, urban planning, the environment, health care, and public health. The public health response to asthma involves a number of actions, all equally important. First, surveillance reveals the distribution and occurrence of asthma. Second, education helps ameliorate the severity of asthma attacks. Third, coalitions that foster collaborative approaches to strategic directions, structure and process in asthma treatment reduce barriers and make goals achievable. Fourth, advocacy addresses the suspected causes of asthma in communities. Finally, interventions – medical, environmental and school-based – create healthier environments and can lead to a decline in the prevalence of asthma. When public health rallies educators, government, industry, and the public to adopt these five steps, asthma begins to be addressed in ways that lead to long-term solutions.

From an environmental standpoint, anyone with asthma – or someone living with a person with asthma – should take preventive measures to control their indoor environment. People with asthma should live with as little dust as possible and should avoid contact with pets that shed hair and dander. The indoor environment should be free from smoke, cockroach and mouse droppings, and mold and mildew. Precautions taken to remove allergens from the indoor environment can reduce the incidence of asthma attacks and can foster other positive personal and public health effects as well.

The public health system can help people create and maintain healthy home and work environments. Looking ahead, outdoor environmental controls that reduce the need for driving offer hope for relieving asthma symptoms. Ideally, the outdoor environment would feature communities friendly to walking and biking with better urban planning and increased access to convenient public transportation. Ideally, highways would be full of automobiles powered by electricity. ► During the Atlanta Olympics in 1996, restricted traffic in downtown Atlanta improved air quality and reduced emergency room visits for asthma by 42 percent. By tightly restricting automobile traffic entering its central business district, Singapore also improved air quality and reduced emergency room visits for asthma.

While some battles in the environmental health arena have been won, as in central Singapore, others still seek effective advocates. The destruction of the World Trade Center towers in New York City in 2001, for example, gave rise to

▼

During the Atlanta Olympics in 1996... restricted traffic in downtown Atlanta improved air quality and reduced emergency room visits for asthma by 42 percent.

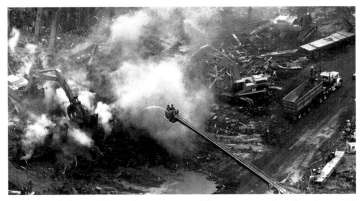

The site of the World Trade Center smoldering six weeks after the attack.

health ramifications for people who worked on rescue and demolition efforts or lived nearby. Evidence continues to mount that increased incidents of RADS – reactive airways dysfunction syndrome – affect rescue workers and residents of the area. The full extent of health problems is not yet known, but many rescue workers will likely face lifelong respiratory illnesses.

Answers to environmental health problems cannot all be known today. Time can be a best friend or a worst enemy when measuring environmental effects. For example, levels of carbon monoxide can be measured in one month and effective countermeasures taken immediately. On the other hand, pesticides in the food chain might take years to measure and can cause great harm before countermeasures are even considered. The effect of climate change on humans, which will take generations to measure, poses a particular challenge for environmental health specialists and other scientists who care about healthy environments. They must convince workers who depend for employment on skeptical industries, and the industries themselves, to accept countermeasures on faith.

How will global change affect future generations? Must environmental problems reach crisis levels before we act? Can we avoid repeating past mistakes? The environmental picture, still murky, is one of threats and advances coexisting. One million people worldwide die of air pollution each year, 90 percent of whom are in developing nations. Industrialization and technology create wealth in the developing world, measured by growth in urban areas and international travel and trade, but at the same time greenhouse gases cause climate change, ecosystems are stressed, chemical hazards multiply, biodiversity is lost and emerging infectious diseases jump continents. Unfortunately, rapidly developing countries contribute to environmental depredation, compounding the problems created by advanced industrial nations. Coral reefs continue to die off, schools of dolphins continue to dwindle, ozone holes continue to widen.

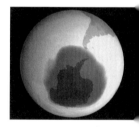

Ozone hole in the Earth's atmosphere.

Government's duty is to prioritize the environmental health agenda. Citizens share a responsibility to become literate about environmental health to help advance the field. Many advances – designated smoking areas, recycling, bicycle paths, greenways – are made possible because the public engages in advocacy, a driver of government change.

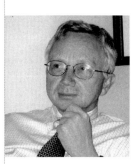

Dr. Richard J. Jackson, former director of CDC's Center for Environmental Health.

Dr. Richard J. Jackson, former director of CDC's Center for Environmental Health, writes about future developments in environmental health: "The current generation now faces its own challenges. One challenge is to better understand the broad impact of our built environment on health and then to build future communities that promote physical and mental health. Public health has traditionally addressed the built environment to tackle specific health issues such as sanitation, lead paint, workplace safety, fire codes and access for people with disabilities. We now realize that how we design the built environment may hold tremendous potential for addressing many of the nation's greatest current public health concerns, including obesity, asthma, injury, depression, violence and social inequities."

Perhaps Jackson best expresses a vision for the future of healthier environments: "Many aspects of the built environment will resist rapid change, even when research has adequately revealed key aspects of healthy communities. Efforts to improve pedestrian facilities, preserve green space and upgrade public transportation are under way in many communities. Whereas our generation may reap some benefits from the new field of the built environment and health, with a little vision and a lot of good science and hard work, our children and grandchildren will be able to walk or bicycle home from their workplaces through attractive communities designed to promote the physical and mental health of all people."

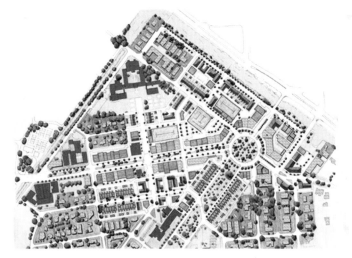

Miami Springs, Florida, site plan—an example of a community planned with plentiful greenery and pedestrian walkways.

Chapter 4

Infectious Disease Control

Looking Back

In the mid-20th century, considered the golden age for antimicrobial advances, Americans came to believe that infectious diseases might be conquered for all time. Vaccines held many scourges at bay in advanced industrial nations, where once-fatal diseases, such as measles, polio and diphtheria, were no longer serious threats. The year 1977 marked success in the global eradication of smallpox, one of the greatest achievements of public health. Some medical researchers grew to believe that an infectious agent only needed to be identified before effective countermeasures could be identified and implemented.

A rude awakening lay ahead, however. The early years of the 21st century have already seen widespread outbreaks of SARS, avian flu, and Ebola virus, debilitating and often fatal emerging infectious diseases. Tuberculosis has re-emerged as a threat to the public's health, the number of HIV infections continues to mount, and growing antibiotic resistance threatens hospitals and communities throughout the United States. ► Who would have thought in the 1950s, as the Salk vaccine effectively eliminated the threat of polio, that so many other infectious diseases would emerge just 50 years later? In an age of rapid global travel and a revolution in the development of therapeutics and public education, we have reached an uneasy standoff between microbes and man's best efforts to create a world free of infectious diseases.

Real advances in infectious disease control began in the second half of the 19th century, but medical care did not become truly transformed until antibiotics were discovered in the 1940s, ushering in dramatic reductions in illness and death from infectious diseases. For example, in 1850 the infant mortality rate in Massachusetts was 130 deaths per 1,000 live-born infants, with many of these deaths due to intra- and postpartum sepsis. By 2003, the infant mortality rate in Massachusetts had dropped to 4.8 deaths per 1,000 live births.

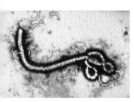

The Ebola virus.

▼

Who would have thought in the 1950s, as the Salk vaccine effectively eliminated the threat of polio, that so many other infectious diseases would emerge just 50 years later?

For a time in the mid-19th century, sanitary reforms helped control diseases. A hygienic movement arose from the squalor of urban slums, trying to eliminate dirt and sewer stenches. While the effort had some effect, it failed to counter diseases spread by fleas and mosquitoes or by personal contact, and it often failed to separate drinking water supplies from sewage. Fortunately, the breakthroughs of Louis Pasteur and Robert Koch and the germ theory of disease were soon to come.

In 1346, the world's most famous scourge, bubonic plague, spread by rats to fleas to humans at first in Asia, migrated to the population centers of Europe with devastating effect. It is thought that as much as half of Europe's population succumbed to the disease in the ensuing years. The disease – a highly contagious, virulent bacteria – caused high fever and attacked the lungs, turning the body black before death. Once the "black death" epidemic died out of its own accord, the relieved but diminished population of Europe moved on to the Renaissance, one of the great ages in human history.

The plague of Florence in the 14th century.

In 1530, the Italian physician Girolamo Fracastoro wrote a poem to express his ideas about the origin of syphilis, positing that this sexually transmitted disease was spread through intimate contact by "seeds." He expanded this early theory of contagion in later writings to include indirect contact, through clothing and even through the air. In giving voice to his ideas, Fracastoro anticipated by 350 years the pioneering work of Louis Pasteur, Robert Koch and their contemporaries in the late 1870s. Their big breakthrough came with the germ theory of disease.

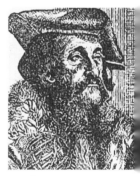

Girolamo Fracastoro

In 1627, Jesuit missionaries in malaria-ridden Peru began carrying the bark of the Cinchona tree back to Europe. They had observed that native Indians used the bark to fight malaria, not yet realizing that the active ingredient, quinine, had anti-malarial properties. When the bark proved to lessen malarial fevers in Europe, quinine gained a spot on the rare list of pharmaceuticals – opium, digitalis, willow bark, and little else – that provided patients some relief prior to the modern era.

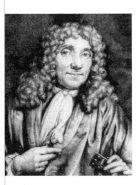

Anton van Leeuwenhoek

In 1683 in the Netherlands, with one of his new microscopes in hand, Anton van Leeuwenhoek visualized bacteria among the *animalcules* – microscopic animals that cannot be seen by the naked eye – he harvested from his own teeth. He was the first to see and describe bacteria, yeast plants, the teeming life in a drop of water and the circulation of blood corpuscles in capillaries. The invention of the microscope opened the way to visualize some of the microbial agents causing contagious diseases, but not until the invention of the electron microscope in the 1930s did the molecular structure of microbes – nucleoids, ribosomes, cell walls and membranes, flagella – become discernible. The electron microscope gave rise to a flourishing era for molecular biology.

In 1796, in Hertfordshire, England, Edward Jenner developed the first vaccine after observing that milkmaids exposed to cowpox were somehow immune to smallpox. Jenner concluded that exposure to a form of the animal infection protects a person from contracting a full-blown – and much more devastating – form of the human disease, and his empirical observation and successful experiments became the basis for vaccines that followed.

The germ theory of disease arose from research by a French chemist, Louis Pasteur, and a German bacteriologist, Robert Koch, which established the sanitary conditions necessary for isolating and studying bacteria. In the

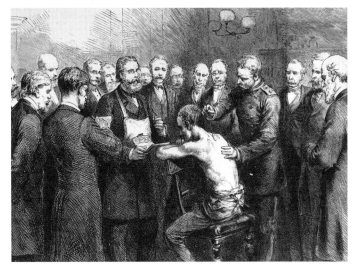

Dr. Koch's treatment for consumption (tuberculosis).

late 1870s, Pasteur invented pasteurization, the process of heating milk to kill dangerous microorganisms, and invented vaccines against anthrax and rabies. Koch's contributions were procedural and have been handed down as "Koch's Postulates," criteria necessary for a particular organism to be proven to cause a particular disease. In 1882, Koch identified the bacterium that causes tuberculosis, and a year later, he did the same for cholera. Koch's discoveries began a golden age of microbiology marked by headlong competition among medical researchers to isolate and identify the microorganisms that cause diseases.

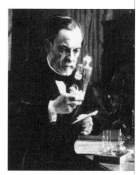

Louis Pasteur works on an experiment.

This germ theory led to advances in treating infectious diseases in western Europe and the United States. By the turn of the century, typhus had virtually disappeared, tuberculosis had started a long decline, and life expectancy began to increase. Nonetheless, annual mortality in the advanced industrial nations remained at two percent, much of it caused by infection. Diseases such as diphtheria, measles, whooping cough, scarlet fever, puerperal fever, tuberculosis and infectious diarrhea remained major killers. In some cases, notably mortality from childhood infectious diseases, such as scarlet fever, little would change until the advent of antibacterial agents in the mid-20th century.

In the 1890s, the Russian microbiologist Dmitri Ivanowski and the Dutch botanist Martinus Beijerinck independently discovered tiny infectious agents that could pass through bacteria-stopping filters. ▶   Too small to be seen with conventional microscopes, these agents were named "viruses." Unlike bacteria, which replicate independently, a virus invades an existing cell and replicates using that cell's genetic code. Research in viruses, thought to cause at least half of human infections, has unleashed a new sphere of competition among microbe hunters.

▼

Too small to be seen with conventional microscopes, these agents were named "viruses."

In the 20th century, great advances in fighting infectious diseases were made possible by the discovery of sulfonamides, penicillin and anti-tuberculosis agents. Vaccine development and smallpox eradication were also great achievements during the century. However, the great infectious disease challenges of the century – influenza pandemics, the HIV pandemic, and failure to control malaria, tuberculosis and worldwide infant mortality – still haunt us at the start of the 21st century.

While antimicrobial agents play an important role in reducing deaths caused by infection, much of this reduced mortality comes from continued improvements in nutrition, housing and environmental hygiene. Vaccination, culminating in the global eradication of smallpox in 1977, also has had a profound impact in reducing the global burden of diseases such as polio, measles, diphtheria and tetanus. Early in the 21st century, polio and guinea worm are very close to eradication, while onchocerciasis and lymphatic filariasis are also targets for elimination.

Approximately 25 percent of physician visits in the United States today are to identify and treat infectious diseases, including HIV infection and related illnesses, with both direct and indirect costs estimated to be $120 billion annually. An estimated 600,000 cases of pneumonia occur each year in the United States and cause as many as 50,000 deaths. In other parts of the world, infectious diseases remain the leading cause of morbidity and mortality.

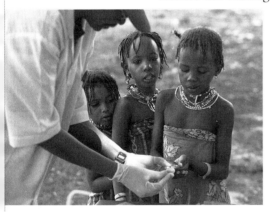

Medical-screening campaign for "sleeping sickness" in Chad.

Each year, malaria claims the lives of more than one million children in sub-Saharan Africa. Worldwide, each year 35 million to 60 million people contract dengue, and approximately 200 million people have schistosomiasis (also called *bilharzia* or snail fever, a tropical disease made widespread through the use of contaminated water, characterized by infection and gradual destruction of the tissues in the kidneys, liver and other organs). In Russia, more than 10,000 cases of diphtheria have occurred since 1993 due to a fall-off in immunization levels. In 1998, the World Health Organization estimated that infectious diseases caused almost a quarter of the 54 million deaths worldwide – over 13 million deaths. Three diseases that had been common in the developed world at the beginning of the 20th century – pneumonia, diarrheal disease, and tuberculosis – accounted for nearly half of these deaths. Still, since the advent of microbiology in the late 19th century, progress against infectious diseases has been remarkable.

The emergence of infectious diseases in this century, despite man's best efforts to eradicate them, comes in part from demographic factors. As people live longer, they are

more apt to be hospitalized in old age and become susceptible to bacterial pathogens lurking on wards. Hospital personnel can spread these pathogens from one patient to
another, causing what are known as "nosocomial infections."
►   Ironically, in the developed world, old people are
most at risk of infectious diseases; while in the developing
world, infants and young children remain most at risk.

Joshua Lederberg, Nobel Laureate in medicine, observes,
"As infectious diseases have assumed lower rankings in
mortality statistics, other killers – mostly diseases of old
age, affluence and civilization – have moved up the ladder.
Heart disease and cancer, for example, have loomed as
larger threats over the past few decades. Healthier lifestyles,
including less smoking, sparer diets, more exercise and
better hygiene, have been important countermeasures.
Prophylactic medications, such as aspirin, as well as medical
and surgical interventions, have also kept people alive
longer." □

▼

Ironically, in the
developed world,
old people are
most at risk of
infectious dis-
eases; while in the
developing world,
infants and young
children remain
most at risk.

Case Study

HIV/AIDS

The mysterious constellation of symptoms that began to appear in gay men in the late 1970s and early 1980s baffled the medical world at first, but not for long. The symptoms consisted of opportunistic infections or cancers – candidiasis in the mouth, pneumocystis carinii pneumonia in the lungs, toxoplasmosis in the brain, Kaposi's sarcoma lesions on the skin and elsewhere, to name a few – that hinted at compromised immune systems as the underlying cause.

The medical community set to work to identify the culprit. Fortunately, each individual infection presenting in gay men had been identified in the early years of the 20th century and by the 1970s, for different reasons, had been linked to an underlying defect of the immune system. Doctors, therefore, understood the complexity and implications of what they now confronted. In New York City and Los Angeles, where the first cases of the new "gay plague" or gay-related immunodeficiency (GRID) were treated, doctors astutely noted that a defect in the immune system was the underlying reason why this constellation of infectious diseases and cancers was occurring.

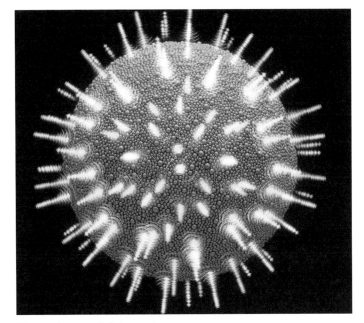

Human immunodeficiency virus.

In 1981, CDC began to formally track cases. The next year, public health officials in the United States began to use the term "acquired immunodeficiency syndrome" (AIDS) to identify the new occurrences of opportunistic infections, cancers and other conditions. In 1983, Drs. Francois-Barre Sinoussi, Luc Montaigner, and colleagues at the Institut Pasteur in Paris isolated and identified the cause of AIDS, a virus they named "lymphadenopathy-associated virus" (LAV). Additionally, discoveries by Dr. Robert Gallo and his colleagues at the National Institutes of Health that same year provided conclusive evidence that this virus indeed caused AIDS. A few years later, the virus was renamed "human immunodeficiency virus" (HIV).

Although the public health community speculated over the years that the source of HIV must be connected to primates in Africa, the origin of the virus in humans was not settled until 1999. That year, a team of researchers reported they had discovered HIV-1 in chimpanzees in west equatorial Africa. HIV-1, the predominant strain of HIV in the developed world, has a cousin, HIV-2, which is a slower-acting strain that occurs primarily in western Africa. The researchers identified a particular subspecies of chimpanzees as the likely original source of HIV-1 and concluded that the virus must have passed to humans from this source.

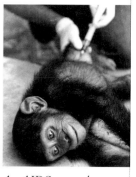

An AIDS researcher drawing blood from a chimpanzee.

The properties of HIV are unique. A retrovirus, HIV replicates by binding to the outer surface of the CD4+ T cell (also known as a helper T lymphocyte, a white blood cell that fights infections and is critical to a healthy immune system). After binding to this cell, HIV enters the cell and remains hidden and protected from other immune system cells. Once inside, HIV copies its RNA, creating a new viral DNA that is integrated into the host cell's DNA. Empowered by the host cell, HIV replicates new virions (single viruses). The new virions leave the host cell to infect others, and the host CD4+ T cell dies. While the body produces about 10 billion new virions daily, the immune system kills and removes most of them, leaving about 100 million virions that are infectious. Although the body creates CD4+ T cells every day, virions kill others off, leading to a struggle for balance of power between HIV and CD4+ T cells.

HIV is transmitted in the following ways:

◆ Sexual contact with an infected partner, including vaginal, anal and oral intercourse; HIV enters the body through the lining of the female and male genitalia, the rectum, and through the mouth (men having sex with men remain the population at highest risk, although the growth rate of HIV infection in women in the U.S. has in some years outstripped that in gay and bisexual men).

◆ Sharing needles or syringes contaminated with infected blood (the number of cases in injected drug users is second only to gay and bisexual men in the U.S.).

◆ From infected woman to fetus during pregnancy or to newborn during birth.

◆ Breast-feeding by infected mothers to newborns.

◆ Transfusion of infected blood or blood products.

Based on available evidence, HIV is not transmitted through saliva, sweat, tears, urine or feces. No transmission has been attributed to biting insects, and only rarely through mucosal or casual contact with blood or body fluids. Casual contact does not include sitting next to someone, shaking hands, hugging, eating in the same restaurant, swimming in the same pool, using the same shower or tub, and using the same toilet seat.

How do people infected with HIV know if they have AIDS? ► When monitoring a person with HIV, two blood tests should be done periodically, a CD4+ T cell count and a viral load count. If the CD4 count drops below 200 cells/mm3, or an AIDS-defining condition develops, the person has AIDS. AIDS-defining conditions, listed below, would be very unusual in someone not infected with HIV.

◆ Candidiasis (known as thrush, a fungus in the mouth)

◆ Invasive cervical cancer in women

◆ Coccidioidomycosis, cryptococcosis, cryptosporidiosis

◆ Cytomegalovirus disease

◆ Encephalopathy (HIV-related)

◆ Herpes simplex (severe infection)

▼

When monitoring a person with HIV, two blood tests should be done periodically, a CD4+ T cell count and a viral load count.

- Histoplasmosis

- Isosporiasis

- Kaposi's sarcoma (a rare skin lesion caused by a type of herpes virus)

- Lymphoma (certain types)

- Mycobacterium avium complex

- Pneumocystis carinii pneumonia

- Pneumonia (recurrent)

- Progressive multifocal leukoencephalopathy

- Salmonella septicemia (recurrent)

- Toxoplasmosis of the brain

- Tuberculosis

- Wasting syndrome

The immediate concern for someone infected with HIV, even before he or she develops AIDS, is treatment. Today, people with HIV should be followed clinically with lab tests to assess their need for antiretroviral therapy and to monitor their progress. The viral load count becomes an important measure in determining when and how to proceed. Generally, anti-HIV medications are called for if the viral load is 100,000 copies/mL or more or if the CD4+ T cell count declines rapidly. Systemic factors also play a role.

Treatment of HIV in the early 1980s consisted mainly of palliative care, since the origins and course of the disease were still a mystery and drugs to fight it effectively had yet to be developed.   ►   Until 1987, when the medication AZT was licensed for use, death usually occurred within 18 months of diagnosis, often from pneumonia after a period of alarming weight loss. Patients often had more than one opportunistic infection or cancer at a time – such as candidiasis, diarrheal disease, Kaposi's sarcoma and, in the end, pneumocystis carinii pneumonia. Not all people with HIV develop symptoms rapidly, however. The median time lag for developing symptoms is estimated to be ten years, but some people infected with HIV develop symptoms very quickly while others stay free of symptoms for many years. Dr. James Curran, dean of Rollins School of Public Health at Emory University and former head of the HIV/AIDS

▼

Until 1987, when the medication AZT was licensed for use, death usually occurred within 18 months of diagnosis....

▼

"Unfortunately, most people in the world with HIV still get no treatment."

unit at CDC, observes, ► "Unfortunately, most people in the world with HIV still get no treatment."

The public health response to the HIV/AIDS pandemic in its early days included education, testing and partner notification. So little was known about the disease that the public clamored for information. Could kissing transmit HIV? Who was most at risk? As CDC began collecting data on every reported case before the discovery of HIV and the availability of testing, new populations surfaced as being potentially at special risk – Haitians, injecting drug users and hemophiliacs. Almost from the start of the epidemic, some hospitals began to separate at-risk populations and AIDS cases and recommended that staff be fully gowned, masked and gloved when treating patients. Since the exchange of blood through needles was known to transmit AIDS, special precautions became necessary for drawing blood.

Some of the more controversial public health measures to address the emerging epidemic included anonymous and voluntary HIV testing, partner notification and blinded seroprevalence surveys. Early on, the public health community encouraged individuals who were at risk of infection to learn about their HIV status through anonymous testing sites that were established at local and state health departments. Individuals who tested positive were encouraged to notify their partner(s). For those who tested positive and were reluctant to notify their partner(s), state and local health departments set up systems for notifying partners, collecting the names and notifying them while shielding the name of the index case. Finally, CDC developed a series of validated or blinded seroprevalence surveys – in pregnant women, in newborns, in STD clinic patients – in order to better understand the epidemic and how it was changing. Controversy developed when states began to feel pressure to identify the positive cases in order to notify them of their HIV status and the need for therapy. In some states, such as New York, the newborn seroprevalence survey has been "unblinded" so that the names of the babies are made known to pediatricians and mothers who are referred for therapy. Since the early 1990s, the U.S. Public Health Services has recommended that all pregnant women in the U.S. receive voluntary HIV testing during pregnancy.

► Today, after concentrated research and development by pharmaceutical companies, the U.S. Food and Drug Administration (FDA) has approved more than 20 anti-HIV medications for adults and adolescents. The U.S. Department of Health and Human Services (DHHS) provides HIV-treatment guidelines to physicians and patients and updates them as the FDA approves new treatment protocols. The guidelines recommend that three or more medications be taken together in a regimen called Highly Active Anti-retroviral Therapy (HAART). Because the choices of combinations of drugs are now numerous, each case requires careful, methodical analysis and periodic adjustment by a physician.

▼

...the U.S. Food and Drug Administration has approved more than 20 anti-HIV medications for adults and adolescents.

Four classes of antiretroviral medications now exist:

◆ Nucleoside Reverse Transcriptase Inhibitors: NRTIs, faulty versions of building blocks needed by HIV to replicate, lure HIV away from normal building blocks and stall reproduction of the virus (first FDA approval: March 1987).

◆ Protease Inhibitors: PIs disable protease, another protein needed by HIV to replicate (first FDA approval: December 1995).

◆ Nonnucleoside Reverse Transcriptase Inhibitors: NNRTIs bind to reverse transcriptase and disable this protein needed by HIV to replicate (first FDA approval: June 1996).

◆ Fusion Inhibitors: FIs prevent HIV from entering cells (first FDA approval: March 2003).

For treatment to be effective, patients must adhere to a strict regimen. They must observe an unwavering daily timetable for ingesting pills and be careful about what they eat and drink. For patients who adhere to the strict regimen, remarkable successes are becoming the norm in keeping HIV and symptoms in check. In fact, AIDS is often now a chronic, treatable disease rather than one that carries an automatic death sentence. However, even now in the United States, over 15,000 deaths from AIDS occur each year, and there is still no cure.

In addition to their focus on providing new antiretroviral medications, pharmaceutical companies have focused on an HIV vaccine since the discovery of the virus. Until a proven vaccine clears the hurdles of clinical trials, however, the only sure method to fight AIDS continues to be prevention. The view of AIDS as a chronic, treatable disease, paired with a current epidemic of methamphetamine use in the gay community, has led many young and middle-aged gay men to resume unprotected sex, a grave concern to the public health community. Public health experts note that messages need to resonate in the teen and young adult population stating that the only sure way to prevent AIDS is abstinence and avoidance of needle-sharing. Although more than two dozen clinical trials of experimental AIDS vaccines are being conducted worldwide, only one has made it to Phase 3 clinical trials. ▶ A viable AIDS vaccine is not yet in sight.

The up and down mood swings felt by the scientific and public health communities and by the public as the AIDS pandemic unfolds – from pessimism and depression to optimism and euphoria and now back to a new realism – accurately capture the repeated cycles of questions that are unique to AIDS. Unlike many other infections, AIDS deals with taboos and denials and a greater amount of fear and uncertainty. Even so, many middle and high schools today openly teach HIV prevention, integrating the latest information about the epidemic into their health and wellness curricula.

Sobering statistics account for the fear and uncertainty. More than 600,000 cases of AIDS have been reported in the United States since 1981. An estimated 850,000 to 950,000 Americans are currently infected with HIV, with African-Americans affected disproportionately. ▶ Included in this estimate are 180,000 to 250,000 people who don't know they are infected. From 1985 to 1996, AIDS cases in women increased threefold. Citing 1999 as the low point in incidence of AIDS, CDC reported in July 2003 that AIDS in gay and bisexual men had increased nearly 18 percent since then. While the rate of HIV infections in the U.S. continues to increase, the number of AIDS cases has fallen dramatically since 1996. In that year, HAART came into common use and the death rate from AIDS in the U.S. began to level off.

The rest of the world is another matter, however. AIDS is now the fourth leading cause of death worldwide and

▼

A viable AIDS vaccine is not yet in sight.

▼

Included in this estimate are 180,000 to 250,000 people who don't know they are infected.

the No.1 cause of death due to infectious disease. AIDS has surpassed malaria as the leading killer in Africa. In 2003, 38 million people were thought to be living with HIV/AIDS and an estimated five million people acquired HIV that year, more than in any prior year. More than three million people were killed by AIDS in 2003, bringing the total number of people who have died from AIDS, since the first cases of AIDS were identified in 1981, to more than 20 million.

Yes, these statistics are sobering. On the other hand, remarkable progress has been made against a disease that emerged from nowhere in 1981. The behavior of gay men in the developed world changed quickly; HIV itself was isolated and identified almost immediately, and new medications and other therapies were discovered and used. The accumulated knowledge of the complex mechanisms of AIDS enabled ever more effective countermeasures to be developed that extend and enrich lives previously viewed as imperiled. In the developed world, AIDS has become an often chronic, treatable condition rather than a rapid death sentence. This progress must be celebrated as a signal achievement of the scientific and public health communities. But as Dr. Curran points out, "We still have a long way to go in the world. There is still neither a cure nor a vaccine. Science and public health cannot rest." ◻

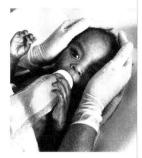

Child receives an aromatherapy massage at an orphanage for children with AIDS.

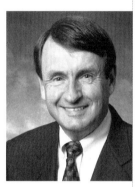

Dr. James Curran, Dean of the Rollins School of Public Health, Emory University.

Vignette

Development of Penicillin

Sir Alexander Fleming discovered penicillin by accident at St. Mary's Hospital in London in September 1928. The story of how he stumbled on an extraordinary advance in public health illustrates the role serendipity can play in the often painfully slow process that accompanies great advances in scientific history.

As he was about to discard a culture plate while cleaning up his laboratory in the Inoculation Department of the hospital, the young Scottish physician noticed something funny. He remembered streaking the plate some weeks before with *staphylococci* and now noticed a contaminant mold growing near one edge of the plate. Around the mold, the colonies of *staphylococci* were translucent and smaller; while further away on the plate, the colonies continued to grow in their normal way, robust and snowy white. Dr. Fleming realized that something in the mold was destroying the disease-causing bacteria.

What was this mold? With the help of the mycology lab one floor below, Alexander Fleming identified it as *Penicillium,* and the sub-

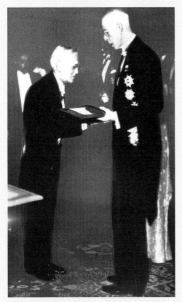

Sir Alexander Fleming receiving the 1945 Nobel Prize for scientific achievement from King Gustav V of Sweden.

stance in it, as penicillin. He began to experiment with penicillin and discovered that its properties also destroyed other disease-causing bacteria. Fleming realized that penicillin would be an effective treatment against infectious diseases, yet other scientists shunned his presentations at scientific meetings and his journal articles. Rather than fight to overcome the skepticism of the scientific community, Fleming turned his attention to other areas of research. He owed much in his work to Sir Almroth Wright, who established the Inoculation Department in 1907 to produce and sell vaccines. The diminutive, reticent Fleming was no match for the brilliant and abundant eccentricities of Wright, but after Fleming earned his degree in surgery, it was Wright who gamely kept

Fleming on staff and encouraged the ingenuity that became a hall-mark of Fleming's experimental techniques.

Twelve years elapsed before Howard Florey and Ernst Chain at Oxford University resuscitated Fleming's findings and vindicated his claims for penicillin. Ironically, it was Alexander Fleming who

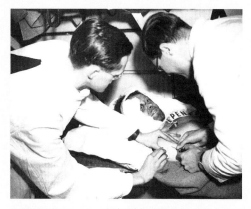

gained fame after penicillin began to be produced commercially in the early 1940s, saving countless wounded on the battle-fields of Europe and Asia with its disease-destroying properties. Fleming had, in fact, become an expert on treating war wounds with antiseptics during his World War I service at Boulogne, France. In 1945, Alexander Fleming was awarded a

In WW II, a wounded soldier is injected with penicillin.

Nobel Prize in medicine, and by staying at St. Mary's Hospital for the remainder of his career, he gained fame for the hospital as the site of his discovery.

Under constant threat of German air raids and a possible invasion, the Oxford group sought help in the United States for continued research and production of penicillin. In the fall of 1942 in Brooklyn, the Charles Pfizer Company dedicated its citric acid production facilities to penicillin. Military demand was paramount, and Pfizer's production eased supply shortages, helping to make penicillin the miracle drug it became on World War II battlefields.

Meanwhile, at Brooklyn's Jewish Hospital, Dr. Leo Loewe and his associates were participating in a clinical trial of penicillin for the treatment of streptococcal subacute bacterial endocarditis, an infec-tion of heart valves damaged by rheumatic fever. The mortality of this disease was 97 percent, and the results for penicillin were not encouraging. Of 17 patients treated, four died, 10 showed no improvement, and two of the three who showed improvement had relapses as soon as treatment stopped. Dr. Loewe now confronted a 34-year-old man for whom his team had tried everything for six months – huge doses of sulfa drugs, artificial fever therapy, heparin, and moderate doses of penicillin. Desperate, they tried a larger dose of penicillin – 200,000 units per day instead of the standard 40,000 units (miniscule by today's standards) – by intravenous drip. The alpha-hemolytic streptococcus disappeared from the patient's blood, reappeared after treatment stopped and disappeared for good after a second several-week course of treatment. Dr. Loewe had proved that endocarditis could be cured with aggressive treatment with penicillin, but he and his associates now faced a shortage of available penicillin, all of it earmarked for the military. Fortunately, the senior executive of nearby Pfizer, John L. Smith, contributed a supply from his research allotment, and another seven patients were treated and cured. Smith visited each of the seven personally and, thereafter, continued to supply Dr. Loewe with penicillin from Pfizer's research allotment, despite the risk of being found in violation of the War Department's requirement that all manufactured penicillin be dedicated to military use.

Fleming's discovery of penicillin was also not without controversy. Others trying to duplicate his experiment failed, and not until 1940, under a microscope at Oxford, was it determined that penicillin worked against microorganisms only when they were actively in the stage of division. What's more, it was later determined that Fleming's serendipitous strain of *Penicillium* happened to be one of the three most effective in its disease-destroying properties. Recent reconstructions of Fleming's discovery have also determined that the weather conditions in September 1928 were ideal – a cold snap followed by warm temperatures – for the phenomena observed by Fleming to occur. Without those ideal conditions, he may never have discovered penicillin. ◻

Looking Ahead
Antibiotic Resistance

Antibiotics, which are also known as antimicrobial drugs, fight infections caused by bacteria. In the decades since their discovery in the 1940s, the antibiotics that normally control bacteria have become less effective as the bacteria have become increasingly resistant. Penicillin – the miracle drug that saved countless wounded on World War II battlefields – today faces the fiercest strain of resistant bacteria.

► In fact, virtually every important bacterial infection in the United States and throughout the world is now becoming resistant, to one degree or another, to antibiotics. For this reason, Centers for Disease Control and Prevention (CDC) considers antibiotic resistance one of its top concerns, and the U.S. Food and Drug Administration (FDA) seeks ways to streamline the approval process for new antibiotics to replace those that have been compromised by resistant bacteria.

Bacteria develop resistance through genetic mutation. No one antibiotic kills every last targeted bacteria. The bacteria that survive, already displaying resistance, pass their genes to a new and more numerous generation, rendering the antibiotic even less effective for the patient the next time it is used. Sometimes, resistant bacteria even exchange their genetic code with unrelated bacteria, causing unforeseen resistance to other antibiotics.

How did this problem develop? The reasons are multifactorial and include the overuse and incorrect use of antibiotics. Parents often request antibiotics to treat their children's colds or ear infections before allowing these conditions to clear up on their own. Against their own better judgment, physicians often acquiesce to a patient's demand for antibiotic treatment. Eager for quick results, physicians sometimes prescribe antibiotics to treat conditions for which they are not appropriate. Both patients and physicians must be educated about the appropriate use of antibiotics.

In 1999, the U.S. Department of Health and Human Services (DHHS) formed a task force among federal agencies to tackle the problem of antimicrobial resistance. CDC,

▼

In fact, virtually every important bacterial infection in the United States and throughout the world is now becoming resistant, to one degree or another, to antibiotics.

FDA and National Institutes of Health co-chaired the task force, which in 2001 issued a plan of action. Known as the Public Health Action Plan to Combat Antimicrobial Resistance, the plan's success depends on the cooperation of state and local health agencies, universities, professional societies, pharmaceutical companies, health care professionals, agricultural producers and the public. ► The plan's primary focus is to facilitate the development of new antimicrobial therapies while preserving the usefulness of current and new drugs.

CDC developed its own Campaign to Prevent Antimicrobial Resistance, which aims to prevent antimicrobial resistance in health care settings. The campaign has four main strategies: prevent infection, diagnose and treat infection, use antimicrobials wisely and prevent transmission. The campaign is developing multiple 12-step programs that target specialty clinicians who treat specific patient populations, including hospitalized children and adults, dialysis and surgical patients and long-term care patients. The campaign is developing educational tools and materials for each patient population.

The American College of Physicians has issued guidelines for patients, physicians and other health care providers.

Guidelines for Preventing Antimicrobial Resistance From the American College of Physicians

For patients:

◆ Insist that antibiotics be prescribed (for yourself or your children) only when they can be useful; know the risks as well as the benefits.

◆ Remember that antibiotics work only against bacteria. Most colds, coughs, sore throats (except strep throat) and runny noses are caused by viruses and cannot be cured by antibiotics.

◆ Don't use antibiotics left over from an old prescription without a doctor's permission, and never share antibiotics with family members or friends.

▼

The plan's primary focus is to facilitate the development of new antimicrobial therapies while preserving the usefulness of current and new drugs.

◆ Wash hands thoroughly with soap and hot water, and teach your children to do the same. Antibacterial soap is not necessary – ordinary soap will eliminate resistant bacteria and help prevent illnesses.

◆ Make sure immunizations are up to date. People older than 65 and people with chronic illnesses should be vaccinated against pneumonia and influenza.

◆ Finish a prescribed antibiotic even if you feel better. By stopping treatment before the full course, some partly resistant bacteria will remain and multiply, making the antibiotic less effective the next time.

◆ Wash fruits and vegetables thoroughly, and avoid raw eggs and undercooked meats, especially ground meats.

For physicians:

◆ Don't overprescribe antibiotics.

◆ Choose narrow- over broad-spectrum antibiotics, using the most specific, narrowly targeted ("narrow-spectrum") antibiotics possible if you know the causal agent. Save the newer, broad-spectrum drugs for infections that resist the older drugs.

◆ Wash hands thoroughly with soap and hot water between each patient visit.

◆ Educate patients about the risks of antibiotic resistance.

◆ Make sure that all patients have the appropriate immunizations.

For hospitals:

◆ Improve infection control.

◆ Use ultraviolet lights, insist on consistent hand-washing by staff, and improve sanitation.

◆ Quickly identify and isolate patients with drug-resistant infections.

For health systems and health departments:

◆ Encourage and facilitate appropriate immunizations for children, adolescents, adults and the elderly.

◆ Monitor overall use of antibiotics to spot possible overuse of broad-spectrum antibiotics.

For the federal government:

◆ Require that product labels on antibiotic drugs contain the most current surveillance information on antibiotic resistance as well as prudent use information.

◆ Adequately fund national surveillance programs. Develop a system of electronic laboratory reporting by hospitals and laboratories. Establish a communication link to public health and medical communities to provide timely updates on aggregate data and their interpretation.

◆ Adequately fund immunization programs.

◆ Strengthen the public health infrastructure to facilitate rapid identification of and response to infectious disease outbreaks. Enhance laboratory capabilities and fund training programs for laboratory, epidemiology and infection control personnel.

◆ Fund research programs to develop new vaccines and antibiotics to prevent or treat diseases resulting from viral, bacterial, fungal and parasitic pathogens.

◆ Fund research programs to study microbial pathogenesis and molecular mechanisms responsible for drug resistance.

◆ Sponsor public health messages to the medical community and the public about the scope of the resistance problem and the prudent use of antimicrobial drugs.

◆ Monitor antimicrobial drug use in food-producing animals in order to protect human health.

For state governments:

◆ Adequately fund state surveillance efforts to study antibiotic resistant and other diseases.

◆ Include in state surveillance programs diseases that are notified nationally, and report collected information to CDC.

For researchers:

◆ Continue to develop and search for new antibiotics or antibiotics that work in new ways.

◆ Develop new vaccines against common microbial diseases to prevent infection in the first place.

For pharmaceutical manufacturers:

◆ On product labels, include messages about antibiotic resistance and information on prudent use of antimicrobial drugs. Discourage unnecessary and inappropriate use of products.

◆ Continue efforts to develop new vaccines and drugs to prevent or treat infectious diseases.

For agriculture:

◆ Reduce widespread use of antibiotics in animal feeds and food production.

For world health:

◆ Develop a global strategy for infectious diseases, and massively increase resources to protect, diagnose and treat people around the world.

◆ Facilitate the development of surveillance in addition to prevention and control measures.

◆ Improve sewage systems and water purity in developing nations.

The FDA is working on a variety of approaches to encourage the development of new antibiotics and new classes of antibiotics and other antimicrobials. One approach is exclusivity rights to protect a manufacturer's drug from generic-drug competition for a specific length of time. The FDA hopes exclusivity will help stimulate new antimicrobial drug development, even while it discourages overuse of antibiotics.   ▶   The FDA also has a variety of existing regulatory tools to help developers of antimicrobial drugs. One of these is an accelerated approval process for drugs that treat severely debilitating or life-threatening diseases; another is for drugs that show meaningful benefit over existing prescription drugs to cure diseases.

The FDA is investigating other approaches for speeding the antimicrobial approval process as well. One approach is to expand the number of clinical trials while reducing the number of participants in each clinical trial program. In

▼

The FDA also has a variety of existing regulatory tools to help developers of antimicrobial drugs.

this way, the FDA hopes to streamline the review process without compromising safety and effectiveness.

Scientists and health professionals generally agree that a way to decrease antibiotic resistance is to use antibiotic drugs more cautiously and to monitor outbreaks of drug-resistant infections. Research is critical to understanding the various mechanisms that pathogens use to evade drugs. Once these mechanisms are understood, new drugs can be designed that are more effective.

To that end, the FDA's National Center for Toxicological Research (NCTR) has been studying the mechanisms of resistance to antibiotic agents among bacteria from the human gastrointestinal tract. These bacteria are known to cause serious infections. The NCTR has also tabulated the amount of antibiotic residues that people consume in food from food-producing animals and has studied whether these residues affect human intestinal bacteria. The FDA is also reviewing drugs for food animals with an eye on assessing the safety of antibiotic drug residues in people. An important mission of CDC is to promote the guidelines noted above to the public and health care provider community. Fortunately, a growing number of public health organizations have joined the chorus in alerting the public to the proper use of antibiotics and basic infection control practices.

Much of the knowledge about antibiotic resistance flows from NIH, the FDA and CDC, the federal agencies that conduct research, develop solutions and educate the public about this emerging problem. As well, these agencies communicate to all levels of the public health infrastructure. The public health work force is committed to educating the public and health care providers about how to reduce transmission of infectious agents and how to use antibiotics appropriately. ► The ability to counteract resistance, however, starts at the individual level. To strengthen the chances for antibiotics to defeat infectious diseases the way they are meant to, each person must use antibiotics wisely and only when they are necessary, practice good personal hygiene and stay current with immunizations. Antibiotic resistance, a phenomenon that's here to stay, can be made more manageable if each person does his or her part. ▫

▼

Our ability to counteract resistance, however, starts at the individual level.

Photo credits

Chapter 5

Cancer

Looking Back

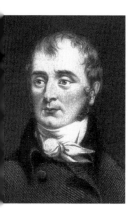

The history of cancer is as old as the history of humankind. Tumors are described in ancient Egyptian writings such as the Ebers papyrus, the Smith papyrus and the Petrie papyrus, all of which date to approximately 1600 BC. Ideas about the causes of cancer originated in Greece, with some of the earliest writings ascribed to Hippocrates. Hippocrates was the first to introduce the term "carcinoma" derived from *karkinos* (crab). He proposed that cancer was a disease caused by an excess of black bile (*atrabilis*), and classified tumors as malignant ulcers and deep-seated or occult tumors. In the second century, the famous Roman doctor Galen codified the Hippocratic theory, proposing that an excess of a body "humor" caused cancer. Galen was the first to use the term "sarcoma" for fleshy tumors and contended that inflammation occurred when the "humor" flowed to any part of the body.

The Smith papyrus approx. 1600 BC.

It wasn't until 1800 that the Frenchman Marie Francois Xavier Bichat proposed that cancer, rather than swollen and inflamed tissue, was instead an overgrowth of cellular tissue. In 1830, after the invention of the microscope, cells were identified as the fundamental unit in tumor tissue. In 1858, Rudolf Virchow, the German pathologist and founder of cellular pathology, first expressed the theory that every cell originates from another cell, a maxim that became the foundation for the modern cellular approach to cancer.

Marie Francois Xavier Bichat

Early in the 20th century, health care advocates began to recognize cancer as a significant problem for society. The American Society for the Control of Cancer (ASCC) was formed in 1913, prompted by the American Medical Association and the American College of Surgeons. Its goal was to educate the American public about cancer and help de-stigmatize the disease. In 1937, Congress established the National Cancer Institute, and in 1945, the ASCC became known as the American Cancer Society.

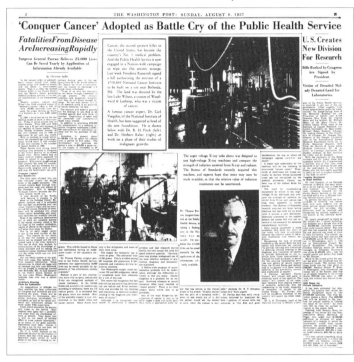

Announcement of the National Cancer Institute on August 6, 1937.

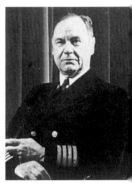

First NCI director Dr. Carl Voegtlin (1938-1943).

Until the 20th century, few cancer patients had any chance for long-term survival. By the 1930s, about one in four patients lived five years post-diagnosis. During the 1940s, cancer claimed 75,000 lives a year in the United States; and by 1970, cancer had become the nation's second-leading cause of death. Fears that cancer was contagious discouraged public discussion, as did the idea that cancer might be inherited. A major step in changing public perceptions about cancer occurred in 1971 when President Richard Nixon signed the National Cancer Act, which has been referred to as the "War on Cancer."

This legislation mobilized the country's resources to fight cancer by accelerating basic research and its translation to treatment. According to Dr. Vincent T. DeVita, one of the country's leading cancer authorities and later the director of the National Cancer Institute, "The National Cancer Act of 1971 was a turning point in the long bitter struggle to defeat the disease." The mandate that was stated in the act itself was "to support basic research and applications of the results of basic research to reduce the incidence, mortality and morbidity from cancer."

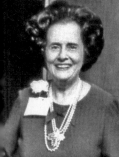

Mary Lasker

The National Cancer Act resulted from the intense lobbying of the late philanthropist Mary Lasker, who lived in New York City, and the unflagging support of Texas Senator Ralph W. Yarborough, who spearheaded the legislative effort in Congress. Mrs. Lasker was a patron and advocate of medical research on cancer, heart disease and blindness. As a volunteer leader of the American Cancer Society in the 1940s, she personally raised the first million dollars the society invested in cancer research. Mrs. Lasker's passionate interest in medicine was fueled in part by the illnesses of people around her and by her concern for her own health; she had painful ear infections repeatedly during her childhood. At the same time, Senator Yarborough sought to make the conquest of cancer a national priority. He led a group of medical experts, cancer advocates and business leaders who explored the issue; the group became commonly known as the "Yarborough Commission." The Yarborough Report became the blueprint for the National Cancer Act.

Lasker and Yarborough argued that government was spending $410 per person per year on defense compared with just 89 cents per person for cancer research, yet the disease had killed 330,000 Americans in 1970 alone. Together, they fought to increase government expenditures in cancer research and treatment, an unprecedented lobbying effort that became remarkably successful. The resulting National Cancer Act of 1971 established as a national priority the goal of conquering cancer and strengthened the National Cancer Institute's ability to lead the national cancer program.

In his May 11 remarks about the 1971 Act, President Nixon explained his rationale for granting special presidential interest to the cancer-cure program: "I have asked Congress to establish a cancer-cure program within the National Institutes of Health, where it can take the fullest advantage of other wide-ranging research. At the same time, it is important that this program be identified as one of our highest priorities and that its potential for relieving human suffering not be compromised by the familiar dangers of bureaucracy and red tape. For this reason, I am asking Congress to give the cancer-cure program independent budgetary status and to make its director responsible directly to the president. This effort needs the full weight and support of the presidency to see to it that it moves toward its goal as expeditiously as possible."

The government directed its actions in the fight against cancer through the National Cancer Institute. After the National Cancer Act passed, the National Cancer Institute became part of the Public Health Service with special independent authority within the National Institutes of Health (NIH). Once housed at NIH, the National Cancer Institute greatly expanded its authorities and resources.

► Since 1971, research funds have grown from less than $1 million annually to nearly $5 billion. The resulting mobilization of resources granted under the 1971 National Cancer Act laid the foundation for building the unparalleled research infrastructure and enterprise that exists today, including a national network of cancer centers that conduct cutting-edge research and deliver state-of-the-art clinical care. The centers support a strong core of cancer research, community-based cancer-prevention programs, and training and continuing education programs for health care professionals. The centers also support clinical trials that offer patients access to new therapies.

▼

Since 1971, research funds have grown from less than $1 million annually to nearly $5 billion.

Cancer: From Fatal to Treatable

Early in the 20th century, the only curable cancers were small and localized enough to be completely removed by surgery. In 1896, a German physics professor, Wilhelm Conrad Roentgen, presented a remarkable lecture titled, "Concerning a New Kind of Ray." He called it the "X-ray," with "X" being the algebraic symbol for an unknown quantity. Worldwide excitement about Roentgen's discovery arose immediately. Within months, systems were being devised to use X-rays for diagnosis; and within three years, radiation began to be used in the treatment of cancer. Radiation was also used after surgery to control small tumor growths that were not surgically removed. In 1901, Roentgen received the first Nobel Prize awarded in physics.

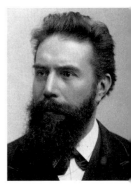

Professor Wilhelm C. Roentgen

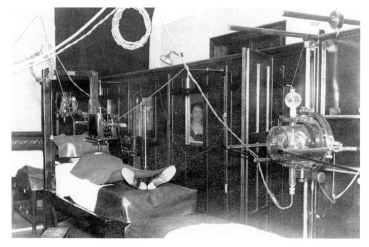

Patient receiving an X-ray in a Roentgen ray apparatus, 1920.

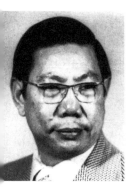

*Dr. Min Chiu Li,
first to cure a form
of metastatic cancer.*

It wasn't until 1956 that the cure of metastatic cancer became possible, when Dr. Min Chiu Li, who worked at NIH, discovered a cure for choriocarcinoma, a cancer that originates in trophoblastic cells of the placenta (afterbirth). Along with other major research advances, Li demonstrated that systemic chemotherapy could result in the cure of a widely metastatic malignant disease.

By the mid-20th century, scientists began to acquire the resources needed to begin exhaustive research on chemical and biological problems presented by cancer. One of these resources was the discovery of the exact chemical structure of DNA by Drs. James Watson and Francis Crick in 1953

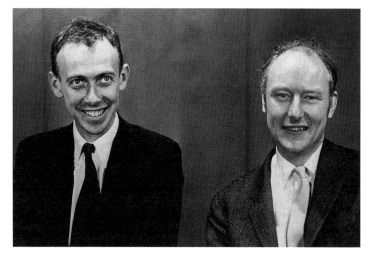

An early photograph of Drs. James Watson and Francis Crick.

in Cambridge, England. This discovery made it possible for scientists to understand how genes worked and how they could be damaged by mutations. As the understanding of DNA and genes increased, scientists determined that it was the damage to DNA by chemicals and radiation or the introduction of new DNA sequences by viruses that often led to the development of cancer. Scientists also discovered that defective genes might be inherited. Offering considerable promise for early screening, these findings on DNA mutation and defective-gene heredity made possible the identification of people who had a higher probability of developing cancer.

Although a cure for cancer has yet to be found, 33 years after the U.S. government declared war on cancer, advances in cancer biology, cancer treatment and prevention have dramatically improved treatment, survival and quality of life for people with cancer. The development and use of chemotherapy drugs have resulted in the successful treatment of many people with cancer. Advances in technology make it possible to aim radiation more precisely than in the past. New surgical procedures allow for more complete removal of many tumors. And a better understanding of the role of environment and lifestyle on cancer development (chemicals, nutrition, physical activity, smoking, sun and exposure) has led to more effective education about prevention. As the former director of the National Cancer Institute, Richard Klausner, MD, said in an interview with *Time* magazine, ▶ "We may not know how to cure cancer yet, but we do know what we need to do to get there. And that's very exciting."

Cancer incidence rates dropped 0.5 percent per year in the last decade of the 20th century (1991-2001), while death rates from all cancers combined dropped 1.1 percent per year from 1993 to 2001 according to the Annual Report to the Nation on the Status of Cancer, 1975-2001.* This report indicates that death rates for 11 of the top 15 cancers in men decreased 1.5 percent per year from 1993-2001, while death rates for eight of the top 15 cancers in women decreased by 0.8 percent per year from 1992-2001. In addition, for men large gains in cancer survival rates (more than 10 percent) were seen in cancers of the prostate, colon and kidney and non-Hodgkin's lymphoma, melanoma and leukemia. At the same time, childhood

▼

"We may not know how to cure cancer yet, but we do know what we need to do to get there. And that's very exciting."

cancers showed some of the largest improvements in cancer survival during the past 20 years, with an absolute survival rate increase of 20 percent in boys and 13 percent in girls. In fact, the current five-year survival rate of over 75 percent confirms the substantial progress made since the early 1970s, when childhood cancers were nearly always fatal. This has been a remarkable accomplishment.

Observes John Seffrin, PhD, chief executive officer of the American Cancer Society: "Advances in our understanding of cancer biology have taught us that cancer is not a single disease that will be conquered with a single 'magic bullet' cure as was believed 30 years ago. ► Today, we know that cancer is far more complex, representing hundreds of diseases, each requiring specialized approaches to treatment. Since its inception, the national cancer program has reaped remarkable returns, revolutionizing the way we prevent, diagnose and treat cancer. We have seen a decline in death rates for many cancers, and more people are surviving than ever before. We have also dramatically improved quality of life for people with cancer." ▫

▼

"Today, we know that cancer is far more complex, representing hundreds of diseases, each requiring special-ized approaches to treatment."

*Cancer-incidence rates and cancer-death rates are measured as the number of cases or deaths per 100,000 people per year and are age-adjusted to the 2000 U.S. standard population. When a cancer affects only one gender – for example, prostate cancer – then the number is per 100,000 persons of that gender.

Case Study
Screening Tools for Cancer Detection

Identifying cancer in its earliest stage, it is widely accepted, leads to improved diagnosis, less radical treatment, decreased mortality and lower health care costs. Today, the health care community is fortunate to have a variety of screening tools available to identify cancers in their initial stage. While these screening methods are not perfect, their use has made early detection, treatment and even prevention possible, especially in four of the most common cancers: cervical, breast, prostate and colon.

Screening for Cervical Cancer

Cervical cancer occurs in the uterine cervix of females. It is often preceded by cervical dysplasia, a precancerous condition caused by the *human papillomavirus* (HPV) and is characterized by a change of cervical cells that can be detected by a Papanicolaou smear and confirmed by biopsy. The Papanicolaou smear is a microscopic examination of cells taken from the cervix. This test was first proposed in 1923 by Dr. George Papanicolaou to diagnose uterine cancer. His proposal was not well received by his colleagues, who argued that the diagnostic method was useless. Undeterred, in 1928 Papanicolaou delivered a lecture called "New Cancer Diagnosis" at the Race Betterment Conference in Battle Creek, Michigan, describing more fully the technique that came to be known as the "Pap smear." The medical profession still paid no attention to his work. His paper, "The Diagnostic Value of Vaginal Smears in Carcinoma of the Uterus," did not appear in the *American Journal of Obstetrics and Gynecology* until 1941. In 1942, he published the technique for staining, which he had developed in his Cornell laboratory; it came to be known as the Papanicolaou stain. In 1954, Papanicolaou published his *Atlas of Exfoliative Cytology,* and this time his peers immediately accepted the monumental work, nearly

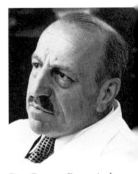

Dr. George Papanicolaou first proposed the "Pap smear" in 1923.

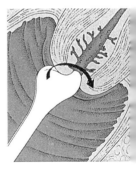

Pap smear technique of taking cells from the cervix.

30 years after his first lecture on the topic. In 1957 the American Cancer Society urged women to demand that Pap tests be included in their annual physicals and, further, earmarked 25 percent of its annual budget for training Pap test technicians and funding Papanicolaou's continued research. Yet it was not until 1988 that the American College of Obstetrics and Gynecology recommended an annual Pap smear to all women who are sexually active or have reached 18 years of age.

▼

The incidence of cervical cancer... has markedly decreased due almost entirely to the advent of the Papanicolaou smear.

► The incidence of cervical cancer, once a major cause of death in U.S. women, has markedly decreased due almost entirely to the advent of the Papanicolaou smear. In fact, between 1955 and 1992 the number of cervical cancer deaths in the United States dropped by 74 percent. The death rate from cervical cancer continues to decline by about two percent a year.

Detecting cervical cancer in its early stages is lifesaving, as survival of cancer of the cervix depends heavily on stage at diagnosis. Unfortunately, elderly, African-American and low-income women are less likely to have regular Pap tests. Similarly, cervical cancer deaths are higher in populations around the world where

American Cancer Society Cervical Cancer Detection Guidelines

Test	Age	Frequency
Pap test	Start 3 years after first vaginal intercourse but no later than 21	Yearly with conventional Pap test or every 2 years with liquid-based Pap test.
	Over 30	After 3 normal results in a row, screening can be every 2 – 3 years. An alternative is a Pap test plus HPV DNA testing and conventional or liquid-based cytology every 3 years.*
	Over 70	After 3 normal Pap smears in a row within the past 10 years, women may choose to stop screening.†
Pelvic exam	Not specified	Discuss with health care provider.

*Doctors may suggest a woman be screened more often if she has certain risk factors, such as HIV infection or a weak immune system.

†Women with a history of cervical cancer, DES exposure, or who have a weak immune system should continue screening as long as they are in reasonably good health.

women do not have routine Pap tests. In fact, cervical cancer is the major cause of cancer deaths in women in many developing countries. These cases are usually diagnosed at an invasive late stage, rather than as pre-cancers or early cancers.

Recognizing the impressive value of the Pap smear as a screening tool for early detection of cervical cancer, Congress passed the Breast and Cervical Cancer Mortality Prevention Act of 1990. This act authorized cervical cancer screening services for underserved women, including older women, women with low incomes and women of racial and ethnic minority groups. In short, when cervical cancer is found early and treated, it has proved to be highly curable. Most deaths from cervical cancer could be avoided, therefore, if women have regular checkups with the Pap test.

Screening for Breast Cancer

Breast cancer is any type of cancerous growth in the breast tissue. It is frequently diagnosed, second only to skin cancer diagnosis in women, and is the second leading cause of cancer death among women in the United States. In 2001, about 192,200 new cases of invasive breast cancer were diagnosed and 40,200 women died of the disease. The incidence of breast cancer has increased in recent years, and much of the increase can be attributed to the detection of smaller, earlier-stage cancers in asymptomatic women using mammography screening. In contrast to the increased detection of breast cancer, death rates decreased annually between 1990 and 2001 by 2.3 percent per year. This decline in breast cancer mortality has been attributed to mammography screening and to improvements in breast cancer treatment.

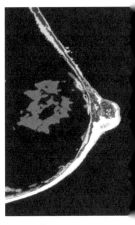

MRI of cancerous breast tissue.

Mammography is one of several screening tools for detecting early breast cancer. Screening mammograms are simply X-rays of each breast. The breast is placed between two imaging plates for a few seconds while the X-rays are taken. In addition to mammograms, other screening tests used to detect breast cancer are clinical breast exams and breast self-exams. A clinical breast exam is an exam done by a health professional to feel for lumps and look for changes in the size or shape of the breasts. A breast self-exam is an exam done by a woman herself. ► Physicians recommend that women do breast self-exams once a month starting in their 20s, about a week after their periods end. In the same way, between the ages of 20 and 39, every woman should have a clinical breast exam every three years, and after age 40 every woman should have a clinical breast exam each year. Although about 15 percent of tumors felt by clinical breast exam cannot be seen by regular mammographic screening, mammograms often detect tumors before they can be felt in clinical breast exams or breast self-exams; they can also identify tiny specks of calcium (microcalcifications) that could be an early sign of cancer. Therefore, a high-quality mammogram with a clinical breast exam is the most effective way to detect breast cancer early.

Several large studies conducted around the world show that breast cancer screening with mammograms reduces the number of deaths from breast cancer for women aged 40 to 69, especially those over age 50. ► Having annual mammograms provides a 20 percent to 30 percent reduction in the breast cancer mortality rate for women 50 years old and older. However, mammography is not without controversy. Cost-effectiveness estimates of mammography screening – based on methodology, population and interval – vary widely; it is estimated that breast cancer screening costs $3,400 to more than $83,000 per life-year saved. However, many experts and health care advocates believe that mammography offers the potential for significant benefits in addition to mortality reduction, including early diagnosis, less aggressive therapy and improved cosmetic results.

Some of the most important contributions toward awareness of breast cancer screening in the United States came in 1974. At that time, three women in the public eye were battling cancer at the same time:

▼

Physicians recommend that every woman do a breast self-exam once a month, about a week after her period ends.

▼

Having annual mammograms provides a 20 percent to 30 percent reduction in the breast cancer mortality rate for women 50 years old and older.

Betty Ford, Susan G. Komen and Rose Kushner. When Betty Ford was first diagnosed, breast cancer was rarely discussed in public and little was known about the disease. The first lady was the first high-profile American woman to publicly discuss her breast cancer, and she gained legions of admirers for the candor with which she faced her disease, as well as for her support of breast cancer awareness, screening and research.

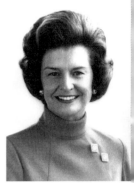

Former first lady Betty Ford in 1974.

Susan G. Komen, also battling breast cancer, asked her sister Nancy before she died to promise that she would do whatever she could to help other women facing breast cancer. In 1982, Nancy Brinker established the Susan G. Komen Breast Cancer Foundation based on that promise. Since then, the Komen Foundation has been instrumental in changing the way people think about breast cancer by inspiring a nationwide movement and rallying millions to the cause. Since its inception, the Komen Foundation has raised $450 million for breast cancer research and community outreach programs; a majority of these proceeds come from the popular Komen Race for the Cure Series, which draws 1.4 million people each year.

Journalist Rose Kushner's discovery in June 1974 of a breast lump that proved to be cancerous changed her life. Finding that there was little information available for the general public, she researched the topic in medical and technical publications and kept notes as she underwent lumpectomy and reconstructive surgery. An article based on her experience appeared in *The Washington Post* and was syndicated in hundreds of newspapers. Her book *Breast Cancer: A Personal History and Investigative Report* (1975) was revised and reprinted twice, as were *Why Me?* (1977) and *Alternatives* (1984). For her books and numerous articles about breast cancer, Rose Kushner received the Medal of Honor (1987) and the Courage Award (1988) from the American Cancer Society. She founded the Breast Cancer Advisory Center in 1975 to provide information and support for breast cancer patients and has frequently testified before Congress on health and cancer topics.

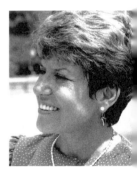

Rose Kushner in 1986.

American Cancer Society Breast Cancer Detection Guidelines		
Test	Age	Frequency
Breast self-exam (BSE)	Over 20	Optional. Women should be told about benefits and limitations of BSE. They should know how their breasts feel normally and report any differences to their health care professional.
Clinical breast exam	20-39	Part of a periodic health exam, preferably every 3 years.
	Over 40	Part of a periodic health exam, preferably every year.
Mammogram	Over 40	Yearly, continuing for as long as a woman is in good health.★

★ Women at increased risk (family history, genetic tendency, past breast cancer) should talk with their doctors about the benefits and limitations of starting mammography screening earlier, having additional tests (such as breast ultrasound, MRI) or having more frequent exams.

Screening for Prostate Cancer

Prostate cancer is the second leading cause of cancer death in men, exceeded only by lung cancer. It accounts for 29 percent of all male cancers and 11 percent of male cancer-related deaths. Modern methods of detection and treatment mean that prostate cancers are now detected earlier and treated more effectively, leading to decreases in death rates in recent years. The most common screening methods are testing the amount of prostate-specific antigen (PSA) in the blood and a digital rectal examination (DRE).

Prostate cancer screening was first implemented in the 1970s with the use of the DRE. However, DRE often detects disease in patients whose prostate cancer has already spread to other organs. The development and application of PSA for early detection and screening has led many patients to be diagnosed at an earlier stage than with DRE screening alone. PSA was first used experimentally in 1979 to monitor patients after prostate cancer treatment as a measure of disease recurrence and/or progression. Beginning in 1989, some evidence of its value in detecting early prostate cancer in men with no symptoms or signs of prostate disease was reported. Moreover, the principal strengths of the PSA test are its superior sensitivity, reasonable cost and high patient acceptance.

Since the use of early-detection tests for prostate cancer became relatively common in 1990, the prostate cancer death rate has dropped. It has been suggested that declines in mortality rates in certain communities reflect the benefit of PSA screening.   ▶   Over the past 20 years, the survival rate for prostate cancer has increased from 67 percent to 97 percent. Among men diagnosed with prostate cancer, 98 percent survive at least 5 years, 84 percent survive at least 10 years, and 56 percent survive at least 15 years. Of the men whose prostate cancers have already spread to distant parts of the body at the time of diagnosis, 34 percent will survive at least 5 years.

▼

Over the past 20 years, the survival rate for prostate cancer has increased from 67 percent to 97 percent.

In 1992, the American Cancer Society published a recommendation that men over 50 years of age be tested annually by DRE and PSA; later, it was modified to recommend that men discuss PSA testing with their physicians and make an informed decision about whether to be tested. In recent years, however, the PSA test has met with controversy. In September 2004, Dr. Thomas Stamey, a professor of urology at Stanford University who championed the test in 1987 as a tool for prostate cancer detection, published a scientific paper stating flatly that "the PSA era is over."

American Cancer Society Prostate Cancer Detection Guidelines		
Test	Age	Frequency
Digital rectal exam (DRE) and prostate-specific antigen (PSA) blood test	Over 50 (average risk)	Should be offered yearly (along with information on benefits and limitations) to men with at least a 10-year life expectancy.
	Over 50 (high risk★)	Yearly (along with information on potential risks and limitations).

★ Defined as African-American men or those with a strong family history (one or more affected first-degree relatives, such as fathers or brothers, diagnosed with prostate cancer at an early age). Men at even higher risk, due to multiple first-degree relatives affected at an early age, could begin testing at age 40. Depending on the results of the initial test, no further testing might be needed until age 45.

Essentially, Stamey wrote that he realized over the years that high PSA levels are merely indicators of prostate enlargement, not prostate cancer. Since then, many doctors and scientists have weighed in, with some taking Stamey's side and others questioning his findings. However, the American Cancer Society continues to recommend that men 50 years and older who have at least 10 years life expectancy with average risk be tested annually with PSA and DRE. Although PSA testing may lead to needless biopsies that remove part of the prostate tissue to make the diagnosis, all men should be made aware of the limitations and benefits of early detection of prostate cancer.

Screening for Colon Cancer

▼

Colon cancer... is the third most common cancer in the United States and the second leading cause of cancer death.

► Colon cancer, a disease in which cancerous cells form in the tissues of the colon, is the third most common cancer in the United States and the second leading cause of cancer death. It is generally accepted that most colon cancers develop from polyps, non-cancerous growths in the colon, which can progress to cancer. Screening reduces colon cancer morbidity and mortality by both diagnosing the disease at a more favorable stage and preventing disease by removing precancerous lesions. There are four common screening tests for colorectal cancer that may be used alone or in combination: fecal occult blood test (FOBT), flexible sigmoidoscopy, double-contrast barium enema (DCBE) and colonoscopy.

FOBT is designed to detect blood in the stool, which may come from either a cancer or, more commonly, large polyps (greater than two centimeters). A positive FOBT is the trigger for a diagnostic work-up of the entire colon with DCBE or colonoscopy to identify the source of bleeding. A sigmoidoscopy allows for direct visualization by the physician of the distal bowel (bowel at the farthest distance), and it is more sensitive and specific for adenocarcinomas and polyps than the FOBT. DCBE is a series of X-rays of the colon and rectum taken after the patient is given an enema, followed by an injection of air. The barium outlines the intestines on the X-rays, allowing many abnormal growths to be visible.

The most successful screening tool for detecting colon cancer, the colonoscopy, has the added benefit of total bowel visualization plus the ability to remove adenomas. A study published in 2000 in the *Journal of the American Medical Association* by Lindsay Frazier, MD of Harvard's Brigham and Women's Hospital, found that ► there would be significantly fewer deaths from colorectal cancer if a single colonoscopy was performed during a person's lifetime. The findings were contained in a cost-effectiveness analysis of 22 screening methods for colon cancer.

▼

...there would be significantly fewer deaths from colorectal cancer if a single colonoscopy was performed during a person's lifetime.

Unfortunately, findings from the National Health Interview Survey, administered by the Centers for Disease Control and Prevention (CDC), indicate that in 2000 only 45 percent of men and 41 percent of women aged 50 years or older had undergone a sigmoidoscopy or colonoscopy within the previous 10 years or had used an FOBT home test kit within the preceding year. Due to the low use of these screening tools, only 38 percent of colon cancers are found in an early stage.

There is a clear need to increase awareness and promote the use of colorectal cancer screening examinations at regular intervals. In 1985, President Ronald Reagan was diagnosed with colon cancer, and the surrounding publicity raised awareness of screening. Since the death from colon cancer in 1998 of Katie Couric's 42-year-old husband, Jay Monahan, the popular television "Today Show" co-host has devoted much of her professional and personal life to raising awareness of the disease. Research completed by the University of Michigan found that awareness efforts had increased colonoscopy rates by 20 percent due to what the researchers called "The Couric Effect."

Currently, CDC and partner organizations are seeking to increase the use of screening tests for colon cancer. For example, CDC and the Centers for Medicare & Medicaid Services have created and implemented "Screen for Life," a multimedia campaign promoting colorectal cancer screening. CDC has also developed a training program for health care providers, titled *A Call to Action*, designed to increase their awareness of and knowledge about prevention and early detection of colorectal cancer. The American Cancer Society has launched an ambitious public awareness campaign to help consumers understand their colon cancer risk and encourage them to discuss testing options with their doctors. ▫

American Cancer Society Colorectal Cancer Detection Guidelines

Test	Age	Frequency
Fecal occult blood test (FOBT) or Fecal immunochemical test (FIT)	Over 50	Yearly
Flexible sigmoidoscopy	Over 50	Every 5 years
FOBT or FIT and flexible sigmoidoscopy	Over 50	Yearly, Every 5 years*
Colonoscopy	Over 50	Every 10 years
Double-contrast barium enema (DCBE)	Over 50	Every 5 years

*Combined testing is preferred over either FOBT or FIT, or flexible sigmoidoscopy every 5 years, alone. People who are at moderate or high risk for colorectal cancer should talk with a doctor about a different testing schedule.

Vignette

Skin Cancer and Sunblock/SPF Products

Skin cancer is the most common type of cancer in the United States. In the past, the public did not perceive exposure to the sun, whether through purposeful sun tanning or through work outdoors, as dangerous. However, more than one million cases of basal cell or squamous cell cancer are diagnosed annually.

Skin cancer is a largely preventable disease if sun protective practices are used consistently. Interestingly, it was only in 1978 that sun exposure was first linked to skin cancer through research. In 1986, a study presented by Dr. Robert Stern, Chief of Dermatology at the Beth Israel Hospital in Boston, found that using sun protection factor SPF 15 sunscreen regularly during the first 18 years of life – when 80 percent of lifetime sun exposure occurs – might reduce by 78 percent a person's lifetime risk of developing nonmelanoma skin cancer. SPF measures a sunscreen's ability to absorb UVB rays and generally indicates how much longer an individual can stay in the sun before burning. After the release of this study, a young child's sunburned shoulders and face, once seen as cute, were viewed as dangerous, and promoting the use of sunscreen became an integral part of skin cancer prevention programs.

Who invented sunscreen is not exactly clear, but this much is known. In the early 1930s, a young chemist in South Australia, H.A. Milton Blake, experimented in a kitchen with some friends to produce a sunburn cream. The University of Adelaide tested the product, gave it a thumbs up, and Hamilton Laboratories was born. In 1936, a French scientist named Eugene Schueller, the founder of L'Oreal, invented the first sunscreen, according to his company's Web site. During World War II, airman and future pharmacist Benjamin Green developed a sun-protective formula for soldiers. Later, in 1944, Green invented a suntan cream called "Coppertone Suntan Cream" in his Miami Beach kitchen. In 1945, he added "Coppertone Suntan Oil" to the line, promoted by the slogan "Don't be a pale face."

In 1972, the Coppertone brand introduced the SPF system in the U.S., but the FDA did not revise its sunscreen regulations until 1993 to state that sunscreens with a high SPF were effective in stopping UVB penetration that might cause skin cancer. In addition to using sunscreen products, sun-safety awareness campaigns have reinforced other preventive measures, such as avoiding the sun between 11 a.m. and 3 p.m. and wearing sun-protective clothing. ◻

Looking Ahead

Genomic Research and Medicine

In 1990, the United States Department of Energy and the National Institutes of Health founded the Human Genome Project, an international collaborative research program. Its goal was the complete mapping and sequencing of all the genes of human beings, and remarkably this goal was fulfilled only a decade later in June 2000. In April 2003, with a high-quality, "finished" sequence completed, the findings on human genomes were made available to researchers and the public. Since then, the medical industry has continued to build upon the Human Genome Project's findings to further understanding of genetic contributions to human health. Specifically, medical professionals from all specialties are turning their attention to investigating the role that genes play in health and disease.

Knowledge of the human genome is being used to prevent and control cancer. ▶ Utilizing new genetic information, scientists have found the mutations in genes or groups of genes that cause many cancers. Scientists have found that diseases such as breast cancer and colon cancer also have hereditary forms. This knowledge enables health care and public health professionals to help people they identify as at risk for developing a cancer, first by studying their genes and then by developing customized prevention or treatment programs that use pharmaceutical or therapeutic approaches.

▼

Utilizing new genetic information, scientists have found the mutations in genes or groups of genes that cause many cancers.

Cancer Gene Identification

Cancer genetics seeks to discover how genomic information can be used to identify cancer-predisposing genes. Identification of cancer-susceptibility genes is important because it will help physicians to make more informed medical decisions in order to restore normal life expectancy of people at a genetically increased risk for cancer. In addition, understanding the mechanisms of cancer growth in inherited cancers will offer insights into common cancer development.

As genes that might cause cancer are identified, it becomes possible to screen for cancer genes through genetic tests.

The American Society of Clinical Oncology recommends that genetic testing be offered under the following conditions.

◆ The individual has a personal or family history of a genetic cancer risk.

◆ Results will help diagnose the cancer or influence the medical care of a patient or family member.

In genetic testing, an affected family member should be tested first for the presence or absence of a specific mutation. If no mutation is found, unaffected family members need not be offered genetic testing. On the other hand, if a mutation is detected in an affected individual, then immediate family members should be tested for the presence or absence of the same mutation. If the mutation is not found, the genes carried by the affected relative do not increase the risk in the unaffected relative. However, these unaffected relatives can still develop cancer later in life, although the risk is usually much less than the risk for the mutation carriers.

The opportunity of identifying individuals in a preclinical state through genetic tests and initiating preventive therapy promises to avert disease treatment costs and suffering. In addition, advances in laboratory technology and in the identification of cancer-susceptibility genes such as BRCA1, BRCA2 and MSH2 will soon make it possible to test large segments of the population for cancer risk. However, the expansion of genetic testing poses other kinds of risks – medical, personal, psychosocial and economic. Public health professionals and medical ethicists will debate how to balance this potentially useful genetic information with the dangers of privacy invasion, insurance denials and employment issues.

Pharmacogenomics

Genomic-sequence information can be used to design highly targeted pharmaceutical therapies. Pharmaceutical genomics or "pharmacogenomics" has evolved as the study of how an individual's genetic inheritance affects the body's response to drugs. This area of study holds the promise that drugs might one day be tailored for individuals and adapted to each person's own genetic makeup. Understanding an individual's genetic makeup is thought to be the key to creating personalized drugs that work safely and with greater efficacy, although environment, diet, age, lifestyle and state of health also greatly influence a person's response to medicines.

Pharmacogenomics might also help to improve the side-effect profiles of cancer-drug therapy. Although chemotherapy is an effective and established treatment, its toxicity is significant. Infections, nausea, vomiting, nerve pain, and hair loss are common and can be an obstacle to completing a patient's recommended course of therapy, reducing its effectiveness. As a result, scientists have begun using the human genome sequence to design specific drugs that maximize therapeutic effects, inhibit malignant-cell growth and decrease damage to nearby healthy cells.

Gene Therapy

Gene therapy is an approach to treating disease that either modifies the expressions of an individual's genes or corrects abnormal genes. The concept of gene therapy was introduced in the late 1970s after the development of recombinant DNA technology. In 1990, Drs. William French Anderson, Michael Blaese and Kenneth Culver, researchers at the National Institutes of Health, performed the first successful gene therapy in humans. The team successfully treated a then four-year-old, Ashanthi DeSilva, for adenosine deaminase (ADA) deficiency, a rare genetic disease in which children are born with severe immuno-

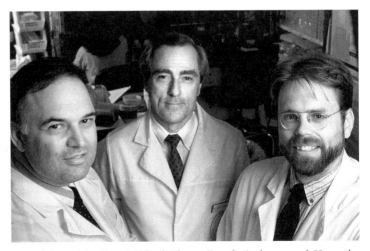

From left to right: Drs. Michael Blaese, French Anderson and Kenneth Culver performed the first successful gene therapy in humans.

deficiency and are prone to repeated serious infections.

With the complete sequencing of the human genome, scientists have more resources to further develop gene therapy. In particular, gene therapy represents a new field of medicine that can potentially cure some forms of cancer. All cancers have a genetic structure, triggered by altered genes in cancer cells, and a different gene or set of genes also controls the progression of a cell from normal to malignant to invasive. Currently, researchers are studying several approaches to treating cancer using gene therapy. Some approaches target healthy cells to enhance their ability to fight cancer, while others target cancer cells to destroy them or prevent their growth.

The Future of Genomics in Medicine

The genomic era is now a reality. Experts have begun to understand the role of genetic factors in health and disease and to use this knowledge in prevention, diagnosis and treatment. The completion of the human genome sequence is impacting public health. In furthering society's interest in good public health, advances in medical applications of genomic research improve the conditions that ensure that people can be healthy. Researchers hope that in the next 10 years, genetic tests for many common conditions will help alleviate inherited risk and that by the year 2020 gene-based designer drugs will be available for many conditions. ► Perhaps the most exciting prediction is that cancer treatment will precisely target the molecular fingerprints of particular tumors, and genetic information will be used routinely to give patients more appropriate drug therapy, avoiding unnecessary side effects and increasing chances of cure. Nevertheless, the ultimate use and interpretation of genetic information raises ethical, social, psychological and political issues. Consequently, public health and governmental authorities need to improve the infrastructure capabilities that will be needed to widely implement genomics' medical applications. Public health and government will also need to create regulatory policy to control the negative implications of genetic information, confronting such issues as privacy, labor and insurance discrimination, ethics and psychological consequences for affected families, among others.

▼

...the most exciting prediction is that treatment will precisely target the molecular fingerprints of particular tumors, and genetic information will be used to give patients more appropriate drug therapy.

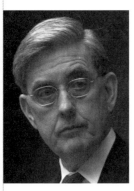

John Seffrin, PhD, chief executive of the American Cancer Society.

As Dr. Seffrin of the American Cancer Society points out, "The public, private and nonprofit sectors must diligently work together to advance groundbreaking cancer research. Prior investments in cancer research have laid the foundation for a period of unparalleled success."

However, current funding constraints allow the National Cancer Institute (NCI) to fund only one in five eligible research projects, forcing the NCI to pass over many exciting cancer research opportunities. With authorities granted under the 1971 National Cancer Act, the NCI director develops a strategic plan for cancer research each year that reflects the best thinking of cancer researchers, patients, clinicians and other constituency groups. As Seffrin explains, "The goal for the nation must be to provide adequate funding to explore the most promising opportunities in cancer research as outlined in this plan. Remarkable achievements such as the mapping of the human genome make new and better cancer treatments inevitable if we invest more of our health expenditures on research and development. Landmark discoveries such as cancer vaccines, targeted therapies and chemoprevention are leading to a paradigm shift in how cancer is treated and to thousands of lives being saved every year."

Seffrin also believes it is critically important to bridge the gap between science and practical application. In arenas where public health has united to drive delivery at the community level, there have been impressive results. "With state-of-the-art cancer care, 67 percent to 80 percent of current cancer patients will survive long-term," explains Seffrin. ► "Tragically, however, nowhere near 100 percent of cancer patients today will receive state-of-the-art cancer care. In fact, only about 60 percent will receive so-called 'standard care.' A cardinal principle of public health states that 'access to the means for the attainment and preservation of health is a basic human right.' In truth, however, full access to our health care system and to the best in cancer care is sometimes available only to a privileged few."

▼

"Tragically, however, nowhere near 100 percent of cancer patients today will receive state-of-the-art cancer care."

To implement a comprehensive cancer control program, according to Seffrin, disparate public health organizations should unite to deliver understandable and actionable cancer prevention and treatment information that increases patients' health literacy. At the same time, medical schools should improve education to enhance delivery of cancer prevention, and early-detection services, hospitals and treatment centers should improve health records systems to help coordinate prevention and screening efforts. Finally, policymakers should require that all insurers cover and reimburse for evidence-based prevention and early-detection services. ▫

Chapter 6

Cardiovascular Disease

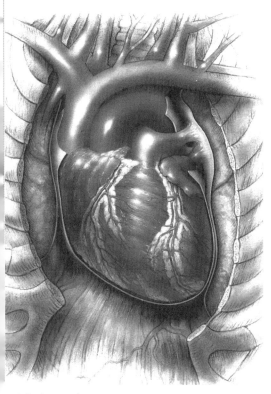

The human heart.

From the moment of birth until death, the human heart pumps continuously. Normally the size of a fist, this incredibly powerful muscle literally is life itself. The heart's form and function have been studied for centuries, leading to incredible advances in knowledge and interventions. However, cardiovascular disease (CVD) remains the leading killer for both men and women among all racial and ethnic groups in the United States. Indeed, cardiovascular disease was the greatest epidemic of the 20th century, outstripping infectious diseases such as polio and AIDS. The epidemic peaked around 1968 in the United States, with an impressive 2.6 percent decline in CVD mortality per year from 1968 to 1990. These declines have been recognized as one of the greatest health achievements in the 20th century.

Despite these declines, one person dies every 30 seconds from CVD, more than 2,600 people every day. Almost one million Americans die of CVD each year, representing 42 percent of all deaths. Of these, 160,000 are individuals between the ages of 35 and 64 years, an indication of how widespread CVD is in the population, not just among older Americans. Heart disease and stroke account for nearly six million hospitalizations each year and cause disability for almost 10 million Americans aged 65 years and older. The costs of treatment approach $329 billion each year when lost productivity from disability is factored in, encompassing physicians, professionals, hospital and nursing home services, medications and home health care. There is evidence that, despite the declines in death rates, the rate of new cases of CVD has not declined. A large proportion of CVD patients are living with their disease. By 2050, an estimated 25 million Americans will carry the diagnosis of coronary heart disease.

Looking Back
A Brief History of Cardiology

One of the earliest physicians, Imhotep (circa 2725 BC), was regarded in ancient Egypt as the god of medicine. He is said to have been the first to connect the pulse rate with the resulting action of the heart. It was not until the time of Hippocrates (460-377 BC), in ancient Greece, that the heart was mentioned again in medical rather than spiritual or mysterious terms. Hippocrates believed that the heart was a strong muscle and understood enough of its structure that he provided theories on the function of the heart's valves.

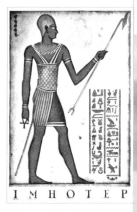

Imhotep (circa 2725 BC).

Roughly another 500 years passed before Claudius Galen (AD 130-201), considered the father of cardiology, studied the heart in detail. An authority on anatomy in ancient Rome, Galen was not allowed to dissect human bodies. Rather, his knowledge of the heart came from dissecting Barbary apes. It was no surprise, therefore, that much of Galen's work proved later to be incorrect. Nonetheless, his interest in the anatomy of the heart laid the foundation of cardiac study in future centuries.

In the 16th century, more progress in understanding the true function of the heart was made. The work of Miguel Servetus (1511-1553), a Spaniard, preceded the discoveries of William Harvey on blood circulation. Unfortunately, his work went unrecognized as he linked his medical views with theological writings that were deemed heretical. Fortunately, Andreas Vesalius (1514-1564), a graduate of Padua University in Italy, enjoyed greater intellectual freedom, leading to the publication in the mid-1500s of his studies on the heart.

Another graduate of Padua University was William Harvey, an Englishman. Harvey was fascinated by the way blood flowed through the human body. In 1628, he published *An Anatomical Study of the Motion of the Heart and of the Blood in Animals*, which explained how blood is pumped from the heart throughout the body, then returning to the heart and recirculated. Harvey's views, controversial at the time, contradicted the belief of many people that the liver and not the heart caused blood to flow. Harvey's work became the basis for modern research on the heart and blood vessels.

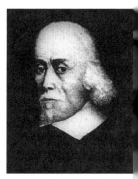

William Harvey explained how the heart pumps and recirculates blood.

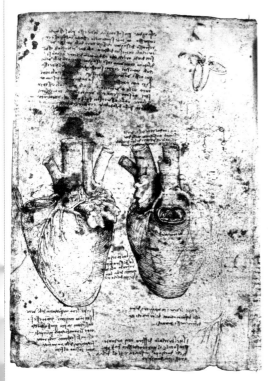

Drawing of the human heart and blood vessels by Leonardo da Vinci.

It is likely that both Vesalius and Harvey were greatly influenced by the anatomical drawings of Leonardo da Vinci (1452-1519) showing the structure of the heart. After injecting a human heart taken from a corpse with liquid wax, da Vinci more clearly illustrated the different components of the organ. Nearly two centuries later, the invention of the microscope by Anton van Leeuwenhock (1632-1723) opened new doors to an understanding of capillaries, small veins and arteries.

In 1714, the English physiologist, chemist and inventor Stephen Hales (1677-1761) conducted the first experiments with blood pressure when he opened an artery of a horse, inserted a brass tube, determined the existence of something called blood pressure and devised a mechanism for measuring it. Hales published his experimental findings under the title *Haemastaticks*. He also discovered that blood pressure varied between veins and arteries and between the contractions and dilations of the heart. Safer methods for measuring blood pressure appeared more than a century later with Marey's wrist sphygmograph, designed in 1857, followed by Dudgeon's, designed in 1882. Both were great steps forward in the search for convenient, simplified ways to measure blood pressure. At the time, Dudgeon's device was so successful that it became standard equipment for the U. S. Navy.

R.T.H. Laënnec, a French physician, first began using a hollow wooden cylinder in the early 1800s, the earliest version of a stethoscope. By the end of the 19th century, flexible, binaural stethoscopes were common. Although some physicians felt the invention of the stethoscope weakened the physician's own powers of diagnosis, the stethoscope offered an immediate diagnosis at a minimal cost.

The invention of the electrocardiograph by Willem Einthoven of the Netherlands enabled physicians to become differentiated as specialists in heart disease.

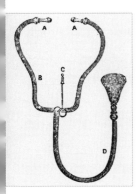

An early version of a stethoscope.

Einthoven received the Nobel Prize for his invention in 1924, the same year the American Heart Association was founded. Through the remaining decades of the 20th century, the field of cardiology became further specialized. Numerous professional organizations and associations were created to accommodate the amazing pace of scientific and clinical discovery related to the heart. ◻

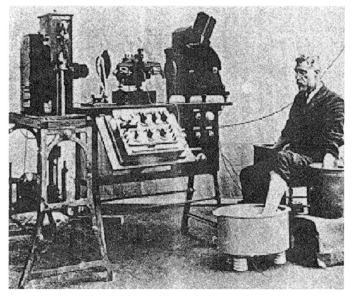

The inventor Willem Einthoven with his electrocardiograph.

Case Study

Risk Assessment

Risk factor screening, accompanied by lifestyle modifications – such as a healthy diet and regular exercise – can lead to early detection of risk and prevention of cardiovascular disease. Cardiovascular disease usually presents as three distinct types: coronary artery disease (CAD), stroke and peripheral arterial disease. Atypical presentations also abound.   ▶   Risk factors include nonmodifiable risks – age, gender, race and family history – and behaviorally modifiable risks, such as obesity, high-fat and high-cholesterol diet, a sedentary lifestyle and smoking. CVD is also caused by physiologic risk factors, such as hypertension, hyperlipidemia and diabetes mellitus (types 1 and 2), which often require pharmacologic treatments in addition to lifestyle modifications.

> ▼
>
> Risk factors include non-modifiable risks – age, gender, race and family history – and behaviorally modifiable risks, such as obesity, high-fat and high-cholesterol diet, a sedentary lifestyle and smoking.

Various tests used to screen for CVD provide a hopeful path to uncovering and treating early cardiovascular disease before it develops into a more serious condition. Physicians can use simple, noninvasive tests, such as risk-factor assessments before moving to more complicated – and usually more expensive and invasive – tests later. Risk factors for heart disease to be assessed in patients over age 20 include:

- ◆ Family history of CVD
- ◆ Smoking status
- ◆ Diet, cholesterol and physical activity
- ◆ Blood pressure
- ◆ Body weight and body mass index
- ◆ Waist circumference
- ◆ Fasting blood lipid profile
- ◆ Fasting blood glucose

These risk factors can be used to calculate a global risk score in people 40 years and older, providing an estimate of the 10-year risk of heart attacks and death from cardiac disease.

Advances in the tests currently available for heart disease continue to evolve. At present, available noninvasive tests include:

◆ Resting electrocardiogram (ECG or EKG)

◆ Signal-averaged electrocardiogram (SAECG)

◆ Chest X-ray

◆ Holter monitor (ambulatory electrocardiogram)

◆ Echocardiogram

◆ Exercise stress test

◆ Computed tomography (CT) scan

◆ Magnetic resonance imaging (MRI)

◆ Magnetic resonance angiography (MRA)

Nuclear imaging tests, which are noninvasive, include:

◆ MUGA scan

◆ Thallium stress test

◆ Technicium stress test

◆ PET test

◆ Stress echocardiography

Other invasive imaging tests include:

◆ Transesophageal echocardiogram (TEE)

◆ Cardiac catheterization ("cath") – also known as coronary angiography

◆ Intravascular ultrasound (IVUS)

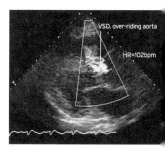

Echocardiogram

Recent developments indicate that high levels of markers of inflammation, such as C-reactive protein (CRP), may also be markers for increased risk of CVD. As a screening tool, blood levels of inflammatory markers may one day become as familiar as cholesterol and blood pressure numbers, but tests with greater specificity need to be developed. In patients presenting with chest pain of unknown cause, measurement of cardiac troponin T can reliably detect damage to the heart from a myocardial infarction within one day after the onset of chest pain, an indication of how continuing improvements in diagnostic tests help identify patients at high risk. Yet another risk factor, fibrinogen, a protein that forms blood clots, is now also thought to be a marker for cardiac risk. Finally, a simple measurement of blood pressure in the arms and ankles provide the ankle-brachial blood pressure ratio. This has been found to be a reliable predictor of CVD in people older than 50 years of age. ◻

Classification and Management of Blood Pressure for Adults Aged 18 Years or Older

BP Classification	Systolic BP* (mm Hg)		Diastolic BP* (mm Hg)	Lifestyle Modification	Initial Drug (Without Compelling Indications)
Normal	<120	and	<80	Encourage	
Pre-hypertension	120-139	or	80-89	Yes	No antihypertensive drug indicated.
Stage 1 hypertension	140-159	or	90-99	Yes	Thiazide-type diuretics for most; may consider ACE inhibitor, ARB, Beta blocker, CCB, or combination.
Stage 2 hypertension	≥160	or	≥100	Yes	Two-drug combination for most (usually thiazide-type diuretic and ACE inhibitor or ARB or Beta blocker or CCB).

From the *Seventh Report of the Joint National Committee on Prevention, Detection, Evaluation and Treatment of High Blood Pressure (JNC VII)*, 2003.

Abbrevations: ACE, angiotensin-converting enzyme; ARB, angiotensin-receptor blocker; BP, blood pressure; CCB, calcium channel blocker. Treatment determined by highest BP category.

*Treatment determined by the highest BP category.

Vignette

Statins

High blood cholesterol is a well-accepted risk factor for CVD. Most cholesterol is carried in the blood in two forms, high-density lipoprotein (HDL) and low-density lipoprotein (LDL), with only HDL considered advantageous for fighting the accumulation of plaque in the blood vessels that leads to CVD. A high LDL level, on the other hand, usually signifies that a patient is at risk for CVD.

Federal guidelines on cholesterol have changed in the last ten years, with stronger recommendations for lowering total cholesterol while maintaining appropriate HDL levels. The current guidelines are:

◆ Patients should consume no more than seven percent of calories from saturated fat (the previous recommendation was ten percent).

◆ Adults are advised to consume no more than 35 percent of calories from total fat (the previous recommendation had been 30 percent), provided that the main source is unsaturated fats, which do not raise cholesterol levels.

◆ Ideal body weight should be attained and maintained.

◆ The new target for dietary cholesterol is less than 200 mg per day (the previous target had been under 300 mg per day).

◆ An optimal LDL-C level is 100mg/dL or less per day for all adults.

The recommendations can be difficult for the average healthy consumer to follow, and ideal LDL-cholesterol levels may be especially difficult for some CVD patients to achieve through diet alone. The development of the class of drugs known as statins has changed the way many physicians manage patients with high cholesterol.

Clinical knowledge of how to counteract elevated blood cholesterol dates back only three decades. Research into inhibitors of HMG-CoA reductase, part of the body's metabolic pathway for the synthesis of cholesterol, began in Tokyo, Japan, in 1971 in the laboratory of Drs. Endo and Kuroda. This team reasoned that certain microorganisms may produce inhibitors of this particular enzyme to defend themselves against other organisms. The first agent to be isolated was mevastatin, a molecule produced by *Penicillium citrinum*. The pharmaceutical company Merck showed an interest in the research in 1976 and isolated lovastatin from the mold *Aspergillus terreus*. Lovastatin would become the first statin to be commercially marketed and would have a dramatic effect on the way high cholesterol is treated.

As of 2005, six statin drugs are on the market in the United States. Studies using statins have reported 20 percent to 60 percent lower LDL-cholesterol levels in patients on these drugs. Statins also reduce elevated triglyceride levels and produce a modest increase in HDL-cholesterol. While most patients tolerate statins well, side effects can include muscle aches and abnormal liver function tests.

Some have questioned the safety of statins, especially given their widespread use in the U.S. When a statin is given at a high dose, the risk for developing abnormalities in liver tests is one to two percent per year. These abnormalities can be reversed, however, by simply reducing the dose or by stopping the drug. Another common side effect, occurring in somewhere between one to two percent of patients, is muscle aches or, more rarely, inflammation of the muscles, called myopathy, in which an enzyme from the muscle leaks into the blood.

Which patients are considered candidates for statin therapy? The list is lengthy.

◆ Those who have had heart attacks or chest pain or those who have undergone bypass surgery or angioplasty, with an LDL-cholesterol greater than 100 mg/dL.

◆ Those with diabetes and those with multiple other risk factors for heart disease with an LDL-cholesterol greater than 100 mg/dL.

◆ Those with evidence of blockage in the arteries carrying blood to the brain (carotid artery disease) or the legs (peripheral vascular disease).

◆ Those with LDL-cholesterol greater than 160 mg/dL and two other risk factors after a therapeutic lifestyle change or those with LDL-cholesterol greater than 190 mg/dL with either one or no risk factors. As research progresses, however, new lipid targets may be recognized.

Statin treatment gained unintended public attention with the emergency heart bypass operation of former president William Clinton in 2004. Some years earlier, an elevated cholesterol count led to the former president's doctor to prescribe a statin to counter what was feared to be incipient heart disease. When the count returned to safe levels relatively quickly, President Clinton chose to discontinue use rather than follow medical advice and continue to take the statin. As the world discovered, that choice may have been a factor in the former president's development of coronary disease, underscoring the rule that once a patient begins a regimen of statins, he should continue that regimen for the rest of his life. ◻

Looking Ahead
Obesity in Young Populations

The growing epidemic of obesity in young people offers the public health community a challenge and an opportunity to prevent disease and instill healthy lifestyles. How to prevent obesity is no secret – a combination of physical activity and wise choices in nutrition can have an immediate impact on weight and foster long-lasting healthy behavior. Reduced weight helps prevent diabetes and cardiovascular disease, among other health threats caused by being overweight. Success in this endeavor does not happen overnight and requires a long-term commitment. An investment made today by the public health and medical communities, along with schools and governments, will pay dividends in future healthy adult populations.

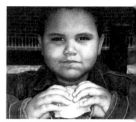

The American Heart Association estimates that the prevalence of obesity has increased by 75 percent since 1991. Metabolic syndrome, perhaps the earliest warning sign of developing health problems, occurs predominantly in people who are overweight. As many as 55 million Americans may meet the diagnostic criteria for metabolic syndrome.

In 1988, Dr. Gerald M. Reavan, an endocrinologist at Stanford University, first described something he called Syndrome X, noting that patients who presented with a cluster of low-level risk factors had a substantially increased risk for heart disease. In 1991, the National Cholesterol Education Program at the National Institutes of Health issued a report that renamed Syndrome X as metabolic syndrome. The report emphasized obesity as a central component of metabolic syndrome and recommended other screening tests that would be easy for primary care doctors to use.

Physicians suspect metabolic syndrome when people present with at least three of the following five criteria: having an increased girth around the abdomen, having moderately high blood pressure, having high blood levels of fats called triglycerides, having low levels of HDL ("good") cholesterol and having above-average blood sugar. It has been estimated that one million U.S. teenagers have been diagnosed with the syndrome, representing four percent of American adolescents. These youths are believed to be at sharply increased risk for developing diabetes when they are still in their 20s, if not before, and heart disease as early as their 40s.

The American Heart Association Council on Cardiovascular Disease in the Young recommends early detection of blood pressure elevation. Management for primary hypertension includes dietary counseling and physical activity prescriptions. Pharmaceuticals are reserved only for children whose blood pressure is consistently very high. Moderation in the use of salt is also recommended, since the diet of the average American child contains much more sodium than is required.

Michael Weitzman and Steve Cook of the American Academy of Pediatrics' Center for Child Health Research and the Department of Pediatrics at the University of Rochester analyzed data on 2,430 adolescents aged 12 to 19 between 1988 and 1994 for the National Health and Nutrition Examination Survey, a nationally representative ongoing federal survey of the U.S. population. The study showed that 4.2 percent of adolescents, or 910,000 teens, met the criteria for metabolic syndrome. The syndrome was found in at least 6.1 percent of males and 2.1 percent of females. The researchers found that nearly 30 percent of those who are either overweight or obese have the syndrome. Fortunately, if this population loses weight, the risk of diabetes and heart disease drops sharply.

▼

One-third to one-half of the population with metabolic syndrome subsequently develops diabetes.

► One-third to one-half of the population with metabolic syndrome subsequently develops diabetes. Even before the onset of diabetes, high blood lipids and other risk factors can cause cardiovascular disease. The earlier mean age of onset for type 2 diabetes of adolescents is startling and disturbing, because CVD development that takes place over many years in adults starts much earlier, potentially leading to onset of CVD in early and mid adulthood. Being overweight is nearly always the trigger for type 2 diabetes (versus type 1 diabetes, which is triggered by abnormalities in insulin production and usually diagnosed in childhood). The onset of diabetes carries with it the distressing probability of cardiovascular disease within two decades, greatly increasing the chances for premature death. Black and Hispanic Americans have nearly twice the incidence of type 2 diabetes as whites and many Native American tribes are experiencing epidemic rates.

► The number of overweight children tripled between 1970 and 2000, reaching 15 percent of those between the ages of six and 19. The highest growth rates have been in African-American and Hispanic youth who live mainly in inner cities, where access to opportunities for physical activity is often limited. In addition, research has shown that adolescents who exhibit high levels of hostility are more prone to becoming obese and developing insulin resistance, two markers of metabolic syndrome that make these youth more likely to develop cardiovascular disease in adulthood. Current research also links sleep disorders with metabolic syndrome.

▼

The number of overweight children tripled between 1970 and 2000, reaching 15 percent of those between the ages of six and 19.

To counter these disturbing trends, the public health community is seeking new ways to communicate the benefits of weight control, healthier eating and physical activity to reinforce even more effectively that improved lifestyle is a key to good health for young adults and children. Training children to live healthy lifestyles can improve cardiovascular health in adult life and is a strategy that must become widespread in schools, especially inner-city schools that serve a high proportion of minority populations.

The health benefits associated with a physically active lifestyle in children include weight control, lower blood pressure, improved psychological well-being and a predisposition to increased physical activity in adulthood. Increased physical activity has been associated with an increased life expectancy and decreased risk of cardiovascular disease. Researchers have also shown that people who eat breakfast every day, especially whole-grain cereal, are far less likely to be obese or have diabetes or heart disease.

A healthy level of physical activity requires regular participation in activities that generate energy expenditures significantly above the resting level and ideally greater than half of maximum exertion. These activities may be accomplished through both recreational pastimes and organized sports. Physical activity in American children, however, has diminished for a variety of reasons. Children rely more on the automobile for transportation, as opposed to walking or bicycling. Growing numbers of children also engage in sedentary entertainment, including television, video games and computers. Unfortunately, participation in organized athletics diminishes greatly after middle school, a special problem for girls.

Although these trends of diminished physical activity are nationwide, socioeconomic factors place certain sub-populations of children at greater risk. ► In large cities, a lack of safe outdoor play areas limits children's ability to participate in active physical play or recreational sports. With tightening school budgets and changes in curriculum, regular physical education in schools has been de-emphasized. The number of families with two working parents or a single parent has increased, with the result that many more parents are limited in their ability to encourage participation.

Federal, state and local health departments are working together to counter these alarming trends. CDC, after much analysis and collaboration, published the following health promotion and disease-prevention strategies aimed at obesity:

♦ Ensure daily quality physical education for all school grades.

♦ Ensure that more food options that are low in fat and calories, as well as fruits, vegetables, whole grains and low-fat or nonfat dairy products, are available on school campuses and at school events.

♦ Make community facilities available for physical activity for all people, including on weekends.

♦ Create more opportunities for physical activity at work sites.

♦ Reduce time spent watching television and in other sedentary behaviors. In 1999, 43 percent of high school students reported watching two hours of TV or more a day.

♦ Educate all expectant parents about the benefits of breast-feeding. Studies indicate that breast-fed infants may be less likely to become overweight as they grow older.

♦ Change the perception of obesity so that health becomes the chief concern, not personal appearance.

♦ Increase research on the behavioral and biological causes of overweight and obesity. Direct research toward prevention and treatment and toward ethnic/racial health disparities.

▼

In large cities, a lack of safe outdoor play areas limits children's ability to participate in active physical play or recreational sports.

◆ Educate health care providers and health profession students on the prevention and treatment of overweight and obesity across the lifespan.

Although it is widely accepted that healthy diets and daily physical activity together help control weight and prevent the onset of CVD, the American population nonetheless suffers from an epidemic of overweight and obesity. Currently 122 million adults are overweight and at risk for hypertension and related conditions that can lead to CVD.

The well-known benefits of physical activity and a healthy diet have not forestalled the epidemic of overweight and obesity in the United States nor the resulting epidemic of diabetes and cardiovascular disease. Unless significant changes are made, today's overweight and obese children will be tomorrow's unhealthy adults. Not only will this affect the health of the U.S. population, it will also become an economic drain on an already overburdened health care system. All of the diagnostic and treatment advances in CVD should mean that this disease is abating. Unfortunately, the incidence of CVD is not declining, and the public health community – in partnership with medical, educational and legislative entities – must find innovative solutions to this challenge.

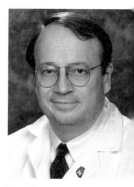

Dr. Thomas A. Pearson, professor of Community and Preventive Medicine at the University of Rochester.

Thomas A. Pearson, MD, MPH, PhD, Professor of Community and Preventive Medicine at the University of Rochester, suggests, ► "The spectacular reductions in cardiovascular disease mortality seen in the 1970s and 1980s are in great danger due to the obesity epidemic. For the first time in U.S. history, experts are warning that the life expectancy of our children may be less than our own. These dire predictions arise from the epidemic of obesity in our children and the return of the CVD epidemic as they become adults. A combined effort of clinical *and* public health strategies to reduce obesity will be absolutely essential. If we fail, the 2010 health goals set for the United States will prove unattainable." ◻

▼

"The spectacular reductions in cardiovascular disease mortality seen in the 1970s and 1980s are in great danger due to the obesity epidemic."

Chapter 7

Safer and Healthier Foods

Looking Back

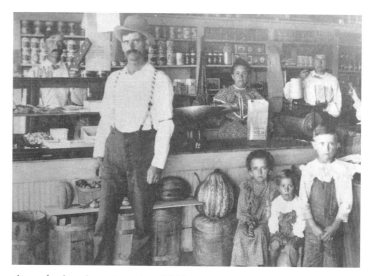

An early American store, circa 1910.

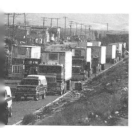

Trucks waiting to enter the U.S. at the Mexican border.

In the past, highly processed foods and beverages were not the mainstay of the American diet as they are today. An American shopping in any supermarket today can choose to ignore fresh produce, fresh meats and fresh baked goods and still purchase foods rich in nutrients. These foods are prepackaged, usually by the manufacturer, and labeled for their nutritional value. These required labels intend to guide consumers toward healthy choices, reassuring them that foods are safe. Foods are not without risk in this country, however, despite the best efforts of the United States Department of Agriculture (USDA), its Food Safety Inspection Service (FSIS), the United States Food and Drug Administration (FDA), the Centers for Disease Control and Prevention (CDC) and state and local health departments. Much of the fresh produce for sale at certain times of year comes across our borders from Mexico, Chile, Brazil and other countries, where safety standards are beyond our control. In 1970, each American ate approximately 175 pounds of fresh fruits and vegetables a year. By 1995, that number rose to 220 pounds per person.

Americans also choose to eat out much more frequently than in the past. Between 1970 and 2004, the percentage of food dollars spent away from home increased from 34 percent to 47 percent. In addition, the very young in day-care centers and the very old in nursing homes are populations at particular risk for foodborne illness, and these populations are growing. Since foodborne illnesses arise most often from fresh produce and from restaurants or other food-service purveyors, growing numbers of Americans are clearly at greater risk for illness. Within the public health community, improvements in systems that protect food safety are still needed.

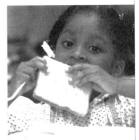

*Lunch at a
day-care center.*

It is estimated that there are 76 million cases of foodborne illness in the United States per year, resulting in patient-related costs in the billions of dollars. Each year, foodborne diseases cause more than 300,000 hospitalizations and an estimated 5,000 deaths. In fact, one of every 100 hospitalizations and one of every 500 deaths in the United States are thought to result from contaminated food. ► It is estimated that from one in three to one in four people will suffer a foodborne illness each year. The full burden may never be known, however, since large-scale studies have yet to be conducted and record-keeping is unreliable. The actual number of illnesses may be much higher because foodborne illness is underreported and often misdiagnosed. Many people with mild cases do not seek medical help. Because symptoms are often nonspecific – nausea, vomiting and diarrhea – food poisoning can be mistaken for the flu or some other common ailment. Even when a victim seeks the help of a physician, many health facilities lack the laboratory technology necessary to identify specific pathogens.

▼

It is estimated that from one in three to one in four people will suffer a food-borne illness each year.

Looking back in history, from the time of Hippocrates 2,000 years ago to the dawn of modern medicine, little distinction was made between food and drugs. Around 460 BC, Hippocrates recognized the essential relationship between food and health. He urged others to study closely the daily dietary regimen he associated with good health. Theophrasus, who lived from 370-285 BC, wrote *Enquiry Into Plants*, the first great botanical treatise that identified plants as sources of food and medicine. But adulteration of food with fillers was noted even in these ancient times. Cato, who lived from 234-149 BC, wrote *On Agriculture*, in which he recommended "the addition to wine of boiled-down must, salt, marble dust and resin" and included a method to determine whether wine "has been watered." Pliny the Elder, the author of *Natural History*, lived from AD 23-79. Not surprisingly, after Cato, he found widespread adulteration in the food supply, describing bread as being full of "chalk, vegetable meals and even cattle fodder." He also found that pepper was often adulterated with juniper berries.

Galen, the renowned Roman physician who lived from AD 131-201, followed the philosophical tradition of the school of Hippocrates. He warned about the common adulteration of food products, but more important, he advocated moderation as the principal rule for a sound diet. Despite all the advances in medical science and nutrition in the intervening centuries, no one has improved on Galen's fundamental rule of sound nutrition.

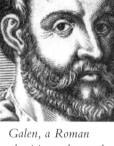

Galen, a Roman physician, advocated moderation for a sound diet.

In Europe during the Middle Ages, the trade guilds regulated food products. The guilds, which dated back to the time of the Norman Conquest, covered every important food category, including bakers, butchers, cooks, grocers, fruiters, poulters and salters. They had the power to search premises and seize unwholesome products, regulating the marketing of food to the public.

By the beginning of the 19th century, advances in chemical analysis provided qualitative methods to detect many common food adulterants. In 1820, a German-born chemist, Frederick Accum, working in England, published his landmark treatise *Adulterations of Food and Culinary Poisons*. The book was an immediate success, gaining widespread publicity in newspapers and capturing the attention of the public. Accum may be the first expert in food safety to achieve hoped-for public education by using the vehicles of mass communication that were then at his disposal.

In 1906, the Pure Food and Drugs Act ushered in the modern era of food safety in the United States. Enacted during the Theodore Roosevelt administration, the act created a Bureau of Chemistry, the agency now known as the Food and Drug Administration, to enforce food and drug laws meant to protect the American people. This act had first been proposed in 1879 by Peter Collier, chief chemist at the Department of Agriculture, and finally came into being only after concerted pressure by organized medicine, women's groups, the press and state public health officials. They were helped in their advocacy by Upton Sinclair's best-selling novel, *The Jungle*, which exposed unsanitary conditions in the meatpacking industry.   ▶   The public became so aroused by those appalling conditions that neither industry nor its supporters in Congress could prevent passage of the Pure Food and Drugs Act.

A part of the Department of Agriculture, the Bureau of Chemistry found agricultural fairs to be a preferred venue for campaigns to educate the public. The chief chemist, Harvey W. Wiley, MD, considered by many to be the founding father of the FDA, tried to separate scientific facts on food safety from scares that were fast becoming a public focus. After the runaway success of *The Jungle*, inflammatory publications fed growing public mistrust, which was further inflamed by congressional hearings. Examples of food safety issues that inflamed the public were the widely used, but unsafe, food preservative borax and the many products labeled "pure" that were in fact counterfeits. Wiley convened a Poison Squad at the Bureau of Chemistry and soon borax, salicylic acid, formaldehyde and copper sulfate were banned as food additives. The operative standard for each food product became a reasonable certainty that it caused no harm.

Food fortification began in the United States in 1924 with the introduction of iodized salt in Michigan. Studies showed that the incidence of goiter, a swelling of the thyroid gland caused by iodine deficiency, declined from 38.6 percent to nine percent; and iodized salt was soon introduced throughout the country, virtually eliminating iodine deficiency as a serious health threat by the 1930s. Perhaps the most famous food-fortification case concerns niacin in breads and cereals. In the early 1900s, pellagra occurred to some extent in every state, and mortality statistics indicated that it was the most severe nutritional deficiency disease ever recorded in U.S. history. Pellagra presents with dermatitis, diarrhea, inflamed mucous membranes and, in severe cases, dementia. It flares up when the skin is exposed to strong sunlight, and in many southern states during the peak incidence years of 1928 and 1929, pellagra became one of the leading causes of death. In 1937, the disease was

▼

The public became so aroused by those appalling conditions that neither industry nor its supporters in Congress could prevent passage of the Pure Food and Drugs Act.

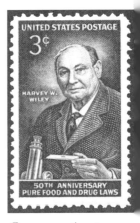

Commemorative stamp honoring Dr. Harvey W. Wiley and the Pure Food and Drug laws.

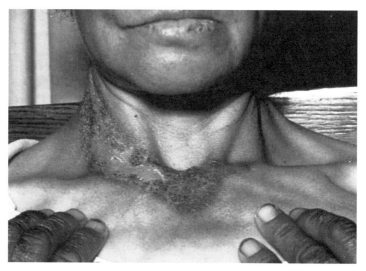

An individual with pellagra.

tied directly to a dietary deficiency in B vitamin niacin, primarily in poor people who lacked animal food – meat, eggs, dairy products – in their diets and subsisted mainly on corn. Bakers began introducing niacin, identified as an anti-pellegra agent, into breads and cereals through yeast, and by 1939, the incidence of pellagra began a rapid decline.

Current controversies in the American diet, namely an overabundance of sugar, overindulgence in processed foods and lack of control in portion size, contribute to epidemics of dental caries, cardiovascular disease, diabetes and obesity.
► Health and dental education in schools and homes can help stem the epidemics, but the real solution comes from individual will power. The Surgeon General issues periodic updates on healthy weights, and the number of overweight and obese people keeps rising, causing real concern in the public health community. Healthy foods and portion control are only part of the solution. Increased physical activity in a society gone sedentary is equally important.

In the United States, the food safety system is based on federal and state laws that are strong, flexible and science-based and on industry's legal responsibility to produce safe foods. The development and revision of regulations occur in an open and transparent process in public, allowing – and even encouraging – participation by the regulated industry, consumers and other stakeholders throughout the

Health and dental education in schools and homes can help stem the epidemics, but the real solution comes from individual will power.

process. Old agency files at the FDA contain elaborate studies conducted with scientists from academia and industry that gathered data that even now serve as the basis of regulations. Not until the late 1970s, when consumer interest in the environment and the food supply began to increase, did this cooperative relationship end. Since the 1970s, the FDA has worked essentially at arm's length from industry in an adversarial environment.

Still, the federal government funds important research centers that are based on university campuses. North Carolina State University, Michigan State University and Rutgers University each hosts an important research center for food safety and technology. Ironically, the federal subsidies that help fund these centers allow the federal government to stretch its own scarce resources.

A Timeline of Food Safety Developments in the U.S. Federal Government, 1879 to the Present:

1879 Peter Collier, chief chemist at the Department of Agriculture, supports a bill to make food adulteration a federal crime; the bill finally becomes law in 1906.

1906 Pure Food and Drugs Act, based on Collier's bill, creates the Bureau of Chemistry within the U.S. Department of Agriculture.

1906 First Meat Inspection Act, allowing "sight, touch, smell" inspection in slaughterhouses to detect unsanitary conditions and adulterated products.

1912 Sherley Amendment to the Pure Food and Drugs Act prohibits false and fraudulent claims; although, the government has to prove intent to deceive, not easily achieved in the face of so many "nostrum makers" expressing faith in worthless goods.

1927 Food, Drug and Insecticide Administration is created from the Bureau of Chemistry, merging the Insecticide and Fungicide Board.

1930 The Food and Drug Administration (FDA) comes into being.

1933-1938 The FDA launches an intensive effort to alert the public to the shortcomings of the 1906 law by high lighting such products as mascara, diet pills and baldness cures that are outside the scope of the 1906 law.

1939 The Federal Food, Drug, and Cosmetic Act.

1940 The FDA moved from USDA to the newly formed Federal Security Agency.

1950 Congress passes the Oleomargarine Act repealing much of the legislation that restricted margarine sales.

1953 The FDA becomes part of the Department of Health, Education and Welfare (HEW).

1954 Miller Pesticides Amendment empowers the FDA to establish tolerances for pesticides.

1957 Poultry Products Inspection Act (PPIA).

1958 Delaney Clause in the Food Additive Amendments to the 1939 Act requires that a food or color additive, once determined to be a carcinogen, not be approved for food use.

1958 Food Additive Amendments require pre-market approval for new food ingredients (before, a marketer could add ingredients without specific FDA approval).

1960 Color Additive Amendment.

1966 The FDA proposes restrictive approach to food fortification.

1966 Fair Packaging and Labeling Act completely restructures American food labels, causing one major food company to change 20,000 labels.

1967 Wholesome Meat Act, amending the 1906 Meat Inspection Act (MIA).

1968 Wholesome Poultry Products Act, amending the 1957 PPIA.

1968 The FDA moves to the Public Health Services within HEW.

1969 President Richard Nixon convenes a White House Conference on Food, Nutrition and Health that recommends fortification of existing and new food products to meet national nutritional needs (this new approach, reversing the 1966 FDA stance, creates new regulations based largely on food-labeling requirements rather than on rigid standards for nutrient composition).

1970 Egg Products Inspection Act, a response to a growing problem of *Salmonella* infection.

1976 Vitamin-Mineral Amendment.

1977 Congress passes the first of several laws precluding FDA action to ban the use of saccharin and directs the FDA not to implement a proposed system for controlling the sanitation of shellfish.

1980 The FDA's department renamed Health and Human Services (DHHS) when Education becomes its own department.

1980 Congress passes the Infant Formula Act, imposing druglike requirements on infant formulas.

1990 Congress passes the Nutrition Labeling and Education Act.

1994 Congress passes the Dietary Supplement Health and Education Act, severely restricting the FDA's authority to regulate human nutritional foods.

1995 CDC, the USDA, and the FDA initiate a Sentinel Site Surveillance project, known now as FoodNet, to collect precise information about the incidence of foodborne illness, especially illness caused by *salmonella* and *E. coli O157:H7*. (Findings from the project show that *Campylobacter* causes the majority of sporadic illnesses associated with meat and poultry products).

1996 The USDA publishes its landmark rule on Pathogen Reduction and Hazard Analysis and Critical Control Points (HACCP), which establishes in-plant performance standards for *Salmonella* and other foodborne pathogens.

1996 The Food Safety and Inspection Service (FSIS) conducts testing for the first time to ensure that these standards are met (the first such performance standard for a broad range of meat and poultry products that are raw).

1997 The President's Food Safety Initiative adds millions of dollars to the nation's food safety budget, improving coordination between food safety regulatory agencies and surveillance for foodborne diseases.

2001 President George W. Bush establishes the Office of Homeland Security.

2002 The Public Health Security and Bioterrorism Preparedness and Response Act, known as the Bioterrorism Act, adds section 304(h) to the 1939 Federal Food, Drug, and Cosmetic Act, allowing the detention of suspect food products.

Protecting public health involves layers of control before food reaches the consumer. The first layer – industry's clear responsibility to prepare safe food – must be monitored by a second layer – regulatory agencies – to ensure that the food industry does its job and produces safe food. In the policymaking arena for food safety in the United States, science and risk analysis are paramount.   ►   The federal government's current efforts focus on the risks associated with microbial pathogens, trying to reduce those risks through a comprehensive, farm-to-table approach to food safety. These efforts follow many years of managing chemical hazards in the food supply by regulating additives, drugs, pesticides, and other chemical and physical hazards considered dangerous to human health. Since biological hazards differ from chemical hazards, the science of food safety has been transformed.

For example, the U.S. government's now-completed risk analysis of *Salmonella enteritidis* in eggs and egg products included the first farm-to-table quantitative microbial risk assessment. The government has also conducted a risk analysis for *E. coli 0157:H7* in ground beef and has entered into a cooperative agreement with Harvard University for a risk assessment of Bovine Spongiform Encephalopathy (mad cow disease) transmission through foods. Yet another risk analysis for *Listeria monocytogenes* in a variety of ready-to-eat foods has also been carried out.

Food safety in the United States is both highly centralized, through the FDA, the USDA and CDC, and decentralized. Each state has its own food, drug and cosmetic act, while the Federal Trade Commission (FTC) regulates advertising of food and food products under the terms of the Federal Trade Commission Act. Some kinds of food, particularly milk and dairy products, are also regulated at the county or city level. Milk shippers cater to differing ordinances that regulate expiration dates on milk products, sometimes in neighboring cities within the same state.

The FDA serves in a public health capacity. In the early 1970s, imported products regulated by the FDA numbered approximately 500,000 formal entries each year (e.g., those valued at $1,250 or more). In 1992, these products accounted for 1.5 million formal entries, of which 78 percent

▼

The federal government's current efforts focus on the risks associated with microbial pathogens, trying to reduce those risks through a comprehensive, farm-to-table approach to food safety.

(1,117,000) were food products. Between 1987 and 1992, detentions of food products nearly doubled from 14,104 to 27,865. Clearly the FDA serves a vital function in protecting public health.

Americans now face a crossroads concerning the issue of safer and healthier foods. Much of the regulatory piece ensuring food safety is in place and working well, although it should never be taken for granted. ▶ What needs work is individual commitment to healthier eating and an active lifestyle. Less sugar, more whole-grain cereals and breads, three to four fresh fruits a day, green vegetables and so on, coupled with exercise routines could make a remarkable difference in the overall health of the American population. ▫

▼

What needs work is individual commitment to healthier eating and an active lifestyle.

Case Study

Jack in the Box *E. coli* Outbreak

Jack in the Box restaurants, founded in San Diego in 1951, popularized the concept of "drive thru" dining, a rite of passage for many American teenagers and a convenience for working parents who have little time to prepare meals. After the founder, Robert O. Peterson, expanded his modest hamburger restaurant into a chain that stretched to Arizona and Texas, Ralston Purina acquired a controlling interest in 1968 and pursued an aggressive expansion strategy. By 1979, there were more than 1,000 "drive thru" Jack in the Box restaurants in 32 states. A period of corporate restructuring followed, including a pullout from the East and Midwest in 1986. Today, Jack in the Box thrives in its intended markets in the West and Southwest, in part because the public in these states admires the way Jack in the Box responded to a serious crisis in Seattle in 1993.

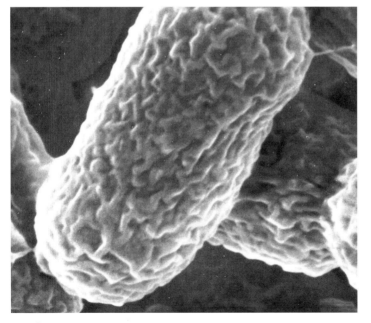

The first Jack in the Box in San Diego in 1951.

That crisis awakened the federal government to the fact that its established inspection systems for food safety had failed to protect the public health. The crisis also introduced the country to a microorganism, *Escherichia coli O157:H7,* which has since become familiar to many.

E. coli 0157:H7

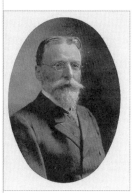

Theodore Escherich first described the bacteria, now called Escherichia coli.

▼

Many patients describe the pain as so severe that it feels like a hot poker searing their insides.

Escherichia coli (*E. coli* for short) was identified in 1885 when the German pediatrician Theodore Escherich first described the bacteria. These rod-shaped bacteria, profuse throughout the digestive system and usually benign, keep disease-causing bacteria from taking over. The *O157:H7* strain, however, is far from benign, as events in Seattle in 1993 were to prove.

Isolated and identified for the first time in 1982, *E. coli 0157:H7* is a problem in red meat, particularly hamburger. The discovery came during an epidemic in Oregon and Michigan caused by undercooked hamburger patties sold in the McDonald's fast food chain. At the time, public health officials viewed the outbreak as an isolated incident, not an omen; in fact, *E. coli O157:H7* is the third most deadly bacterial toxin, after the bacteria that causes tetanus and botulism. Its distinctive symptoms are bloody diarrhea and fierce abdominal cramps. ► Many patients describe the pain as so severe that it feels like a hot poker searing their insides.

During an *E. coli* outbreak, between two and seven percent of patients – mostly young children and the elderly – develop hemolytic uremic syndrome (HUS), which can lead to death. HUS sets in when Shiga toxins, emitted by *E. coli O157:H7*, ravage cells lining the intestines and cause bleeding. The bleeding permits the toxins to enter the circulatory system, and when this happens, the damage is very similar to that of rattlesnake venom. The toxins tear apart red blood cells and platelets, and the victim becomes vulnerable to brain hemorrhaging and uncontrolled bleeding. Clots form in the bloodstream and block the tiny blood vessels around the kidneys, the heart's middle layer and the brain. As the kidneys give out, the body swells with excess waste fluids, and complications ripple through all major organ systems. Stroke, blindness, epilepsy, paralysis and heart failure can result. Although doctors know how to manage HUS symptoms and are researching new ways to stop the toxin, there is currently no cure or effective treatment.

In 1993, Jack in the Box restaurants promoted its most popular menu item, the Monster Burger, as "So good it's scary." Eleven years after undercooked hamburgers at McDonald's caused outbreaks of *E. coli O157:H7* in

Michigan and Oregon, a much graver crisis struck Seattle. A Jack in the Box restaurant served undercooked Monster Burgers and killed four children among more than 700 people who became ill.

When the Jack in the Box tragedy struck, 22 previous out-breaks of *E. coli O157:H7* had already killed 35 people in the United States. Not until the Seattle outbreak, however, were fast food hamburgers, a staple of American culture, viewed for the first time as potentially lethal. Public health investigators from Seattle/King County Department of Health, aware of the previous *E. coli* outbreaks, zeroed in immediately on undercooked hamburgers as the outbreak's likely cause and quickly identified the particular Jack in the Box restaurant in Seattle as the source.

Tracing where the contaminated meat came from, however, was no easy task. A single carcass, when shredded for ham-burger, has the potential to pollute up to eight tons of ground beef. ►   In the Jack in the Box outbreak, investigators quickly identified the supplier but found that the ground beef contained meat from 443 different cattle that had come from five slaughterhouses served by farms and auction in six states.

How does meat become contaminated? Cattle produce abundant feces, which contain bacteria; when the feces are passed back and forth in crowded feedlots, as they inevitably are, microorganisms like *E. coli* spread. Cattle fed on grass seldom carry the organism. However, cattle fed on corn, the staple of the feedlot, develop acid in their stomachs. *E. coli* has learned to thrive in acid environments and are now principally a feedlot microbe, very common in the manure of feedlot animals.

When cattle arrive at the meatpacking plant and pass through the door on their way to becoming food, they are caked with manure that comes from sleeping and resting in very tight quarters. Unless the hides are carefully separated in a way that minimizes contact with the meat, *E. coli O157:H7* in the manure can contaminate the meat. Bacteria present in the intestinal tract can also contaminate the meat. Unfortunately, when *E. coli* then passes into human stomachs through undercooked meat, the bacteria's tolerance for acidity means that gastric shock won't kill it.

▼

...the (contami-nated) ground beef contained meat from 443 different cattle that had come from five slaugh-terhouses served by farms and auc-tion in six states.

It is thought that as few as 10 bacteria can kill a person once they release their lethal toxin. When Jack in the Box became aware of this danger, the company attempted to set things right. The company hired Dave Theno, a food safety expert, to overhaul the company's system of food preparation. His advice was simple: "Make sure the meat products are fresh, look good, are cold, not discolored or things like that; keep them refrigerated and cold; follow shelf-life information, coded information. And then when you cook them and prepare them, make sure you wash and sanitize your hands. Clean your utensils. Ground beef should not be served medium rare or rare. Juices should run clear. Internal temperatures should be over 155. Rare hamburgers need to be a thing of the past."

After the Jack in the Box outbreak, the federal government proposed a new inspection system – known as "HACCP" (Hazard Analysis and Critical Control Points) – that required microbial testing for the first time to detect harmful bacteria such as *E. coli* and *Salmonella*. Since the start of this new system in 1996, the USDA has reported a drop in *Salmonella* contamination of ground beef, while the CDC has seen a decrease in the incidence of other foodborne illnesses.

Americans may still face serious risks, however. Increasing evidence indicates that the modern meat industry's widespread use of antibiotics to promote growth and keep livestock healthy results in infectious bacterial strains that resist treatment with antibiotics. ► Meanwhile, with global trade, the risk that diseased cattle or beef will enter the United States and decimate the livestock population increases.

A recent court ruling may also threaten food safety. In 2001, a Texas meat-grinding company, Supreme Beef, filed a lawsuit against the USDA after it was effectively shut down for failing three bacterial contamination tests in succession. One test found that nearly 50 percent of its meat was contaminated with *Salmonella*. Supreme Beef sued the government over its right to shut down operations simply because the company failed to meet USDA *Salmonella* standards. The National Meat Association supported Supreme Beef's claim, pointing out that contaminated cattle were the source of *Salmonella*, not the plant, and the shutdown

▼

Meanwhile, with global trade, the risk that diseased cattle or beef will enter the United States and decimate the livestock population increases.

was, therefore, unnecessarily punitive. In March 2002, a federal appeals court ruled in favor of the company.

Per-capita annual meat consumption in the United States peaked in the early 1970s at 85 pounds and has since fallen; in 1995-97, it was down to 64 pounds. In 2001, more than 100 million pounds of bad meat had to be recalled. The meat industry's response to the Seattle outbreak and contamination incidents since has been a series of high-tech solutions, such as sprays. A spray based on milk appears to kill *E. coli*. Another solution, passing meat through steam cabinets in bags of hot water, kills most of the bacteria. Finally, irradiation appeals to the meat industry because it is cost effective. Even with the highest standards for sanitary processing, some manure may still be in the meat. Irradiation eliminates the threat posed by manure.

Another, much simpler solution is possible, recommended by James Russell, a researcher at Cornell University. By putting cattle on grass or hay for the last several days of their lives, changing the pH balance in their stomachs, the *E. coli* population plummets by as much as 80 percent. The industry resists this solution, however. To them, it is costly and impractical – shipping so much hay to feedlots is a disincentive, as is lost gain – that is, cattle losing pounds just before slaughter.

The politics of meat are instructive for effective advocacy. The key associations – American Meat Institute, National Meat Association, and National Cattlemen's Beef Association – target their lobbying activities to a few key lawmakers and regulators. ▶ Despite a relatively low level of financial contributions, the industry usually succeeds at preventing, weakening or delaying new meat safety initiatives. Now that Tyson, the largest poultry producer, has purchased IBP, the largest beef producer, the politics of meat safety initiatives favor the industry even more.

One demonstration of the meat industry's lobbying muscle came in 1995. Two years after the Jack in the Box disaster in Seattle, the USDA proposed HACCP, the new food-safety regulations for *E. Coli* and *Salmonella* testing in beef. The meat industry, objecting to new testing, convinced a member of a key appropriations committee in the House of Representatives to introduce an amendment to stop the rule-making process, calling for the USDA to conduct

▼

Despite a relatively low level of financial contributions, the industry usually succeeds at preventing, weakening or delaying new meat safety initiatives.

more extensive hearings. This move effectively delayed the implementation of the new regulations. The meat industry has in fact fought food-safety inspection from the start, not wanting to be held accountable. Even in the face of the Jack in the Box evidence and ensuing meat safety standards, the beef industry pushed its supporters to counter that the standards were unscientific and did not improve meat safety. The industry claims that the incidence of *E. coli* in beef is less than one percent.

The good news for government regulators, however, is that food-safety inspections, backed by testing, work. PulseNet, a newly created testing system based at CDC, demonstrates how testing brings benefits to everyone. PulseNet is a network of state public health laboratories throughout the country that are now fingerprinting *E. coli* O157 and other foodborne bacteria on a routine basis. *E. coli* O157 has many different fingerprints, and usually no two will match in a given period of time. If a state public health department sees a string of cases in which fingerprints match or CDC learns of cases in different states that have matching fingerprints, victims of the outbreak clearly have something in common. Investigations can then focus on those people, using fingerprinting to analyze what they have in common. With the technology up and running at all state public health laboratories, comparisons can be made through the Internet. Connections through matching fingerprints can be made between *E. coli* infections in as many as 22 states, a real advantage in identifying outbreaks sooner and in greater detail than ever before.

► The Jack in the Box *E. coli* outbreak in 1993 informed the public and scientific and public health communities that standards for meat safety needed strengthening. Regrettably for the victims, warning signs had been overlooked. Once the threat was understood, however, the company itself responded with new food-preparation systems that mitigated the threat. Government also played its part, requiring testing of raw meat for invisible bacteria for the first time and upgrading meat-inspection systems. The public health and scientific communities are collaborating in tracing genetic fingerprints of foodborne pathogens, building knowledge in particular of the mechanisms of *E. coli* O157:H7. Since the outbreak in Seattle in 1993, much progress has been made. ▫

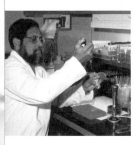

A technician at PulseNet working to identify fingerprints of foodborne bacteria.

▼

The Jack in the Box *E. coli* outbreak in 1993 informed the public and scientific and public health communities that standards for meat safety needed strengthening.

Vignette

Nutrition Labeling on Food Packaging

Grocery store aisles could easily become classrooms for greater knowledge about nutrition and healthy eating. Under the FDA and Food Safety and Inspection Service (FSIS) regulations, food labels now offer more information than ever before. The challenge has been to educate consumers to read the labels carefully, analyze the information and make healthier food choices. Despite improvements in food labeling, the growing rates of obesity, diabetes, high cholesterol and other chronic conditions indicate that people do not always use food label information in their own best interest. The need for the public health community to continue educating the public about the use of food labels is still imperative.

Start here →

Check calories

Limit these nutrients

Get enough of these nutrients

Footnote

Nutrition Facts

Serving Size 1 cup (228g)
Servings Per Container 2

Amount Per Serving

Calories 250	Calories from Fat 110

	% Daily Value*
Total Fat 12g	18%
Saturated Fat 3g	15%
Trans Fat 3g	
Cholesterol 30mg	10%
Sodium 470mg	20%
Total Carbohydrate 31g	10%
Dietary Fiber 0g	0%
Sugars 5g	
Protein 5g	

Vitamin A	4%
Vitamin C	2%
Calcium	20%
Iron	4%

* Percent Daily Values are based on a 2,000 calorie diet. Your Daily Values may be higher or lower depending on your calorie needs.

	Calories:	2,000	2,500
Total Fat	Less than	65g	80g
Sat Fat	Less than	20g	25g
Cholesterol	Less than	300mg	300mg
Sodium	Less than	2,400mg	2,400mg
Total Carbohydrate		300g	375g
Dietary Fiber		25g	30g

Quick guide to percent of daily values

5% or less is low

20% or more is high

Sample label for macaroni and cheese.

Today's food labels intend to offer consumers:

◆ Nutrition information about almost every food in the grocery store.

◆ Distinctive, easy-to-read formats that enable consumers to more quickly find the information they need to make healthy food choices.

◆ Information on the amount per serving of saturated fat, cholesterol, dietary fiber and other nutrients of major health concern.

◆ Nutrient reference values, expressed as "% Daily Values," to help consumers see how a food fits into an overall daily diet.

◆ Uniform definitions for terms that describe a food's nutrient content – such as "light," "low-fat" and "high fiber" – to ensure that these terms mean the same for any product.

◆ Claims about the relationship between a nutrient or food and a disease or health-related condition, such as calcium and osteoporosis, and fat and cancer, which are helpful to people concerned about eating foods that may help keep them healthier longer.

◆ Standardized serving sizes that make nutritional comparisons of similar products easier.

◆ Declaration of total percentage of juice in juice drinks, to help consumers know exactly how much juice is in the product.

In November 1990, President George H. W. Bush signed the Nutrition Labeling and Education Act (NLEA). The act required the FDA to issue proposed regulations within 12 months and final regulations within 24 months. By November 1991, the FDA had published 26 proposals and the FSIS had published a parallel proposal for the nutrition labeling of meats and poultry.

In January 1992, the FDA and FSIS called a public hearing on the proposals and received 92 comments in person from food industry representatives, the scientific community and consumer groups. More than 40,000 comments were received in writing, the largest number ever received in response to an FDA proposed regulation. Of these, 75 percent were form letters from organized campaigns. Meanwhile, the FSIS received more than 1,100 comments, most of which requested that FDA and FSIS labels be consistent with one another.

Most requirements arising from the NLEA raised troublesome issues, such as evaluating health claims related to certain nutrients and setting serving sizes. Foods were grouped into 139 categories, with serving sizes determined by establishing reference amounts that represented the amount of food customarily eaten per occasion. Health claims for certain nutrients were another matter, because little research existed for most claims, whether they were very specific or broad. The FDA strove to come up with a general set of principles that could be applied across all claims, and after lengthy and complicated evaluations, in the end, approved seven of ten relationships between diet and health.

Another challenge was agreeing on definitions. The difference between "lean" and "extra lean," for example, had to be determined across product lines. The American Heart Association helped determine these definitions based on different levels of fat, saturated fat, and cholesterol for all of the meat products regulated by the FDA, including fish and game meat.

The final regulations arising from the NLEA can be modified in the future as required. Industry can petition for changes, as can anyone else, and the FDA will set up a fair and open evaluation process. New processed foods come on the market all the time, eating habits change, and the next diet fad lies just around the corner. In fact, the food pyramid recommended by the USDA, representing dietary guidelines for healthy eating, changes with some regularity. In a sense, the NLEA created a process that never ends.

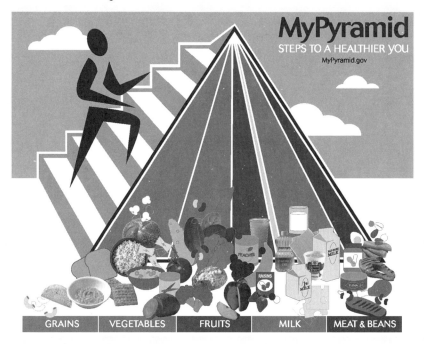

The latest USDA food pyramid.

The latest USDA food guide pyramid, which introduced the most dramatic changes ever, offers consumers easy-to-use tips on how to maintain a healthy diet. For example, completely avoiding foods that are high in fat, saturated fat, cholesterol and sodium is unnecessary, provided the consumer calculates average intake over several days. If one meal contains high-fat food, it should be countered with several subsequent meals that contain low-fat foods. In general, limiting intake of processed foods that contain fat and added sugars is a good idea. The USDA now posts a customized My Pyramid on its Web site, balancing nutrition and exercise for people of varying age, weight and physical condition. The site offers the following general advice:

◆ Eat at least three ounces of whole-grain breads, cereal, crackers, rice or pasta daily.

◆ Vary your vegetables; eat more dark green and orange vegetables daily, and eat more dry beans and peas.

◆ Eat a variety of fruit daily (fresh, frozen, canned or dried will do), and don't overdo fruit juices.

◆ Get fats from fish, nuts and vegetable oils, and limit solid fats, like butter, stick margarine, shortening and lard.

◆ Milk is important for getting calcium-rich foods, but favor low-fat or fat-free milks (lactose-free, if necessary).

◆ Choose low-fat or lean meats and poultry (baked, broiled or grilled), and vary your choices with more fish, beans, peas, nuts and seeds. ◻

Looking Ahead

How to Ensure a Safe Food Supply

A safe food supply depends on improvements and innovations in inspections, irradiation, genetic engineering and regulations. For example, the use of fingerprinting *E. coli O157:H7* through PulseNet helps to quickly analyze outbreaks. In the Jack in the Box outbreak, it was just such fingerprinting that helped limit the tragedy.

A safe food supply depends on the detention of suspect food products as they enter or are shipped within the country. Suspect food products can even be held in their country of origin, as Guatemala agreed to do when raspberries harvested there in 1996 were found to be the source of an outbreak due to *Cyclospora* in the United States. ▶   Under the provisions of the 2002 Bioterrorism Act, the USDA must collaborate with the Office of Homeland Security both in protecting the public from suspect foods and in securing the mammoth food infrastructure of this country. Farms, fields, processing plants, distribution and storage facilities and supermarkets are all vulnerable to bioterrorism attacks. Such attacks might consist of microorganisms, toxins or chemicals intentionally spread to harm the food supply or crops, or of a pest infestation. The challenge for the USDA, given the scope and size of the food industry infrastructure, is immense.

Irradiation offers another solution for food safety. Irradiation of ground beef and of other high-risk meats will likely be an important public health tool, much as pasteurization of milk has been. The irradiation process used for meats induces no radioactivity in the meat. Except for the bacteria it kills, irradiation introduces no important changes in the meat at all. After irradiation, nutritional values are identical to what they were before, and the safety of meat after irradiation should be no issue at all.

Genetic engineering is yet another promising solution for food safety and productivity. In Hawaii in the mid-1990s, the papaya ring spot virus (PRSV) threatened to decimate the state's second-largest fruit crop. By 1998, however, Hawaiian farmers were planting seeds of PRSV-resistant papaya made possible by genetic engineering. A team of

▼

Under the provisions of the 2002 Bioterrorism Act, the USDA must collaborate with the Office of Homeland Security… in protecting the public from suspect foods….

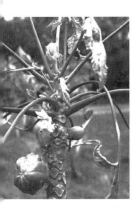

Papaya crop destroyed by the papaya ring spot virus.

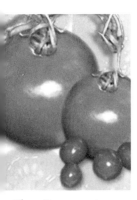

Flavr Savr tomatoes, the first genetically engineered product marketed in the U.S.

researchers from academia, industry and the government had isolated and copied a virus gene, then used a gene gun to shoot the gene into cells of the papaya plant. The papaya cells integrated the virus gene into their own chromosomes, making the papaya and subsequent generations resistant to the virus. While food products derived from genetic engineering remain controversial, the Hawaiian papaya farmers have qualms neither about the process nor the products. Genetic engineering saved their livelihoods.

The first genetically engineered product in the United States went on the market in May 1994 when the FDA approved a new tomato that could be shipped vine-ripened without rotting. The FDA determined that the genetically engineered tomato was as safe as other commercially grown tomatoes. Called the Flavr Savr, the tomato has gained wide acceptance in this country, especially during times of the year when fresh-picked tomatoes are unavailable. In the European community, however, genetically modified foods have caused much greater controversy and are actively discouraged by regulators. On the other hand, American consumers have found that genetic engineering offers a greater variety of reliably safe foods, broadening the range of available nutrients during nongrowing months.

Regulation offers other solutions for food safety. The doses of subtherapeutic antibiotics administered by farmers to poultry, swine and penned fish in overcrowded facilities, to diminish incidence of disease and encourage faster growth, result in resistant strains of *Salmonella* and other foodborne pathogens. A particularly aggressive strain of resistant *Salmonella* has been identified as *DT 104*. Although policy decisions must rely on accurate research, it is already apparent that regulation of feedlots and other overcrowded animal facilities must be stepped up. The overcrowding, itself a problem, is often compounded by reckless use of antibiotics, and farmers need to be held to account if resistance is to be controlled. Regulators also need to look to the food industry in general – processing plants, food distributors, restaurants and supermarkets – to bring the problem under control. The use of antibiotics by farmers, a response to the imperative of controlling costs, can be mitigated if the links higher up in the food industry and, ultimately, the public insist that cattle, eggs, pigs, poultry and sheep be raised to market readiness in humane conditions without undue use of antibiotics. To this point, the food industry witnessed a "Save the Dolphins" campaign that became so popular that tuna-fishing methods changed in response.

Education, another important avenue for improving food safety, must encourage fundamental research on the natural history of human pathogens in animals. How do these microorganisms develop disease resistance and how is it that they produce toxins? Educating those involved in producing, transporting and preparing food, including consumers, can help stem the threat of serious foodborne illnesses.

► Food behavior must first change with individuals in their homes and can be as simple as keeping perishable food refrigerated, keeping food cold before preparation and cooking food properly. For hamburgers, chicken and pork, this means using a food thermometer to determine that the meat is thoroughly cooked. If restaurants followed these simple rules, the incidence of foodborne illnesses would decline dramatically.

▼

Food behavior must first change with individuals in their homes and can be as simple as keeping perishable food refrigerated, keeping food cold before preparation and cooking food properly.

The U.S. Department of Transportation (DOT) regulates conditions for the transport of edible products. In July 1994, Congress passed a transportation bill that contained provisions addressing the sanitary transportation of food. The regulations, still going through an approval process, will address proper temperature in refrigerated trucks among other issues. For now, the FSIS has no comprehensive regulatory program that governs the handling of meat, poultry and egg products once they leave a regulated plant. As of now, a mishmash of state and local regulations govern the transportation of these perishable goods from the time they leave the plant to the time they reach the consumer.

CDC's ability to monitor foodborne illness outbreaks improved significantly with the President's Food Safety Initiative of 1997. CDC now operates some 20 surveillance systems, including the two main systems, FoodNet and PulseNet. FoodNet is an "active" surveillance system that encompasses a population of 20.5 million Americans in nine geographic areas. The system collects outbreak information on nine foodborne pathogens, toxoplasmosis, HUS, and Guillain-Barre syndrome. Once information is collected, FoodNet estimates the burden of illnesses, monitors trends, and names specific foods that carry risks. CDC also now funds nine Environmental Health Specialist (EHS-Net)

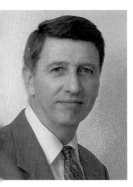

Dr. Ernest Julian, chief of the Office of Food Protection, Rhode Island Department of Health.

states where research is conducted on the factors that most often cause illness and the best means to prevent illness in food service operations.

According to Ernest Julian, PhD, Chief of the Office of Food Protection at the Rhode Island Department of Health, many states, but not all, have mandatory training and certification for managers of food service operations. A recent study conducted by CDC found that establishments without a certified manager were more likely to be associated with foodborne outbreaks than those with a certified manager. Similarly, the FDA found that establishments without a certified manager were statistically more likely to have certain risk factors present that are associated with foodborne outbreaks. Julian observes, "These studies provide a sound basis for all health departments to require mandatory food manager training and certification. While food manager certification is a critical component, inspections are still needed to ensure that the establishment has a certified manager as required and to make certain that there is compliance with other required food safety practices."

▼

If federal food-safety responsibilities were consolidated into a single agency...the attention accorded food safety would be much more focused and unified.

In the current federal food-safety system, 12 different agencies enforce 35 different statutes, which can lead to bureaucratic conflicts that undermine both enforcement and prevention efforts. ► If federal food safety responsibilities were consolidated into a single agency – from farms and feedlots to truckers to processing plants to retailers – the attention accorded food safety would be much more focused and unified. Consolidation would also strengthen prevention efforts. Such consolidation remains only a dream, however, and perhaps unrealistic in the face of many special interests in the food industry. While the public health community puts public health first, the food industry – farmers, processing plants, food distributors and supermarkets – have a different concern, putting their goods first. Hence, the public health community and government regulators, despite noteworthy advances in food safety, must remain wary. ▫

Photo credits

Page 123: Early American store, © Bettmann/CORBIS.

Page 123: Trucks lined up for NAFTA border inspection, © Steve Starr/CORBIS.

Page 124: Lunch at a day care center, © Annie Griffiths Belt/CORBIS.

Page 125: Galen, courtesy The National Library of Medicine.

Page 126: Dr. Harvey W. Wiley stamp, © FDA/CFSAN.

Page 127: Pellagra victim, © Lester V. Bergman/CORBIS.

Page 132: E. coli, © Gary Gaugler / Visuals Unlimited.

Page 137: PulseNet technician, courtesy Centers for Disease Control
and Prevention.

Page 140: MyPyramid, courtesy of www.MyPyramid.Gov.

Page 143: Papaya ring spot virus, courtesy Carol and Dennis Gonsalves, from the
article *Transgenic Virus-Resistant Papaya*.

Page 143: Flavr Savr tomatoes, courtesy www.agbios.com, Agriculture &
Biotechnology Strategies (Canada), Inc.

Chapter 8

Advances in Maternal and Child Health

Looking Back

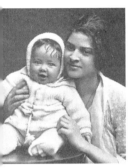

Advances in maternal and child health have been one of the greatest public health achievements of the 20th century. According to the U.S. Department of Labor and the National Center for Health Statistics, in the early 1900s about one in 10 infants died before his/her first birthday. Between 1915 and 1997, this figure fell by more than 90 percent. Maternal mortality rates have also experienced a significant decline, from approximately 850 deaths per 100,000 live births in 1900 to only 7.7 deaths per 100,000 live births in 1997. Although improvements in medical care were the main force behind these declines in infant and maternal mortality, public health interventions also played an important role. These include environmental interventions, improvements in nutrition and living standards, better surveillance and monitoring of disease and higher education levels.

Maternal Mortality Rates

Maternal deaths are defined as those that occur during a pregnancy or within 42 days of the end of a pregnancy and for which the cause of death is listed as a complication of pregnancy, childbirth or the puerperium. In 1900, one out of every 100 pregnant women died. Maternal death rates were highest from 1900 to 1930, caused mainly by home deliveries performed either by midwives or general practitioners with poor obstetric education who knew little about aseptic techniques. In fact, sepsis accounted for 40 percent of the deaths, one half after vaginal deliveries and one half after illegally induced abortions. The remaining deaths were due to hemorrhage and high blood pressure. Within this period, some 916 deaths were due to the flu epidemic of 1918. Another cause of maternal deaths can be linked to common medical practice in the 1920s, which included excessive surgical and obstetric interventions such as induction of labor, forceps, episiotomy and cesarean deliveries. For example, Dr. J.B. DeLee of Chicago

published an account of his "prophylactic forceps operation" in which full anesthesia, delivery by forceps and manual removal of placenta was routine for all women, except
those who evaded his plan by having a quick and sponta-
neous delivery. Following such examples, obstetricians with
insufficient skills undertook difficult surgical procedures,
often with fatal results.

After 1933, maternal mortality rates started to decrease.
During that year, the Report on the White House Conference on Child Health Protection, Fetal, Newborn, and
Maternal Mortality and Morbidity demonstrated a connection between poor aseptic practices, excessive operative

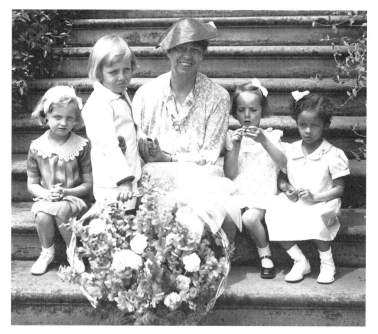

Eleanor Roosevelt at the White House on Child Health Day.

deliveries and high maternal mortality. During the 1930s
and 1940s, the government developed guidelines defining
physical qualifications needed for hospital delivery privi-
leges. These policies were aimed to have an accredited
specialist obstetrician deliver every baby in a hospital.
As a result, a shift from home to hospital deliveries
occurred between 1938 and 1948, and the proportion of
infants born in hospitals increased from 55 percent to 90
percent. The shift from home to hospital deliveries and
improvements in aseptic conditions in hospitals led to a
71 percent reduction in maternal mortality by 1948.

During the 1950s and 1960s medical advances brought about further declines in maternal mortality. These advances included the use of antibiotics, oxytocin to induce labor, safe blood transfusion and better management of hypertensive conditions. Furthermore, legalization of induced abortions led to an 89 percent reduction in deaths from septic illegal abortions between 1950 and 1973. The national maternal mortality rate continued to decrease until 1982, when it reached a plateau. Since then, maternal mortality rates have fluctuated between seven and eight maternal deaths per 100,000 live births. As a result, the goal proposed in 1987 for *Healthy People 2000* of 3.3 maternal deaths per 100,000 live births has not been achieved. At the same time, the current maternity mortality rate of 7.2 per 100,000 – a 99 percent decrease since 1900 – cannot be underestimated.

Some experts argue that the U.S. has reached a level in maternal mortality that cannot be reasonably lowered any further, but the World Health Organization estimates that 20 countries have reduced their maternal mortality rate below that of the United States. The 21st century offers an opportunity to continue the decrease of maternal death rates, as approximately 59 percent of all U.S. maternal deaths can be prevented through early diagnosis and appropriate medical care of pregnancy complications. However, obstacles exist to reducing this rate. In 1996, approximately 10 percent of all pregnant women received inadequate or

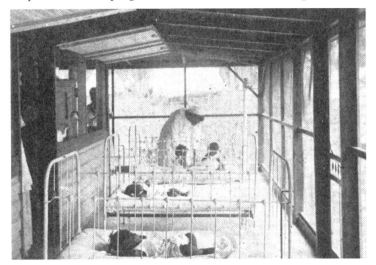

"Baby shack," Washington, D.C., circa 1927.

no prenatal care. Historically, the maternal mortality rate has always been higher for black and minority women than for white women. For example, in 1920 the maternal mortality rate for white women was nearly half that of black women. Currently, the maternal mortality rate is 5.5 per 100,000 live births for white women compared with 23.3 per 100,000 for black women and 7.9 per 100,000 for Hispanic women. Interventions must be designed to create awareness of the importance of prenatal care and to apply strategies to reduce persistent differences in mortality rates between white and minority women.

Infant Mortality Rates

The decline in infant mortality is unparalleled by any other mortality reduction in the 20th century. Today, less than one in 100 American babies die in infancy. A century ago, as many as one in six infants died. This incredible change results from a process that has roots in the 1850s when infant mortality was first recognized as a social problem.
▶   During the first 30 years of the 20th century, public health, social welfare and clinical medicine collaborated to combat infant mortality. These partnerships began improving living conditions and the environment in urban areas, upgrading the quality of commercial milk and improving mothers' abilities to carry, bear and rear healthy infants. At the beginning of the last century, the first steps to decrease infant mortality were established. First, the establishment of sewage disposal and safe drinking water were particularly important in reducing infant mortality rates during these years. Second, milk pasteurization, first adopted in Chicago in 1908, contributed to the control of gastrointestinal infections from contaminated milk supplies. Third, infancy and maternity programs secured federal funding, specifically to establish the National Children's Bureau in 1912, which was proposed by Martha May Elliot, among others.

Martha May Elliot (1891-1978) is considered a pioneer in maternal and child health. A graduate of Johns Hopkins University, she was a leading pediatrician and an important architect of programs for maternal and child health. Elliot directed the National Children's Bureau Division of Child and Maternal Health from 1924 until 1934. During her tenure, this institution became the primary government agency to work toward improving maternal and infant welfare. As early as her second year of medical school,

▼

During the first 30 years of the 20th century, public health, social welfare and clinical medicine collaborated to combat infant mortality.

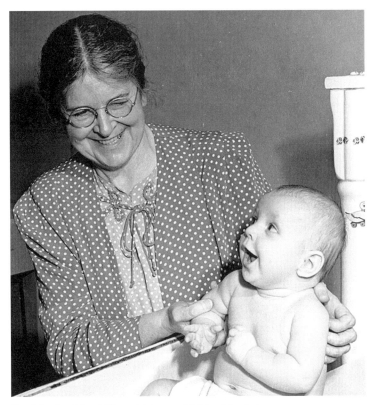

Dr. Martha May Elliot visiting a child health clinic in Washington, D.C., 1945.

Elliot hoped to become, in her words, "some kind of social doctor." While leading the Children's Bureau, she helped establish government programs that implemented her ideas about social medicine. The Children's Bureau advocated comprehensive maternal and infant welfare services, including prenatal, natal and postpartum home visits by health care providers. By the 1920s, the integration of these services changed the approach to infant mortality from one that addressed infant health problems to one that included infant and mother. The new approach focused on prenatal-care programs to educate, monitor and care for pregnant women. Even more significant changes in infant mortality were still to come, however.

The advent of antimicrobial agents (sulfonamide in 1937 and penicillin in the 1940s), the development of fluid and electrolyte replacement and safe blood transfusions accelerated the decline in infant mortality rates during the 1930s and 1940s. From 1950 through 1964, infant mortality declined more slowly. Increasing rates of infant death were attributed to prenatal causes that occurred among high-risk neonates, especially low birth weight (LBW) and preterm babies. This led to renewed efforts in the 1950s and 1960s to improve access to prenatal care, especially for the poor, and to concentrate efforts to establish neonatal intensive care units and to promote research in maternal and infant health. This research included technologies to improve the survival of LBW and preterm babies. In the late 1960s during the advent of Medicaid and other federal programs, infant mortality declined substantially. From 1970 to 1979, neonatal mortality plummeted 41 percent due to technologic advances in neonatal medicine and the regionalization of perinatal services.

During the early to mid 1980s the downward trend in U.S. infant mortality slowed again. In the early 1990s, infant mortality declined slightly faster due to the widespread introduction of artificial pulmonary surfactant to prevent and treat respiratory distress syndrome in premature infants and to the increased use of maternal steroids. From 1991 to 1997, the decrease in infant mortality continued, in part, because of reduced mortality from sudden infant death syndrome (SIDS). ►   Thanks to public health authorities recommending that infants be placed on their backs to sleep, SIDS rates declined greater than 50 percent during this time. Overall, the infant mortality rate today represents a 90 percent decrease from that experienced at the beginning of the 20th century. Despite this incredible achievement, medical and public health problems in maternal and child health remain to be resolved, among them birth defects, currently the leading cause of infant mortality. Yet the causes for 70 percent of birth defects remain a mystery.

▼

Thanks to public health authorities recommending that infants be placed on their backs to sleep, SIDS rates declined greater than 50 percent during this time.

Birth Defects

A birth defect is an abnormality of structure, function, or metabolism present at birth that results in physical or mental disability. Birth defects can be fatal and are the leading cause of infant mortality in the U.S., accounting for more than 20 percent of all infant deaths. Of 120,000 U.S. babies born each year with a birth defect, 8,000 die during their first year of life. According to a report by the National Academy of Sciences, nearly half of all pregnancies today result in the loss of the baby or a child born with a birth defect or chronic health problem. The leading birth defects associated with infant death are heart defects (31 percent), respiratory defects (15 percent), nervous system defects (13 percent), multiple abnormalities (13 percent) and musculo-skeletal abnormalities (7 percent). Birth defects contribute substantially to childhood morbidity and long-term disability and are also a major cause of miscarriages and fetal death.

The true incidence of birth defects is very difficult to determine because of inconsistent and incomplete national data gathering. Although surveillance systems are vital for monitoring and detecting trends in birth defects, there has never been an effective nationwide data system on birth defects. The Pew Environmental Health Commission recently reviewed this issue, finding that while the incidence of some birth defects is increasing rather dramatically, ► one-third of all states have no system for tracking birth defects, and systems are inadequate in most others. Moreover, even in states with birth defect registries, most do not include children whose defects do not become apparent until months or years after birth.

▼

...one-third of all states have no system for track-ing birth defects, and systems are inadequate in most others.

In the late 1960s, the Centers for Disease Control and Prevention (CDC) started the first birth-defects surveil-lance system in the United States, but that system was limited to the metropolitan area of Atlanta, Georgia. Since 1967, the Metropolitan Atlanta Congenital Defects Program (MACDP) has been monitoring all major birth defects in five counties of the metropolitan Atlanta area (Clayton, Cobb, DeKalb, Fulton and Gwinnett) with approximately 50,000 annual births in a population of about 2.9 million. For some time, CDC used the newborn hospital discharge summary and vital statistics to monitor birth defects nationwide, but both of these systems proved to be extremely inaccurate because many structural con-genital anomalies were not accurately identified at birth. In 1983, the California Birth Defects Monitoring Program began an active surveillance system in the five counties around the San Francisco Bay area. Founded by Drs. John Harris and Richard Jackson in conjunction with Califor-nia's legislature and governor, this program became a model for surveillance in other states and a worldwide leader in birth defects research. Adding new counties to its surveillance area, statewide coverage was achieved in 1990. The program is now the leader in birth defects surveillance and prevention with more than 250 published findings, ongoing monitoring of 334,000 births per year and trailblazing research.

► Perhaps the most important advance in the registry and prevention of birth defects data came in 1996, when the Congress directed CDC to establish the Centers for Birth Defects Research and Prevention (CBDRP). Formalized with the passage of the Birth Defects Prevention Act of 1998, CDC was authorized to: (1) collect, analyze and make available data on birth defects; (2) operate regional centers that conduct applied epidemiologic research for the prevention of birth defects; and (3) provide the public with information on preventing birth defects. Currently, CDC has established centers in Arkansas, California, Iowa, Massachusetts, New York, North Carolina, Texas and Utah. The centers were established in states whose existing birth defects programs were nationally recognized for expertise in birth defects surveillance and research.

▼

Perhaps the most important advance in the registry and prevention of birth defects data came in 1996, when the Congress directed CDC to establish the Centers for Birth Defects Research and Prevention.

The ultimate goal of tracking and research is to develop and implement effective programs to prevent birth defects and developmental disabilities. Even without an accurate national birth defects tracking system, it has been possible to implement prevention campaigns to decrease birth defects. One example of a success in this area is the national folic acid education campaign led by the March of Dimes, CDC and its partner organizations, such as the Spina Bifida Association. President Franklin Roosevelt founded the March of Dimes in 1938 as a national voluntary health agency to help combat birth defects. This new multiyear national education campaign aims to increase the number of women who take folic acid daily, and it is known to have had an impact. A study published in the *Journal of the American Medical Association* in 2001 showed that neural tube defects in newborns decreased 19 percent between 1995 and 1999 in the wake of this campaign. Furthermore, advances in neonatal technology have improved the survival rate of preterm babies who weigh less than five pounds, eight ounces at birth.

Today, birth defects loom as the No. 1 cause of infant death. The fact that one in 28 babies is born with a birth defect should give the public health community pause. Advances in medical treatments will continue to improve the survival rate of babies with birth defects and may continue to shift mortality associated with these deaths from infancy to later stages of life. However, increased funding for surveillance and research will be necessary to develop effective programs to prevent the tragedy of birth defects, which occur in 150,000 American families every year.

Family Planning

The hallmark of family planning in the United States in the 20th century has been the ability to achieve desired birth spacing and family size. Smaller families and longer intervals between births have contributed to the better health of infants, children, and women and have also improved the social and economic role of women. However, access to effective and legal contraception has not always been available to women. In 1900, it was illegal under federal and state laws to distribute information and to counsel patients about contraception and contraceptive devices. Some sectors of society rejected this law, and the modern contraceptive movement began.

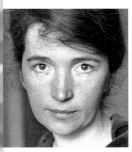

Margaret Sanger in 1916.

In 1912, Margaret Sanger initiated efforts to circulate information about and provide access to contraception. Sanger was a public health nurse concerned about the adverse health effects of frequent childbirth, miscarriages and abortion. In 1916, Sanger challenged the laws of the day and opened the first family planning clinic in Brooklyn, New York. The police closed her clinic, but Sanger continued to promote family planning by opening more clinics and challenging legal restrictions during the 1920s and 1930s. The court challenge established a legal precedent that allowed physicians to provide advice on contraception for health reasons, and physicians gained the right to counsel patients and to prescribe contraceptive methods. By the 1930s, a few state health departments (such as North Carolina) and public hospitals had begun to provide family planning services. By 1933, the average family size had declined from 3.5 to 2.3 children.

During the 1940s and 1950s, new efforts arose to create effective contraceptive methods. In the early 1950s, John Rock, a highly regarded obstetrician and gynecologist, who graduated from Harvard University, and Gregory Pincus, a biologist, who graduated from Cornell University, worked together to create an oral contraceptive. They tested their version of an oral contraceptive pill in preliminary trials in

Boston in 1954 and 1955. After the success of the preliminary trials for the Pill, Rock and Pincus were confident they had created an effective contraceptive method. But without large-scale human trials, the drug would never receive FDA approval necessary to bring the drug to market.   ►   In the summer of 1955, Pincus visited Puerto Rico and discovered a perfect location for these human trials. Puerto Rico had no anti-contraceptive laws on the books and had an extensive network of birth control clinics already in place.

The base for the first trial was a clinic in Rio Piedras, Puerto Rico. The Rio Piedras trials got off the ground quickly in April 1956. In no time, the trial was filled to capacity, and expanded trials began at other locations on the island. The pharmaceutical company G.D. Searle manufactured the pills for the trial. Rock selected a high dose of Enovid, the company's brand name for its synthetic oral progesterone, to ensure that no pregnancies would occur while test subjects were on the drug. Later, after discovering Enovid worked better with small amounts of synthetic estrogen, that active ingredient was added to the Pill as well.

Dr. Edris Rice-Wray, a faculty member of the Puerto Rico Medical School and medical director of the Puerto Rico Family Planning Association, supervised the trials. After a year of tests, Rice-Wray reported good news to Pincus. The Pill was 100 percent effective when taken properly. However, she also informed him that 17 percent of the women in the study complained of nausea, dizziness, headaches, stomach pain and vomiting. So serious and sustained were the side effects that Rice-Wray told Pincus that a 10 milligram dose of Enovid caused "too many side reactions to be generally acceptable."

Rock and Pincus quickly dismissed Rice-Wray's conclusions. Confident in the safety of the Pill, Pincus and Rock took no action to assess the root cause of the side effects. As a result, in later years, Pincus' team would be accused of deceit, colonialism and the exploitation of poor women of color. The women had been told only that they were taking a drug that prevented pregnancy and were not told that they were involved in a clinical trial, that the Pill was experimental and that potentially dangerous side effects were possible. Pincus and Rock, however, believed they

▼

In the summer of 1955, Pincus visited Puerto Rico and discovered a perfect location for these human trials.

were following the appropriate ethical standards of the time. To this day, questions linger over whether Pincus and Rock, in their rush to bring an effective pill to market, overlooked serious side effects from the original high-dosage Pill during trials. The current dosage of oral contraceptives has been dramatically lowered, and the incidence of serious side effects has been greatly reduced.

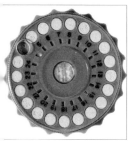

In 1960, the era of modern contraception began when both the birth control pill and the intrauterine device (IUD) became available. These effective and convenient methods resulted in widespread changes in birth control and social behavior. By 1965, the Pill had become the most popular birth control method, followed by the condom and contraceptive sterilization. Meanwhile, the IUD fell out of favor following reports that sterility might result if the device was improperly implanted or monitored. In fact, lawsuits caused bankruptcy of the manufacturer of the popular Dalkon Shield. It would be decades until newer, safer IUDs were reintroduced to the market as a contraceptive option.

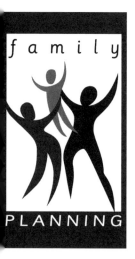

1960 contraceptive pills.

In 1970, federal funding for family planning services was established under the Family Planning Services and Population Research Act, which created Title X of the Public Health Service Act. During this period, the Supreme Court finally struck down state laws prohibiting contraceptive use by married couples. Medicaid funding for family planning was authorized in 1972. Services provided under Title X grew rapidly in the 1970s and 1980s; after 1980, public funding for family planning continued to shift to the Medicaid program. Since 1972, the average family size has leveled off at approximately two children, and the safety, efficacy, diversity, accessibility and use of contraceptive methods have increased. In the late 1990s, legislatures in 19 states mandated partial or comprehensive insurance coverage for reversible methods of contraception. Access to high-quality contraceptive services will continue to be an important factor in promoting healthy pregnancies and preventing unintended pregnancy in this country. ◻

Case Study

Folic Acid

Each year, spina bifida or anencephaly, the two most common forms of neural-tube defects, occurs in one in 1,000 pregnancies in the U.S. Anencephaly and spina bifida, which affect approximately 4,000 fetuses each year, are important factors in fetal and infant mortality. All infants with anencephaly are stillborn or die shortly after birth; whereas, many infants with spina bifida now survive as a result of extensive medical and surgical care. However, infants with spina bifida who survive are likely to have severe, lifelong disabilities. In addition to the emotional cost of spina bifida, the estimated monetary cost is staggering. In the U.S. alone, the total cost of spina bifida over a lifetime for affected infants born in 1988 was almost $500 million or $249,000 for each infant.

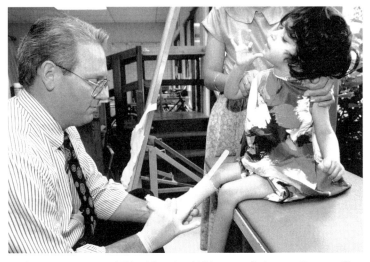

A doctor examines a child with spina bifida at a clinic near Brownsville, Texas, on the U.S.-Mexico border.

Although these severe conditions have been recognized since antiquity, never before has progress been as fast and substantive as in the last three decades, particularly in the area of prevention. During that time, evidence mounted that vitamin supplements in the early stages of pregnancy could prevent neural-tube defects. In 1976, Dick Smithells and colleagues in the United Kingdom reported that women who gave birth to babies with neural-tube defects

▼

...among women who had previously had an affected pregnancy, those who took a multivitamin during the early stages of pregnancy had an 86 percent lower risk of having another affected fetus or infant than those who did not take the multivitamin.

had low serum levels of micronutrients, including some vitamins. These findings led them to propose a randomized controlled trial of vitamin supplementation. ► As a result, in 1983 they reported that among women who had previously had an affected pregnancy, those who took a multivitamin during the early stages of pregnancy had an 86 percent lower risk of having another affected fetus or infant than those who did not take the multivitamin. However, because Smithells and colleagues had not been permitted to randomly assign the use of the multivitamin among participants in their study, their finding did not lead to public action.

In fact, action was delayed until the publication of two randomized, peer-reviewed studies a decade later. In 1991, a randomized controlled trial funded by the British Medical Research Council demonstrated that folic acid supplementation before pregnancy and during its early stages markedly reduced the risk of neural-tube defects in newborns. This finding led the Public Health Service and CDC in 1992 to recommend that all women who are planning to become pregnant take folic acid supplements beginning before pregnancy and continuing through its early stages. CDC directs its recommendation at women of childbearing age, because as many as 50 percent of pregnancies in the U.S. are unplanned. The evidence suggests that folic acid supplementation must begin before pregnancy to protect against neural-tube defects.

Public health officials have considered three approaches to achieving CDC's recommendation for a daily folic acid intake of 0.40 milligrams (mg): (1) promoting daily use of vitamin supplements that contain folic acid, (2) promoting dietary intake of foliate-rich foods, and (3) fortifying food with folic acid. A landmark public health decision by the Food and Drug Administration allowed the third approach to be implemented in January 1998. The FDA mandated that all enriched grain products, such as flours and pastas, must also be fortified with 140 micrograms (μg) of folic acid per 100 grams grain. The measurement was based on the estimate that the average American woman of reproductive age would consume about 100 μg of folic acid per day from foods containing enriched grain products. This public health decision has proved to be a success. The addition of folic acid to commonly eaten foods has dramatically reduced by 50 percent the incidence of spinal bifida in newborns. More important, the cost of fortification is small. In the U.S., it costs about one cent per person per year, or about $1,000 per neural-tube defect prevented, which represents less than one percent of the total cost of spina bifida over a lifetime for each infant affected.

Regardless of the method chosen to increase folic acid intake, the full potential of preventing neural-tube defects can be realized only if women increase their intake of folic acid supplementation at the correct time of pregnancy. In 1998, according to Gallup surveys commissioned by the March of Dimes, most women were taking folic acid too late to reduce their risk of having a baby with a neural-tube defect. The surveys showed a steady increase in the number of women who had heard of folic acid, but no increase in the number of women taking a multivitamin every day. However, this trend has changed with time and the hard work of organizations seeking to increase women's intake of folic acid. According to the March of Dime's latest survey published in a September 2004 *Morbidity & Mortality Weekly Report*, ► a record 40 percent of American women of childbearing age reported taking a daily multivitamin containing folic acid in 2004, up from 32 percent in 2003, and the highest level since the March of Dimes began surveying women in the 1990s.

Dr. Jennifer L. Howse, president of the March of Dimes, recently said that the latest survey shows that women today seem to understand the importance of folic acid to the health of babies. This means that women who might become pregnant in the United States are aware of the benefits of folic acid intake and are taking this preventive approach. Increasing folic acid intake represents a major step in reducing infant mortality and morbidity and is one of the 20th century's clearest public health successes. ▫

▼

...a record 40 percent of American women of childbearing age reported taking a daily multivitamin containing folic acid in 2004....

Vignette

Amniocentesis

The tapping of amniotic fluid has been practiced for more than 100 years. Transabdominal amniocentesis in the third trimester of pregnancy was first reported in the literature in 1877. For today's pregnant woman, having amniocentesis, or "amnio," is an important decision that she must make between 15 and 18 weeks of pregnancy. Amniocentesis is the most common prenatal test used to diagnose chromosomal and genetic birth defects and has an accuracy rate of between 99.4 percent and 100 percent in diagnosing chromosomal abnormalities. Amnio is recommended for women over age 35 because the risk of chromosome disorders increases with maternal age. The test is also recommended to women who have had a previous child with a birth defect that amniocentesis can diagnose, a family history of a genetic disorder or an abnormal triple-screen blood test result.

In 1956, in their seminal article in the journal *Nature,* F. Fuchs and J. Riis reported the first use of amniotic fluid examination in the diagnosis of genetic disease. They determined fetal sex from cells found in amniotic fluid, based on the presence or absence of the Barr body (an inactive X-chromosome found in the nuclei of somatic cells of most female mammals). That same year in the United Kingdom, John Edward also discussed for the first time the possibility of the "antenatal detection of hereditary disorders." The determination of fetal sex led to the prenatal management of patients with *Haemophilia A* in 1960 and Duchenne muscular dystrophy in 1964.

In their paper in *The Lancet* in 1966, the researchers M. W. Steele and W. R. Breg demonstrated that cultured amniotic fluid cells were suitable for karyotyping. In 1972, David J.H. Brock and Roger Sutcliffe discovered that excessive amounts of alpha-fetoprotein (AFP) were present in the amniotic fluid of pregnancies with neural-tube defects. But a study in *The New England Journal of Medicine* in 1970 by Henry Nadler and Albert Gerbie was the real impetus in genetic amniocentesis and diagnosis. Following the publication of their article, "Role of amniocentesis in the intrauterine diagnosis of genetic defects," genetic laboratories for analysis of amniotic fluid became prevalent and included the detection of chromosomal abnormalities, X-Linked conditions, inborn errors of metabolism and neural-tube defects.

Thanks to advances in technology, amniocentesis today is a safe test for both mother and fetus; although, a small risk of miscarriage (one in 200 or less) exists. However, a recent study by the National Center for Human Genome Research and the Agency for Healthcare Research and Quality found that amniocentesis can be "cost-effective at any age or risk level" and should be offered to all pregnant women. Using ultrasound as a guide, the health care provider inserts a thin needle through the mother's abdomen. A small amount of amniotic fluid (the fluid that surrounds the baby) is removed and tested. A positive diagnosis indicates, with near 100 percent certainty, a specific genetic abnormality in the fetus.

Fortunately, advances in prenatal therapy now make it possible to treat some birth defects before birth. For example, biotin dependence and MMA (methylmalonic acidemia), two life-threatening inherited disorders of body chemistry, can be detected by amniocentesis and treated in the womb, resulting in the birth of a healthy baby. However, if a fetus has a condition for which prenatal treatment is not yet possible, prenatal diagnosis may help parents prepare emotionally for the birth and plan the delivery with their health care provider. Parents can discuss their options with genetic counselors as well as with their health care providers.

A framework for the role public health can play in prenatal screening such as amniocentesis, was best presented by the Institute of Medicine in *The Future of Public Health* (1988). The framework identifies the following four essential public health components:

1. Surveillance and population-based epidemiologic studies to assess how risk for disease and disability is influenced by the interaction of human genetic variation with modifiable risk factors.

2. Evaluation of policies and quality of genetic testing to ensure the appropriateness and quality of population-based genetic testing.

3. Intervention development, implementation, and evaluation to ensure that genetic tests and services are incorporated into programs that promote health and prevent disease and disability.

4. Communication and information dissemination to provide timely and accurate information to the general public and professional audiences on the role of genetics in health promotion and disease prevention.

Based on the experience with amniocentesis and advances in genetics, genetic screening will challenge the field of maternal health in the near future. ▫

Looking Ahead

Genetic Screening

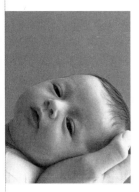

State newborn screening systems were the first genetics programs for children, and they remain the largest. Nationwide, state public health programs screen an estimated four million infants annually for genetic disorders. Each year approximately 3,000 babies with severe disorders are detected due to newborn screening programs. Undetected and untreated abnormalities can result in mental retardation, severe illness and premature death. State newborn screening programs involve testing, follow-up, diagnosis, treatment and evaluation.

As public health initiatives, newborn screening programs focus resources on treatable conditions that occur relatively frequently. Currently, tests are available for 29 genetic and metabolic diseases, but most babies are not tested for all of these disorders because policies regarding genetic testing vary from state to state. Advances in technology, particularly in genetics and metabolic research, will enable testing for numerous abnormalities. These disorders include: carnitine uptake defect (CUD), congenital adrenal hyperplasia (CAH), cystic fibrosis (CF), hearing deficiency, maple syrup urine disease (MSUD), phenylketonuria (PKU) and sickle cell anemia (SCA).

Genetics is growing in importance as the public becomes more knowledgeable and more demanding of genetic services, and as the knowledge of our genes and their functions permits more effective strategies for treatment and especially for prevention, the special responsibility of public health. As genetic research yields vast information about sequences, mutations and variation, the public health sciences will be called upon to interpret clinical significance in the context of environmental, metabolic, nutritional and behavioral risk factors.

The prevention of human disease is a time-honored and honorable goal of public health professionals. What might it mean, however, to use the special tools and authorities of public health agencies to attempt to prevent genetic disease? Many approaches to prevention are possible, but attempts to locate them within traditional public health categories like "primary, secondary and tertiary" prevention have been confusing. It is important to distinguish between two definitions of "prevention" that are often used in public health genetics: "phenotypic" prevention and "genotypic" prevention.

Phenotypic prevention describes medical efforts to delay or stop the clinical manifestations of a genetic disease in an at-risk patient, such as newborn screening and dietary treatment for PKU. Genotypic prevention, on the other hand, describes efforts to avoid the transmission of particular genotypes from one generation to the next. Genotypic prevention can include pregnancy termination or the decision not to have children. ► These decisions have a profound impact on prospective parents as individuals and as part of society, as they can affect the incidence of a disease in the larger population.

From a public health perspective, the ethical issues surrounding genetic counseling include:

1. Autonomy. The right of individuals to act freely with adequate information.

2. Non-Malfeasance. The concept of "do no harm."

3. Beneficence and Justice. Information should be helpful and available to all.

4. Confidentiality. All information is private and not to be shared with others.

In 1997, CDC created the Office of Genomics and Disease Prevention to highlight the emerging role of genetics in the practice of public health in the United States. The office provides internal coordination and promotes external partnerships in activities related to genetics, disease prevention and health promotion. Prevention includes the use of medical, behavioral, and environmental interventions to reduce the risk of disease among people susceptible because of their genetic makeup. This office supports the responsible use of genetic tests and services, including adequate family history assessment and genetic counseling, to promote health and prevent disease in different communities.

▼

These decisions have a profound impact on prospective parents as individuals and as part of society....

The public health approach to genetic screening places major emphasis on preventing the occurrence or manifestation of a particular disorder. If this proves not to be feasible, a secondary approach is to identify high-risk individuals and institute a program of early screening followed by active treatment to minimize any critical expression of the condition. This model works reasonably well and is ethically acceptable when the disorder to be treated will have serious, irreversible or possibly lethal effects in the individuals affected. In these situations, the risk/benefit ratios will more than likely benefit the individuals identified as at-risk or affected.

The same cannot be said of the person screened if the disorder identified will not manifest itself for a number of years, if the treatment available may be of questionable value or if no effective intervention is known. The issue becomes even more complex when the screening result places the individual merely in a category of increased risk to develop the condition.

Dr. Allen Rosenfield, dean of the Mailman School of Public Health at Columbia University and noted authority on maternal and child health, observes, "20th century medical advances, together with universal access to maternity care, can now prevent the most common labor complications from becoming life-threatening.   ▶   These advances have dramatically improved the lives of women in the United States, sparing them the unnecessarily high risk of death and disability that women in many resource-poor countries in Africa, Asia and Latin America still face." Rosenfield continues, "While current state-of-the-art advances have been of great importance, basic interventions can help women experiencing complications when more sophisticated options are not available. Programs have been developed in resource-poor countries to provide access to emergency obstetric care, including cesarean sections, treatment of postpartum hemorrhage and infection, and management of the complications of unsafe abortions to women whose complications would otherwise cause death or disability."

In other words, advances in maternal and child health owe as much to sound public health practices as to new technologies. In order to realize its promise, genetic screening

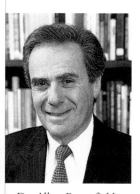

Dr. Allen Rosenfield, dean of the Mailman School of Public Health, Columbia University.

▼

"These advances have dramatically improved the lives of women in the United States, sparing them the unnecessarily high risk of death and disability that women in many resource-poor countries in Africa, Asia and Latin America still face."

will need to be partnered with good public health practices. It is these practices that have brought such astounding
success to reducing maternal and child mortality. Genetic
screening itself will inevitably become a powerful new
public health practice, transforming yet again the field
of maternal and child health, as long as proven practices
continue to be faithfully observed. ◻

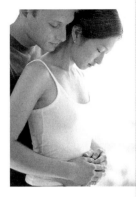

Photo credits
Page 147: Mother with baby, courtesy New York Public Library Digital Gallery.
Page 148: Eleanor Roosevelt with children, © Bettmann/CORBIS.
Page 149: "Baby shack" 1927, courtesy New York Public Library Digital Gallery.
Page 151: Dr. Martha May Elliot, © Eileen Darby Images, Inc.
Page 155: Margaret Sanger, © Bettmann/CORBIS.
Page 157: The Pill contraceptive, © SSPL/The Image Works.
Page 157: Family Planning, courtesy Washington State Department of Health.
Page 158: Doctor examining child, © Annie Griffiths Belt / CORBIS.
Page 163: Newborn baby, © CORBIS.
Page 166: Man and pregnant woman, © CORBIS.

Chapter 9

Oral Health

Looking Back

The mouth is a mirror, reflecting the health of the rest of the body. Associations between the mouth and diseases elsewhere in the body – in the heart and lungs, for example – are well-documented. Still, people don't always recognize oral health as a key measure of overall health. Despite notable advances in reducing the prevalence of dental caries, or tooth decay, during the past century, the United States still has a long way to go to make good oral health, and the improved quality of life it promotes, a public health priority.

Poor oral health remains a silent epidemic. Disadvantaged populations are disproportionately the victims of oral diseases, resulting in great societal costs. From missed hours

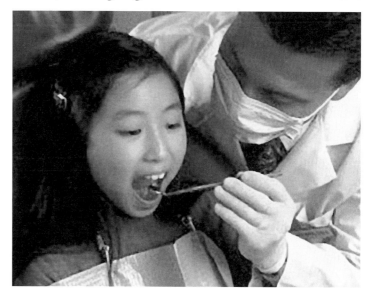

at school and work, to periodontal disease that leads to premature low birth-weight babies, to heart disease and stroke associated with oral infections, the costs quickly mount. In 1994, low-income children had almost 12 times more days of missed school due to dental problems than higher income children. Early childhood caries (ECC), also called "baby bottle tooth decay," occur most often in the upper anterior primary teeth when a baby is regularly given a bottle with sugary liquid at bedtime or naptime. Prevalent in lower-income families, ECC can cost as much as $6,000 per child to treat because general anesthesia and an operating room are often required. Clearly, teaching parents and caregivers how to avoid ECC would be more cost-effective and would help prevent unnecessary pain and infection.

Dentistry Becomes a Profession

The mouth has historically been disconnected from the rest of the body in health sciences, education and practice. With the founding in 1840 of the world's first dental school, the Baltimore College of Dental Surgery, dentistry became a separate profession from medicine. Dentistry could have become a medical specialty had the Maryland legislature not rejected a request, due to attendant costs, to incorporate dentistry as a department at the University of Maryland's medical school. Thus, dentistry set its own course.

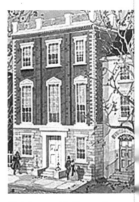

Baltimore College of Dental Surgery

Dr. Chapin A. Harris, the father of American Dental Science and co-founder of the Baltimore College of Dental Surgery, was born in 1806 in Pompey, New York. He moved West as a young man to Madison, Ohio, where he joined two of his brothers, one a physician, to study medicine. In 1824, he passed the Ohio Board of Medical Censors and began the practice of medicine and surgery in Greenfield, Ohio. Having taken up the study of dentistry in 1828, he moved to Baltimore in 1833 to pursue further dental studies with Dr. Horace H. Hayden. In 1839, after establishing an itinerant dental practice throughout the South, Harris founded the world's first dental journal, *The American Journal of Dental Science*, and remained its chief editor and publisher until his death in 1860. Also in 1839, he published *The Dental Art: A Practical Treatise on Dental Surgery*, which in 1845 became *The Principles and Practice of Dental Surgery* and remained the most useful dental textbook of that century through 11 editions dating to 1896. In 1840, Drs. Harris and Hayden organized the American Society of Dental Surgeons, the first national dental organization. In 1845, Harris published his second book,

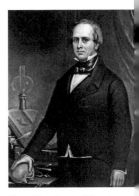

Dr. Chapin A. Harris

Dictionary of Dental Science, which saw five editions dating to 1898.

In 1840, as co-founder of the Baltimore College of Dental Surgery with Hayden, Harris became its first dean and a professor of practical dentistry, then the school's second president upon Hayden's death in 1844. The Baltimore College of Dental Surgery was later to merge with the University of Maryland School of Dentistry in 1923. Between 1840 and 1867, nine more autonomous dental schools were founded in the United States using the Baltimore model. In 1867, Harvard established the Harvard School of Dental Medicine in association with the Massachusetts General Hospital, becoming the first university-affiliated dental school.

By 1870, only 15 percent of the 8,000 practicing dentists in the United States had graduated from dental schools; the rest were trained under preceptor arrangements or simply proclaimed themselves as dentists. Dental infections and complications from tooth extractions were among the most common causes of death. Indeed, the Bills of Mortality listed dental infections and complications as leading causes of death from the 1600s through the 1800s. ► In the late 1800s, the preceptor model of dental training shifted dramatically, as a growing number of schools of dentistry were founded in the United States and as graduates began to predominate in the ranks of practicing dentists. In 1894, the University of Michigan School of Dentistry became the first dental school to offer graduate courses in dentistry. By the mid-1920s, less than three percent of practicing dentists had trained under preceptor arrangements. In the 1920s, after the transforming Flexner Report of 1910 on medical education, the Carnegie Foundation funded Dr. William J. Gies of Columbia University to study existing dental schools, most of which were merely trade schools unaffiliated with universities. In 1926, Gies published what came to be known as the Gies Report. The report advocated for incoming dental students to have at least two years of university education and for the teaching of the basic biology of oral structure and the pathology of oral-facial disease. Widely adopted, the report's recommendations began transforming American dental education into an oral specialty of medicine. With the growing interest

▼

In the late 1800s... a growing number of schools of dentistry were founded in the United States and graduates began to predominate in the ranks of practicing dentists.

in dental education, more university-based dental schools and newly formed dental societies took hold. They continued to operate separately from medical schools and medical societies, however, and as a consequence, many health care professionals were never fully educated on the impact of oral diseases on overall health.

The dental health profession consists of dentists, dental hygienists, dental assistants and dental laboratory technicians. Nine dental specialties – dental public health, endodontics, oral and maxillofacial surgery, oral pathology, orthodontics, pediatric dentistry, periodontics, prosthodontics and radiology – are joined by other oral health specialties within medicine. Endocrinologists deal with salivary glands, neurologists address the mouth's nervous system, and orthopedic surgeons correct musculoskeletal defects.

► Dramatic improvements in oral health occurred once dentistry became a profession in 1839. For the next 100 years, the United States led the world in research and innovations and paved the way for preventive dentistry. Although dental caries and periodontal diseases were far more prevalent a century ago, today the silent epidemic of tooth decay continues unabated. This is especially true in low-income, inner-city and rural populations and among developmentally disabled people and other underserved groups, such as the homeless, homebound and medically compromised. Preventive dentistry's success story has yet to reach everyone who can benefit, and until it does, poor oral health remains a neglected epidemic.

▼

Dramatic improvements in oral health occurred once dentistry became a profession in 1839.

The Beginnings of Oral Health

Dental infections were a common cause of death in ancient peoples, often the result of extensive dental caries. Rates of dental caries correlated largely to diet. Diets heavy on meat tended to lower caries rates, while diets rich in vegetables tended to increase them. In pre-Columbian America, for example, pre-contact Zuni Indians had high vegetable diets and a caries rate of 75 percent. Pre-contact Eskimos, on the other hand, with a diet rich in meat, had the lowest rate of dental caries – about one percent. Once refined sugar was introduced to their diet, however, the caries rate among Eskimos soared.

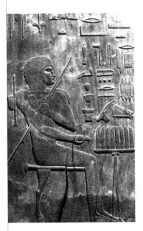

Hesi-Re, earliest-known dentist.

Archeologists in Egypt discovered that lower-class people in ancient Egypt show a very low caries rate while royalty, with diets rich in carbohydrates, show an 80 percent caries rate. In Egypt, ancient skulls have been found with small holes drilled through the jawbone, thought to be a way to alleviate the pressure of abscesses, a secondary complication of dental caries. The earliest known dentist, Hesi-Re, dates from the Zoser dynasty in Egypt around 2600 BC. In addition to ancient Egypt, written records of oral health care have been handed down by ancient civilizations in China, India, Mesopotamia, Greece and Rome and by more recent civilizations in the Islamic Middle East and Medieval Europe and in Mexico and Central America. In ancient Mesopotamia, dentistry was part of medicine, its history preserved by the Sumerians as far back as 2800 BC through ideograms, later to be translated by Assyrian and Babylonian students and copied on clay tablets with cuneiform writing. The Code of Hammurabi (1900 BC) shows that as far back as 2500 BC the government regulated the medical profession, and with it, dentistry.

Milestones in Dental Innovations

Toothbrushes

Chewsticks, the first toothbrushes, were borrowed from the Chinese and Babylonians and first mentioned as a common method for cleaning the teeth by the Romans. They are still common today in many parts of Africa and many Islamic countries. In Islam, oral hygiene is part of the

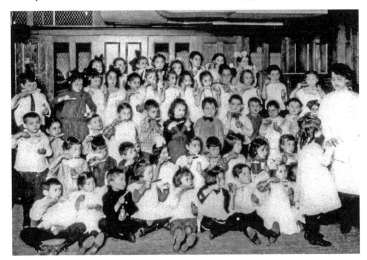

Toothbrush drill in New York City, 1913.

religion, and the use of the chewstick, called the Miswak or
Siwak, is a daily ritual. Any stick of fibrous material, smaller
in diameter than a pencil and about six inches long, will
do. One end is chewed until the fibers separate and these
are then used to clean the surfaces of teeth, one at a time.
Early bristle toothbrushes, invented by the Chinese, were
made from the neck bristles of cold-climate pigs. In modern times, nylon toothbrushes date only from 1938, when
DuPont introduced them. It was only after World War II
that tooth-brushing became a daily routine for most
Americans, when returning soldiers kept up an enforced
military discipline. In fact, the rejection rate of draftees

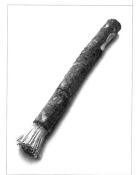

*A chewstick called
a Miswak.*

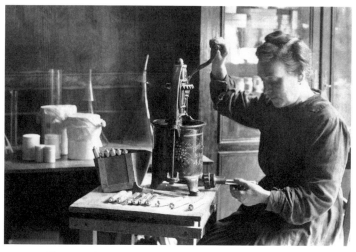

Women filling toothpaste tubes in the 1890s.

during World War II due to poor oral health had been so
high that standards had been lowered to meet targets.

Toothpaste

The roots of toothpaste can be traced to ancient China
and India as far back as 500 BC. Toothpaste more similar
to what we know today began to be developed in the
1800s. In 1824, Dr. Peabody added soap to toothpaste;
and in the 1850s, Dr. Harris added chalk. In 1873, Colgate
began to mass-produce scented toothpaste in a jar. In
1892, Dr. Sheffield's Creme Dentifrice, the creation of
Dr. Washington Sheffield of Connecticut, became the first
toothpaste put into a collapsible tube. In 1896, Colgate
Dental Cream became the first toothpaste packaged in
collapsible tubes to become widely available, and it was

not until 1986 that the pump dispenser, introduced from Europe, began to compete with the collapsible tube. Colgate's research led the way to introducing fluoride to toothpaste, but Procter & Gamble and its Crest brand were first out of the gate with fluoride toothpaste in 1956. For toothpaste to be effective in preventing tooth decay, it must have fluoride. Without fluoride, toothpaste can help prevent gum disease but not tooth decay.

Mouth Rinses

Another means for cleaning teeth, discovered by the Romans, was the mouth sponge. Long branches and vines were collected, scorched to remove the bark and then woven into a tight ball. When a bite of this sponge was chewed, it released a foaming substance, an astringent that was alternately rinsed and spit out during the 20 minutes the chewing normally took.

Novocaine

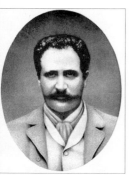

In 1905, the chemist Alfred Einhorn researched easy-to-use and safe anesthesia for dental procedures. He refined the chemical procaine until it was effective and named it Novocaine. This synthetic local anesthetic had none of the addictive properties of cocaine, which had been introduced as an ophthalmologic anesthetic in 1884 by Dr. Carl Koller, a colleague of Sigmund Freud in Vienna, and as a blocking agent in oral surgery by the American surgeon, Dr. William Halsted.

Alfred Einhorn

Dental Floss

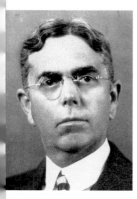

Dental floss has existed in one form or another since ancient times. The creator of modern dental floss, a New Orleans dentist named Levi Spear Parmly, was born in 1790 and died in 1859. In 1815, he began to promote flossing with a string of silk thread. It was not until 1882 that a company in Randolph, Massachusetts, began to manufacture unwaxed silk floss for home use. The Johnson & Johnson Company of New Brunswick, New Jersey, patented dental floss in 1898 and continues to be the major manufacturer today. Dr. Charles C. Bass developed nylon floss during World War II and made flossing the important part of oral hygiene it is today.

Dr. Charles C. Bass

High-Speed Drill

In 1957, John Borden introduced a high-speed, air-driven, contra-angle hand piece for drilling teeth. Called the Airotor and an immediate commercial success, the drill obtained speeds of up to 300,000 rotations per minute and launched a new era of high-speed dentistry.

The Major Oral Diseases

Dental Caries

The three general types of tooth decay are coronal (on the crowns of teeth), root surface (on the roots of teeth) and recurrent (reoccurring tooth decay). The elderly are especially vulnerable to root surface decay, but 84 percent of 17-year-old school children have had tooth decay, with an average of eight affected surfaces; and 99 percent of adults aged 40 to 44 have had tooth decay, with an average of 30 affected surfaces.

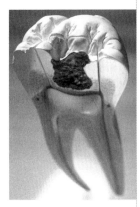

Coronal tooth decay.

Gum Diseases

Gingivitis and periodontitis are the two common infections of the soft tissues (gum) surrounding teeth. Gingivitis, a localized infection or inflammation of the soft tissues characterized by swelling and bleeding of the gums, disproportionately affects certain populations, especially Native Americans and Alaskan Natives, Mexican Americans and low-income individuals. Periodontitis, also an infection or inflammation of the soft tissues, involves the supporting alveolar bone around teeth with loss of periodontal attachment. Its prevalence increases with age, and it disproportionately affects immunosuppressed individuals, such as those with HIV/AIDS.

Oral Cancer

A serious epidemic, oral and pharyngeal cancers affect more than 30,000 Americans each year, and about 7,800 die annually. Men over 40 years of age are most at risk due to tobacco and alcohol use, which are associated with over 70 percent of oral and pharyngeal cancers. Oral cancer incidence may increase in the future due to the growing use of smokeless tobaccos, especially among teenagers. Of all cancers, oral and pharyngeal cancers show the largest discrepancy in five-year survival rates between Euro-Americans (56 percent) and African-Americans (36 percent).

Other Oral Diseases

► Complete tooth loss, or edentulism, was once much more widely prevalent than it is today. Still, of those aged 65 and older, 30 percent have no teeth at all. Crooked teeth, another widespread epidemic, cause severe or very severe malocclusion in an estimated 29 percent of adolescents. Finally, cleft lip and palate affect one out of 700 Americans born each year. ◘

▼

Complete tooth loss, or edentulism, was once much more widely prevalent than it is today.

Case Study

Fluoridation

The link between fluoride and healthy teeth is the great discovery and success story for better oral health in the past 100 years. Community water fluoridation is one of the great preventive health measures in history. Who first linked fluoride in drinking water with decreased dental caries, and how was the discovery applied to the public's health?

Fluoride, whether present in tap water, toothpaste and oral rinses or as a topical application administered by dentists or oral hygienists, has become an integral part of better oral hygiene for most Americans. Fluoride occurs naturally in all drinking water, in greater or lesser concentrations according to geological features, and is odorless, colorless and tasteless at the recommended level.

The fluoridation movement can be traced to the early years of the 20th century, when dentists began to focus on naturally fluoridated water for its preventive action on dental caries, or tooth decay. The most famous example was named the Colorado Brown Stain phenomenon by its discoverer, Frederick S. McKay, a young dentist who established his practice in Colorado Springs. In 1908, Dr. McKay began to investigate why people in particular communities in Colorado had severe tooth discoloration, known as dental fluorosis, or more popularly, mottled enamel. In 1909, he enlisted the collaboration of a renowned dental researcher, Dr. G. V. Black of Northwestern University, who was lured to Colorado by a report of the Colorado Springs Dental Society showing that nearly 90 percent of the city's locally born children were subject to the blight of mottled enamel. Together, Black and McKay determined that children waiting for their secondary teeth to erupt were at high risk of Colorado Brown Stain, while adults whose teeth had calcified without the stain were no longer at risk. Before Black's death in 1915, the two also realized that teeth afflicted with Colorado Brown Stain were inexplicably resistant to decay.

In 1923, McKay's hunch that the Colorado Brown Stain phenomenon might result from an ingredient in water was

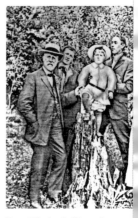

Drs. Black (left) and McKay (right) visit Colorado Springs to investigate brown stain phenomenon.

given a boost in Oakley, Idaho. Parents in Oakley were alarmed by a sudden onset of severe tooth discoloration in their children and invited McKay to investigate. The community had recently constructed a communal pipeline to a warm spring five miles away. McKay evaluated this new source of water and while it appeared normal according to his tests, he nonetheless advised the community to cease using the pipeline and begin using a nearby spring instead. Over the next few years, he determined that the new water source had the effect of ending new cases of mottled enamel in children and that affected children were also relieved of the blight when their secondary teeth erupted.

Separately, also in 1909, Dr. F.L. Robertson realized that people drinking water from a newly dug well in Bauxite, Arkansas, were showing signs of severe mottled enamel. The blight became so widespread that the well was closed in 1927. McKay, hearing of the trouble in Bauxite, a company town owned by the Aluminum Company of America, traveled there with Dr. Grover Kempf of the U.S. Public Health Service to investigate. They were surprised to learn that mottled enamel was nonexistent in a town five miles away, but their tests with the available technology failed to determine the causative agent for the children's mottled enamel in Bauxite. Their report reached the desk of H.V. Churchill, ALCOA's chief chemist in Pennsylvania, who had spent years defending aluminum cookware from charges it was poisonous. In 1930, to avoid yet another controversy, he ran a photospectrographic analysis on water from the Bauxite well. ► The results showed a high presence of naturally occurring fluoride, something he could not believe, having never heard of fluoride in water. He tested a second sample from the well with the same result. He immediately wrote a letter to McKay, inviting him to send water samples from Colorado. McKay sprang to action, and Churchill's photospectrographic analyses of the Colorado water samples also showed fluoride as the agent causing discoloration.

▼

The results showed a high presence of naturally occurring fluoride, something he could not believe, having never heard of fluoride in water.

In 1931, McKay finally knew that fluoride was the natural element in drinking water that caused the Colorado Brown Stain phenomenon. His single-minded investigation over several decades proved that naturally abundant fluoride in the water supply would mottle tooth enamel but at the same time inhibit dental caries. To McKay, the question was how to harness fluoride at a dosage that would inhibit both dental caries and mottled enamel.

In the 1930s, McKay collaborated with Dr. H. Trendly Dean of the U.S. Public Health Service to determine if fluoride could be added to drinking water to prevent cavities. They collaborated on several classic studies, one an epidemiologic study involving 32 communities with naturally fluoridated water supplies, and established a community fluorosis index. Their associates conducted further studies that predicted the optimal amount of fluoridation for preventing both tooth decay and discoloration. In effect, they were searching for an adjusted fluoridation standard that would have the benefit of reducing dental caries while avoiding tooth discoloration, and they concluded that the standard should be one part per million (1 ppm).

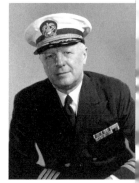

Dr. H. Trendly Dean

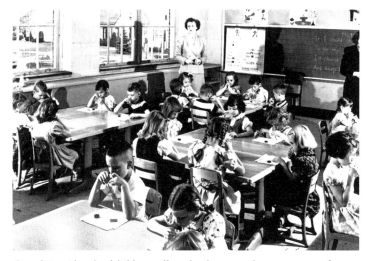

Grand Rapids schoolchildren collected saliva samples once a year from 1945 to 1960 to help dentists study the effects of fluoridation.

World War II interrupted further studies, but on January 25, 1945, Grand Rapids, Michigan, became the first city in the world to adjust its water fluoride concentration to the new adjusted fluoridation standard. [The 60th anniversary of fluoridation was observed, therefore, in early 2005.] Newburgh, New York, added sodium fluoride to its water supply in June 1945, and later that month, Brantford, Ontario, did the same. In February 1947, Evanston, Illinois, fluoridated its water supply. Four nearby communities with similar demographics were used as the control group – Muskegon in Michigan, Kingston in New York, Sarnia in Ontario, and Oak Park in Illinois. Careful tracking of rates of dental caries ensued over 15 years, and the studies concurred that one part fluoride per million parts of a community's drinking water was the optimal standard, giving maximum protection against dental caries with minimum staining of the teeth.

Emboldened after just five years by the success of these studies, the U.S. Public Health Service in 1950 recommended community water fluoridation as a public health measure. The American Dental Association seconded that recommendation six months later. In the initial studies dating from 1945 conducted by the U.S. Public Health Service, the prevalence of caries decreased 48 percent to 70 percent among 12- to 14-year-olds who had lived in the four original fluoridated communities their entire lives. In other communities studied, the prevalence of caries decreased 45 percent to 94 percent (median 58 percent) among children who had been exposed to fluoridation for ten years. By the early 1980s, epidemiologic evidence indicated that the prevalence of dental caries was declining throughout the United States. ► Three national surveys completed between 1971 and 1987 showed that children demonstrated a continued decrease in caries prevalence.

▼

Three national surveys completed between 1971 and 1987 showed that children demonstrated a continued decrease in caries prevalence.

Today, 60 years after Grand Rapids led the way, 170 million people live in fluoridated communities in the United States, including an estimated 10 million who live in communities with water supplies that are naturally fluoridated at the optimum level (1 ppm). Another 30 to 40 million people are estimated to live without public water supplies, depending on such sources as drilled wells or natural springs. Despite conclusive proof that community water fluoridation at the accepted standard benefits oral health, with no known side effects, the remaining population of the United States live in communities without fluoridated water supplies. Only a few of the top 50 cities in the U.S. have yet to be fluoridated, including Portland (Oregon), San Antonio (Texas) and San Jose (California). Tucson, Arizona, voted to fluoridate in 1992, but as of early 2005 had not yet fluoridated, a case in point for how long it can take to fluoridate a community. San Diego and the surrounding counties, involving 100 water districts and nearly 18 million people, approved fluoridation in 2003 but allowed 30 months for it to take effect.

While the benefits of fluoridation to the public's health are incontrovertible and not at all controversial to scientists and public health professionals, the notion of community water fluoridation still sparks controversy among people who oppose any form of government intervention in private lives and who regard it as forced medication and a violation of personal freedom. Although opponents often base their counterclaims to fluoridation on quack science, masked by the twin complaints of safety and effectiveness, adverse publicity has succeeded in delaying community fluoridation. In 1980, for example, 41 fluoridation referenda were held in the U.S. but only eight were approved. In the period between 1977 and 1982, approximately 25 percent of fluoridation referenda passed. In both 2002 and 2004, 26 communities across the country voted in referenda for fluoridation, while in 2003, 14 communities voted for fluoridation. Most communities (91 percent) fluoridate administratively through local or state government.

► Fortunately, the furor caused by opponents of fluoridation has dissipated slowly in the past two decades, with the underlying science holding sway more and more. Since 1980, however, progress in fluoridating the water in communities with central water supplies has been disappointing. Only 11 states, the District of Columbia and Puerto Rico have passed laws that require fluoridation, usually only in communities of a certain size (California, Connecticut, Delaware, Georgia, Kentucky, Illinois, Minnesota, Nebraska, Nevada, Ohio, South Dakota). In the last great tumult, in California in 1995, opponents of fluoridation suffered a stinging defeat when the state legislature mandated fluoridation in communities with public water systems serving more than 10,000 households. Nonetheless, many opponents have persisted with legal challenges. Michigan, for example, changed the wording in its law and made fluoridation voluntary rather than mandatory. In the 30 years from 1954 to 1984, more than a dozen cases reached the U.S. Supreme Court. None of the cases were actually heard by the court;

▼

Fortunately, the furor caused by opponents of fluoridation has dissipated slowly in the past two decades, with the underlying science holding sway more and more.

they were dismissed either for lack of a substantial federal question or because they were simply not commented upon.

Long-range studies show conclusively that children who grow up from infancy until age six drinking fluoridated water are much less prone to dental caries and other oral diseases, perhaps for the rest of their lives. The United States led the way in harnessing fluoride as a natural preventive for dental caries and leads the way with the largest number of people in the world living in fluoridated communities. In 2002, more than 67 percent of the U.S. population who lived in communities with public water supply systems received fluoridated water. Still, much work remains to be done to ensure that the greatest possible number of people benefit from community water fluoridation. Because oral health impacts the quality of everyone's life, and because fluoridation can be shown to help keep students in school, learning, and workers at work, working, every community without water fluoridation should carefully consider the evidence. Overwhelmingly, the evidence shows that communities with fluoridated water supplies have reduced the prevalence of dental caries in their populations. ◻

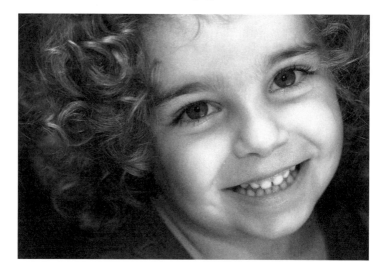

Vignette
Dental Sealants

Dental sealants are thin plastic coatings placed as liquid plastics on the pits and fissures of the chewing surfaces of teeth and then polymerized. While fluorides are most effective at preventing decay on the smooth surfaces of teeth, sealants effectively prevent decay on the chewing surfaces of teeth. Applying dental sealants is painless and noninvasive and does not require anesthesia or the cutting of tooth structure. Children aged six to eight and 12 to 14 years should be targeted for the procedure, just as the six-year and 12-year molars erupt. These molars are the most susceptible to decay.

The origins of dental sealants lie in the work of Dr. Michael Buonocore who, in 1955, discovered the properties required to bond resins to tooth enamel. The process involves applying a phosphoric acid solution to the tooth surface for 30 seconds, then rinsing and applying shortly afterward an acrylic resin on the same surface. Buonocore experimented first on extracted teeth and then on volunteers to determine the right amounts and adhesion times. His discovery first led to composite fillings for anterior tooth surfaces, especially fractured incisors, and then evolved into the preventive dentistry of fissure sealants. The application of fissure sealants, an effective method to prevent fissure caries in permanent molars, relies on the acid etching and bonding to enamel perfected first by Buonocore in 1955.

Currently, more than 85 percent of school-aged children lack dental sealants. The simple efficacy of fissure sealants in preventing fissure caries – people with sealants suffer six times less tooth decay – calls for their widespread application in young children. Effective school-based prevention programs should combine fluorides and sealants, to protect both the smooth and pitted surfaces of teeth. For children who live in communities without fluoridated water, an alternate approach would be to apply fluoride topically to the smooth tooth surfaces. Fluoride application is most preventive in children when first and second molars erupt, between the ages of six and eight and 12 and 14, respectively. As it happens, these are the precise times when the application of fissure sealant is also most preventive. Sealants, together with community water fluoridation, represent major milestones in preventive dentistry and improved oral health and promise to spare millions of children the discomforts of dental caries and gingivitis. ◻

Looking Ahead

Oral Diseases, Still a Neglected Epidemic

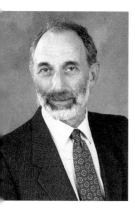

Dr. Myron Allukian, former director of Oral Health, Boston Public Health Commission.

Oral health must become a higher priority at the local, state and national levels if oral health disparities are to be improved and resolved. Dr. Myron Allukian, a retired director of oral health at the Boston Public Health Commission and a former president of the American Public Health Association, says, "Fluoridation and community-based prevention must be the foundation for better oral health." In 2000, the U.S. Surgeon General issued its first-ever *Report on Oral Health*, with a call to action that has yet to be realized. Among the report's recommendations, local and state health departments and every other level of the public health system are called upon to emphasize oral health to a much greater degree and to create dental health programs with properly trained staff to address a neglected epidemic.

Report on Oral Health by the U.S. Surgeon General

The major findings of the report are as follows:

1. Oral diseases and disorders in and of themselves affect health and well-being throughout life.

2. Safe and effective measures exist to prevent the most common dental diseases – dental caries and periodontal diseases.

3. Lifestyle behaviors that affect general health such as tobacco use, excessive alcohol use, and poor dietary choices affect oral and craniofacial health as well.

4. There are profound and consequential oral health disparities within the U.S. population.

5. More information is needed to improve America's oral health and eliminate health disparities.

6. The mouth reflects general health and wellness.

7. Oral diseases and conditions are associated with other health problems.

8. Scientific research is key to further reduction in the burden of diseases and disorders that affect the face, mouth and teeth.

Concerns for the Future

◆ Currently, at the federal level about a dozen oral health specialists work within the CDC and just a handful remain in the Health Resources Services Administration (HRSA), which once had 300. Just one oral health professional works at the Centers for Medicaid and Medicare, the largest health-related program in the federal government. The federal government could show a greater commitment to fighting oral diseases by boosting the number of oral health specialists in its key agencies.

◆ At the state level, 39 percent of states do not have full-time state oral health directors, and some states are eliminating them.

◆ In 2004, only 152 of the 160,000 practicing dentists in the U.S. were board-certified in public health. About 1,600 dentists work in public health roles, but only 600 have at least two years of advanced education. While a clinician may see 800 patients a year on average, public health dentists reach millions of people. Unfortunately, training in public health is perceived to diminish earnings potential, a perception that can be changed only if government at every level validates the work of public health dentists.

◆ Currently, only 2.2 percent of practicing dentists in the United States are African-American, as compared with a 12 percent share of the total population. Hispanics and Native Americans are similarly underrepresented, and this is cause for concern in lower-income communities.

◆ According to a Government Accounting Office (GAO) study in 1998, only 20 percent of children in Medicaid receive dental care, even though Medicaid includes dental services aimed specifically at children through the Early Periodic Screening Diagnosis and Treatment (EPSDT) Program. In the same vein, the oral component of the Children's Health Insurance Program (CHIP) needs to be upgraded. Meanwhile, in an unfortunate response to deficits, many states have eliminated dental care from adult Medicaid.

◆ Of people in the United States older than 40 years, 93 percent have not had an oral cancer exam in the past year. Oral cancers are more prevalent than cervical cancer, yet most women receive pap smears routinely.

- Of nursing home residents in the United States, 81 percent have not had an annual oral exam. For the 19 percent who did, the exam often comes only after the resident has been rushed by ambulance for emergency care.

- Currently, only about half of the United States population has some form of dental insurance. If a diabetic person presents with a leg ulcer, medical insurance would cover care, but if that same individual presents with a mouth ulcer, his care would not be covered without dental insurance.

- As a percentage of total health expenditures, dental service expenditures have decreased 28 percent, from 6.4 percent in 1970 to about 4.6 percent today.

The most vulnerable in the population are most at risk for oral diseases and suffer their worst effects. Studies show that up to 97 percent of homeless people need dental care; over half of Head Start children in some locations have had early childhood caries (ECC); almost half of abused children have orofacial trauma; and so on. Jonathan Kozol, the education critic and author of *Death at an Early Age*, winner of the National Book Award in 1968, and *Savage Inequalities*, a best-seller published in 1992, writes, ▶ "Bleeding gums, impacted teeth and rotting teeth are routine matters for the children I have interviewed in the South Bronx. Children get used to feeling constant pain. They go to sleep with it. They go to school with it. …Children live for months with pain that grown-ups would find unendurable."

Since 1997, with the introduction of the State Children's Health Insurance Program (SCHIP), nearly every state has begun to offer dental benefits to low-income children. In most cases, SCHIP affords both preventive and diagnostic care, providing a new vehicle to reach a large segment of the U.S. population previously underserved with dental care. In 2003, seven states had already exceeded Healthy People 2010 goals, while many others were quickly approaching the goals. By providing dental care to low-

▼

"Bleeding gums, impacted teeth and rotting teeth are routine matters for the children I have interviewed in the South Bronx. Children get used to feeling constant pain.…"

income people, usually for the first time, SCHIP saves growing numbers of children from unendurable pain. More important, SCHIP also provides families with peace of mind.

Public-Private Partnerships

Partnerships between the public sector and private industry can provide access to quality dental care for underserved children. One such approach is the Crest "Healthy Smiles 2010" campaign initiated by Procter & Gamble in 2001 with the backing of the American Dental Association, the Boys & Girls Clubs of America and the American Academy of Pediatric Dentistry. "Healthy Smiles 2010" aims to reach 50 million children this decade to alleviate the silent epidemic of tooth decay, the most common chronic child-hood disease. Tooth decay in children is five times more prevalent than asthma and seven times more prevalent than hay fever. Key initiatives in the campaign are "Give Kids a Smile" Day in February, the Crest First Grade Program, and Crest "Smile Shoppes," full-service dental clinics established in Boys & Girls Clubs in six U.S. cities. As well, more than 1,000 Boys & Girls Clubs throughout the country have become "Cavity-Free Zones" thanks to an oral health curriculum for children in grades K-3 set up in on-the-spot education centers in the clubs.

Perhaps most critical, Crest won the commitment of dental schools throughout the country to send dental students into schools in their communities to provide preventive treatment and oral health instruction to children, especially underserved and at-risk children.
► "Creating public-private partnerships can help affect change in the oral health of our country. These collective efforts can help educate both the public and health profes-sionals, as well as provide the health care services and oral care tools needed to help end the current disparity in our nation's oral health," said Dr. David Satcher who, as U.S. Surgeon General, oversaw the publication of the *Report on Oral Health* in 2000. The Crest "Healthy Smiles 2010" campaign distributes millions of toothpaste tubes and toothbrushes to children free of charge every year, and children learn how and when to brush their teeth, critical steps to good oral hygiene.

▼

"Creating public-private partner-ships can help affect change in the oral health of our country."

A Sealant Success Story

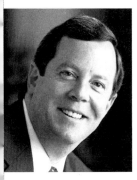

Dr. Edward M. Hundert

Another example of public-private partnerships is the Case Western sealant program in Cleveland, Ohio. The president of Case Western Reserve University, Dr. Edward M. Hundert, came from the medical school at the University of Rochester, where as dean, he focused on public health and eliminating disparities in care among ethnic groups. After he arrived at Case Western Reserve in 2002, Hundert moved quickly to involve students in Cleveland. His constant refrain has been to give students real-life experiences by helping the community. To this end, Case Western dental students currently apply sealant to the teeth of 15,000 second- and sixth-graders in the Cleveland Public Schools every year. "Our philosophy is that the external things we're doing are the things that will set our university apart," Hundert said.

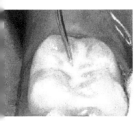

Applied dental sealant.

For now, the dental sealant program symbolizes most visibly Case Western's engagement with Cleveland and, for dental students, has become the high point of their year. "It's a wonderful thing on all sides," said Dr. James Lalumandier, the chairman of community dentistry. "In this country, 80 percent of dental disease is in 20 percent of the children, and these are the 20 percent. Students arrive at the medical school and dental school with a desire to help people, and if you get them into clinical work quickly, they don't lose that desire."

"When you sit down for the first time to use a probe in the mouth, it's a big moment," said Oliver Thuernagle, a student from Idaho. "I'm from a place where you don't lock the door when you go on vacation, and here I am at schools where you sign in and they check you for guns," Thuernagle said. "We saw children whose teeth had erupted only five months ago and were already rotten to the core. You refer them to someone who will take care of the cavities. But you wish you were there five months ago."

The Challenges Ahead

To address oral health needs, the number one priority of public health policymakers should be to extend community water fluoridation as widely as possible. As Dr. Allukian says, "Fluoridation is nature's way to prevent tooth decay." The second priority should be to make school-based dental sealant programs as widely available as possible to high-risk children whose first molars have fully erupted (ages six to eight) and again when second molars have erupted (ages 12 to 14). Children without deep crevices and who show no sign of tooth decay would not be deemed high-risk. Aside from good oral hygiene, which must be taught systematically in schools, these two measures – community water fluoridation and school-based dental sealant programs – would together, if fully implemented, address the neglected epidemic of oral disease. The most effective preventive measures, focused on school-aged children, require the full engagement of government in fostering public-private partnerships.

Government can engage by supporting the dental public health infrastructure. More minorities need to be recruited to careers in oral health, more local and state oral health directors need to be named and funded, and more public-private partnerships need to be cemented to provide care when it counts most, when first and second molars erupt. Successful sealant programs require follow-up a year later to be sure that the initial applications were done carefully. The Robert Wood Johnson Foundation, which announced a $19 million program to recruit minorities to careers in medicine and dentistry, could also fund outreach to minorities for public health training.

► Why shouldn't there be a national movement for community-based prevention? As Allukian says, "There's never been one and there should be." Mouth guards should be required for all contact sports. Every second-grader should receive sealants. Every community's water supply system should be fluoridated. Boston's fluoridation process took eight years and involved approvals from 33 separate communities, but thanks to Allukian's persistence, it got done. Everywhere he goes in Greater Boston, Allukian can take satisfaction from the fact that the teenagers he encounters won't suffer as in the past from oral diseases that cause debilitating pain.

A final word from Allukian: "Oral diseases are a neglected epidemic in our country, and the oral health disparities of the underserved are shameful. We need to reconnect the mouth to the rest of the body." ▫

▼

Why shouldn't there be a national movement for community-based prevention? As Allukian says, "There's never been one and there should be."

Photo credits

Page 167: Dentist examing a girl's teeth, © Peter Beck/CORBIS.

Page 168: Baltimore College of Dental Surgery, courtesy the National Museum of Dentistry.

Page 168: Dr. Chapin A. Harris, courtesy the National Library of Medicine.

Page 171: Hesi-Re, © Archivo Iconografico, S.A./CORBIS.

Page 171: Toothbrush drill, 1913, courtesy the National Library of Medicine.

Page 172: Miswak stick, © 2005 Reiner Lubge/Warhaftig Associates.

Page 172: Filling toothpaste tubes, © Bettmann/CORBIS.

Page 173: Dr. Charles C. Bass, courtesy of Rudolph Matas Medical Library of Tulane University.

Page 174: Coronal tooth decay, © Fotosearch, LLC.

Page 176: Drs. Black and McKay, courtesy of the CDC Public Health Image Library.

Page 178: Dr. H. Trendly Dean, courtesy of the CDC Public Health Image Library.

Page 178: Grand Rapids schoolchildren, courtesy of the National Institute of Dental and Craniofacial Research.

Page 181: Smiling child, © CORBIS.

Page 187: Dr. Edward M. Hundert, courtesy Case Western Reserve University.

Chapter 10

Addiction

Looking Back

Addiction – whether to tobacco, alcohol or prescription or illicit drugs – does not discriminate on the basis of social class, education, economic level or geography. Many families in the United States and across the world deal privately with some form of addiction as part of their daily lives.

▶ As many people know too well, addictions transcend the user and can have negative physical and emotional effects on family, friends and the community.

Nicotine addiction, caused by tobacco use, adversely affects the health of cigarette smokers and those around them through second-hand smoke, leading to exacerbation of asthma and otitis media (ear infections) in children. Alcohol addiction causes extensive liver damage and organ system failure and creates mental and physical challenges for those around alcoholics. The deadly combination of drinking and driving causes injury and death for hundreds of innocent victims each year. Substance abuse of illegal psychoactive drugs – marijuana, cocaine, LSD and opiates, among other mood-altering drugs – leads users to crimes such as burglary and prostitution to support a habit and can further lead to wholesale wars between rival drug-dealing gangs.

The challenge for public health in changing addictive behavior is further complicated by shifting public attitudes toward drug and alcohol use and by the impact of advertising and peer pressure. It is not unusual for one generation to come of age without direct experience of an addiction that an older generation knows too well. For example, during the 1800s opiates and cocaine were both thought to have beneficial health effects for users. They seemed palliative, easing symptoms of ill health; the public viewed them positively, despite their addictive properties, and began using them widely. In fact, when the soft drink Coca-Cola was invented in the late

▼

As many people know too well, addictions transcend the user and can have negative physical and emotional effects on family, friends and the community.

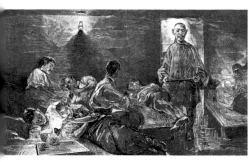

An opium den in New York, 1881.

1880s, many thought that the coca plant was one of its original ingredients.

By the early to mid-1900s, however, the public's view of psychoactive drugs changed. Addictive properties of the drugs were now frowned upon, and the public began to clamor for stricter controls. Alcohol, too, was viewed negatively by a public acutely aware of its addictive properties, and in 1919, under the leadership of Carrie Nation, the Temperance Movement achieved the prohibition of alcohol

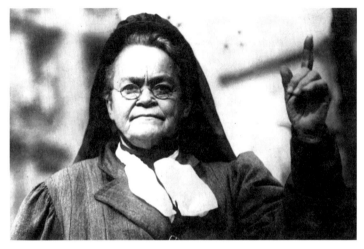

Prohibitionist Carrie Nation

through the 18th Amendment to the U.S. Constitution's Bill of Rights (the 21st Amendment reversed Prohibition in 1933). ► After World War II and especially in the 1960s and the 1970s, the public became more tolerant of such psychoactive drugs as marijuana, not fully aware that marijuana often opens doors for users to try much more addictive and debilitating drugs, such as cocaine. The heavily publicized drug excesses of the last decades of the 20th century, however, have shifted public opinion in the early 21st century back toward intolerance.

How do addicts differ from occasional or even frequent users of the same substances? What makes an addict? The American Psychiatric Association defines someone with an addiction as meeting at least three of five criteria. The first is tolerance, the need for markedly increased amounts of the substance to achieve the desired effect or, with continued use of the same amount, a markedly diminished effect. The second is withdrawal. When the user stops taking the

▼

...the public became more tolerant of such psychoactive drugs as marijuana, not fully aware that marijuana often opens doors for users to try much more addictive and debilitating drugs, such as cocaine.

substance for a time, uncomfortable or dangerous symptoms result. For example, tobacco users experience irritability, lack of concentration, fatigue and hunger when they go without nicotine. The third is loss of control, when a user takes more of a substance over a longer period of time than was intended. Again, using tobacco as an example, 70 percent of smokers would like to quit, but less than half actually do. The fourth is preoccupation, leading a user to spend a great deal of time obtaining and using a substance or recovering from the effects. ► The final criterion is continuation despite adverse consequences, which finds users sacrificing the full dimensions of life – social, occupational and recreational – to satisfy cravings for the substance.

▼

...which finds users sacrificing the full dimensions of life – social, occupational and recreational – to satisfy cravings for the substance.

What gives substances their addictive properties? Researchers have studied the effects of psychoactive drugs on the brain for decades. Drugs cause short-term surges in dopamine and other brain messengers that signal pleasure or reward. Pleasure and reward lead to cravings that become fixed in memory, making it difficult for a user to

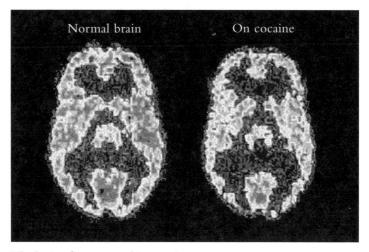

The brain of a person taking cocaine.

resist the lure. Meanwhile, as the brain's pleasure circuits adapt to the deluge of short-term surges, they become desensitized and can suffer withdrawal once the binge is over. A perplexing aspect of addiction – that drugs usually don't induce as much pleasure after prolonged use – is due, in part, to the phenomenon of tolerance. Despite the reduced pleasure, addicts keep taking their drug of choice even as they consciously try to abstain. Positron emission tomography (PET) scans show that parts of the nervous system are unusually active when people experience cravings. Cravings can be provoked by the slightest stimulation – the whiff of a remembered odor, the flashback of a place, a remembered pleasurable activity or piece of drug paraphernalia. An addict's cravings are awakened by stimuli in the same way Pavlov's dogs salivated. Relapses, the core clinical problem of addiction, are frequent, even years after the last dose. The brain's demand for the pleasure "fix" usually overcomes any rational thoughts to the contrary.

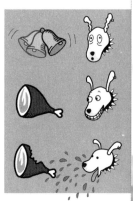

Pavlov's dog.

Before researchers came to understand addiction more fully, "inebriety" was viewed by the health professions as a functional disease thought to be triggered by an underlying mental disturbance. An individual could inherit or acquire a weakened, nervous constitution and be more susceptible to addictive behavior than another individual viewed as neurologically normal. Rather than a vice, as the general public might view it, the public health community viewed addictive behavior as a disease that affected susceptible people for whom there were risk factors, environmental triggers and potentially successful treatments if identified early.

Purified cocaine became commercially available in this country in 1884, and its use spread rapidly. Cocaine affects the central nervous system powerfully, creating a sense of euphoria. The pharmaceutical company Parke-Davis supplied cocaine in 15 forms, from coca cigarettes to cocaine for injection to cocaine for sniffing, all of which were legal at the time. Marijuana, on the other hand, entered the U.S. through Mexico during a time of drug intolerance in the 1920s and spread more slowly. Not until the public mood shifted once again toward drug tolerance in the 1960s did marijuana become widely used.

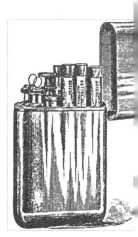

An 1894 emergency kit, readily available to the public, carried cocaine, morphine, atropine and strychnine.

It is estimated that more than half of all smokers suffer serious health consequences from tobacco addiction – foremost, premature death from lung cancer – and innocent bystanders also suffer health consequences from exposure to secondhand smoke, known as environmental tobacco smoke (ETS). The legislative accomplishments of cities and towns in outlawing smoking in public places, a public health phenomenon of the 1990s and continuing into the present, offer a vivid contrast to the laissez faire attitude of earlier generations toward this health hazard.

Alcohol abuse and dependence continue to be major health problems in the United States. Unlike other drugs, alcohol is legal, advertised widely and sold in the retail market. Alcohol finds uses in religious ceremonies, happy events such as weddings, and sad gatherings such as wakes; it is often a gift given to commemorate special occasions. Nonetheless, nearly 14 million Americans – one in 13 adults – are either alcoholics or abuse alcohol heavily. Alcohol abuse also occurs among teenagers who may indulge in the extremely dangerous habit of binge-drinking by consuming, within several hours, more than five alcoholic drinks at one sitting. The body metabolizes alcohol at approximately one drink per hour, so an amount that exceeds that causes intoxication and can lead to potential complications.

In 2000, more than 18,500 deaths in the United States resulted from alcohol abuse. ► In 1990, the economic costs were estimated to exceed $98 billion, and alcohol involvement was implicated in nearly half of all traffic crash deaths. In 1988, alcohol-related deaths numbered 107,800, or five percent of the total mortality in the United States. One-fifth of these deaths were directly attributable to alcohol abuse and dependence – involving liver cirrhosis, for example. The remaining four-fifths were alcohol-related, representing 35 percent of all accidental fall fatalities; 28 percent of all suicides; 45 percent of all accidental fire fatalities; 38 percent of all accidental drownings; and 50 percent of all deaths due to cancers of the lip, oral cavity, pharynx and esophagus. Clearly, the costs of alcohol abuse, whether direct or indirect, are staggering.

Alcoholism, also known as alcohol dependence, is a chronic, progressive and potentially fatal disease. Many more Americans are addicted to alcohol than to illicit drugs. Researchers at the University of Colorado Health Sciences Center in Denver have identified 41 genes that help determine whether a person becomes an alcoholic. Alcoholics display the following characteristics:

◆ Drinking excessive amounts frequently.

◆ A strong need or compulsion to drink.

◆ Inability to limit one's drinking on any given occasion.

▼

In 1990, the economic costs were estimated to exceed $98 billion, and alcohol involvement was implicated in nearly half of all traffic crash deaths.

◆ Inability to curb drinking despite medical, psychological or social complications.

◆ Increased tolerance to alcohol.

◆ Withdrawal symptoms, such as nausea, sweating, anxiety and shaking after stopping drinking.

Alcohol is classified as a depressive drug because it causes relaxation, sedation, and if a sufficient quantity is consumed, coma and even death. Among the major health problems that result from alcohol abuse are damage to the digestive system, including stomach irritation, gastritis and ulcers and cirrhosis of the liver, which results from alcohol decreasing the liver's ability to metabolize fat. Other health problems include enlargement of the heart leading to coronary heart disease, high blood pressure, and psychiatric problems that include irritability, hyperactivity, paranoia and hallucinations. ▶ Women who drink alcohol during pregnancy run the risk of miscarriages and infant death, and pregnant women who are alcoholics run the risk of delivering infants with fetal alcohol syndrome.

Women have often been outliers with regard to substance abuse. Historically, women were much less likely to use tobacco, viewing it as masculine, and local ordinances often forbade bars and liquor stores from selling alcohol to women. During the Victorian era, society strove to preserve an image of purity in women. Women who used and abused alcohol, in saloons or elsewhere, were commonly viewed as prostitutes. In fact, divorce law in many jurisdictions allowed "intemperance" on the part of the wife to be grounds for divorce. Today, women are nearly as likely as men to smoke, and alcohol abuse knows no gender. The fact that more women than men die from cardiovascular disease, a common complication of smoking, shows that women have equalized the playing field of substance abuse.

The late 1800s in America gave rise to progressivism, a political movement seeking to redress the wrongs and excesses of industrial capitalist society. Progressivism in turn gave rise to the Temperance Movement, led by women whose goal was to save their husbands from alcohol abuse. The Temperance Movement reached its pinnacle in 1919 when the 18th Amendment to the Bill of Rights passed, outlawing the distribution and sale of liquor. A prominent

▼

Women who drink alcohol during pregnancy run the risk of miscarriages and infant death.

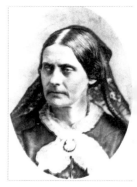

Susan B. Anthony

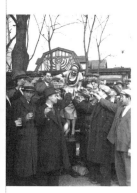

*Prohibition ends,
April 1933.*

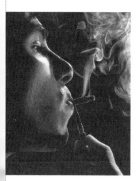

*Young man smoking
marijuana.*

leader of the Temperance Movement, Susan B. Anthony, also led the fight for women's suffrage, and while she did not live to vote herself, her life's work achieved its goal in 1920 when the 19th Amendment, giving women the right to vote, quickly followed Prohibition. It was no coincidence that the amendments introducing Prohibition and women's suffrage passed in consecutive years; women who wanted to save men from the ravages of drink and chauvinism were energized enough to influence the nation's politics. Although Prohibition had at its core the goal of eliminating alcohol abuse in men and saving families, its enforcement became such a problem that the 21st Amendment was passed in 1933, repealing Prohibition and ending the brief age of the "speakeasy."

In the 1960s, when the Haight Ashbury district of San Francisco gave rise to a psychedelic movement, the word "hippie" came to define a generation. This restless, resistant generation, raised in relative affluence by fathers who were World War II veterans and mothers who stayed at home, made its presence felt in anti-war politics. Ironically, as the Johnson administration launched a far-reaching, ambitious War Against Poverty to right economic disparities in American society, the Vietnam War tore the generations apart. "Never trust anyone over 30" became a mantra. One of many dividing lines was tolerance for psychotropic drugs. While alcoholic, nicotine-addicted World War II veterans filled Veterans Administration hospitals, many Vietnam War veterans returning from an unpopular war to a tumultuous society continued to use marijuana, hashish and other psychotropic drugs that had been readily available in Vietnam. This generation had a high tolerance for illicit drugs and suffered from their addictive properties. The public health community, prominent in the ranks of those fighting the War Against Poverty, was late in recognizing the public health implications of excessive drug use.

To gain traction against addiction, the public health community often has to overcome public misperceptions – the hippie celebration of psychotropic drugs is an example – and to sway government to intervene to regulate health hazards. The federal government and the cumbersome legislative machinery of Congress often enter the fray last. Effective legislation usually takes place first at the state and local level, and Congress benefits from being able to observe local activism at its best. ► The National Center on Addiction and Substance Abuse (CASA) at Columbia University has found that children who reach the age of 21 without smoking, using illegal drugs or abusing alcohol are virtually certain never to do so. In 1984, Congress passed legislation denying highway funds to states unless they mandated a minimum legal drinking age of 21. Most states have also outlawed tobacco sales to teens under 18; in some states, new laws have raised that age to 19. While states vary in sentencing guidelines for those convicted of the sale and distribution of illicit drugs, legal penalties have generally toughened over time. In combating the health hazards of addictive substances, the public health community has, in the end, found government to be a willing and necessary ally. ▫

▼

...children who reach the age of 21 without smoking, using illegal drugs or abusing alcohol are virtually certain never to do so.

Case Study

Tobacco

Dr. Julie Gerberding, the director of the Centers for Disease Control and Prevention (CDC) in Atlanta, wrote in a recent report: "In the four decades following the release of the first Surgeon General's *Report on Smoking and Health*, we have seen dramatic progress in reducing tobacco use in this country. Adult-smoking rates have been cut nearly in half between 1965 and 2001, from 42.4 percent to 22.8 percent, and per-capita consumption of tobacco products has fallen more than half, from 4,345 cigarettes in 1963 to 1,979 cigarettes in 2002. But, tragically, smoking remains the leading preventable cause of death and disease in the United States, claiming the lives of more than 440,000 Americans each year. The good news is that we know what works to curb tobacco use: comprehensive programs combining school, health care, community, media and policy efforts."

In 2001, 46.2 million adults in the United States were current smokers and an estimated 8.6 million people had serious smoking-related illness. Tobacco's enormous toll on the health of the public causes 4.8 million deaths world-wide. The World Health Organization projects that by the year 2030, the use of tobacco will kill 10 million people annually, including seven million in developing countries. Just as in the United States, tobacco use will become the rest of the world's leading cause of preventable death.

▶   Excluding adult deaths from exposure to secondhand smoke, adult males and females in the United States lose an average of 13.2 and 14.5 years of life, respectively, if they smoke. Among adults, between 1995 and 1999, most deaths caused by tobacco use were from lung cancer (124,813), ischemic heart disease (81,976) and chronic airway obstruction (64,735). Estimates show that smoking causes $82 billion in lost productivity and $75 billion in excess medical expenditures annually. The costs are estimated to be about $4,391 per smoker per year. Each cigarette pack sold in the U.S. costs the nation an estimated $7.18 in medical care costs and lost productivity.

Joseph A. Califano, Jr., director of the National Center on Addiction and Substance Abuse, observes, "Cigarette

▼

...adult males and females in the United States lose an average of 13.2 and 14.5 years of life, respectively, if they smoke.

smoking is Public Health Enemy Number One in the United States. People who smoke are committing slow-motion suicide. The economic cost of smoking in health care, fires, accidents and lost productivity tops $150 billion. The cost in grief and sadness for the children and families of the victims is beyond calculation."

▶   Every day, more than 4,000 young people try cigarettes for the first time. From 2000 to 2003, tobacco use among high school students declined significantly, from 34.5 percent to 28.4 percent, continuing a downward national trend since 1997. There were no significant declines among middle school students, however.

The demographics of tobacco use have been changing. For the first time, smoking prevalence among black men is similar to that among white men. During the period 1965–2001, smoking declined faster for non-Hispanic blacks aged 18 years and older than for non-Hispanic whites of the same age. In 2001, among racial and ethnic groups, smoking prevalence was highest among American Indians/Alaska Natives (32.7 percent) and lowest among Hispanics (16.7 percent) and Asians (12.4 percent). In 2002, the prevalence of smoking in the United States stood at 25.5 percent among men and 21.5 percent among women, down from the peaks of 57 percent among men in 1955 and 34 percent among women in 1965. The decline in rates of smoking reached a plateau in 1990 that has persisted, however.

In 2001, 41 percent of smokers stopped smoking for at least one day because they wanted to quit.   ▶   The success rate is daunting, however – less than five percent of smokers who quit for one day are able to do so for three to 12 months.

Smoking and mental illness are closely linked. Smoking rates have been reported to be over 80 percent among people who have schizophrenia, 50 percent to 60 percent among people with depression, 55 percent to 80 percent among those who have alcoholism, and 50 percent to 66 percent among those who have other substance-abuse problems. In one study, smokers with coexisting psychiatric or substance-abuse disorders were estimated to account for 44 percent of all cigarettes smoked in the United States. This percentage reflects both the high prevalence of smoking in connection with these conditions and the fact that patients with these disorders are likely to be very heavy smokers.

▼

Every day, more than 4,000 young people try cigarettes for the first time.

▼

The success rate is daunting, however – less than five percent of smokers who quit for one day are able to do so for three to 12 months.

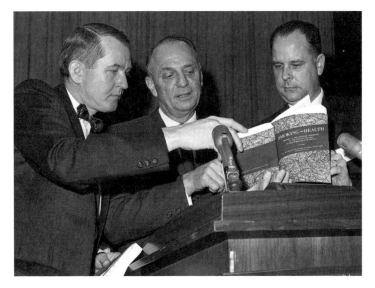

In 1964, looking over the Surgeon General's Report on Smoking and Health are (left to right): Dr. James Hundley, Dr. Luther L. Terry and Dr. Eugene H. Guthrie, all members of the Advisory Committee.

On January 11, 1964, Luther L. Terry, Surgeon General of the U.S. Public Health Service, released the report of the *Surgeon General's Advisory Committee on Smoking and Health*, commonly known as the first *Surgeon General's Report on Smoking and Health*. This landmark document was America's first widely publicized official recognition that cigarette smoking causes cancer and other serious diseases. Spurred to action by the report, Congress enacted in 1965 the Federal Cigarette Labeling and Advertising Act, requiring warning labels on cigarette packs. In 1969, Congress passed the Public Health Cigarette Smoking Act, strengthening the warning label to read "Warning: The Surgeon General has determined that cigarette smoking is dangerous to your health." This is the label that is still in effect. Starting in 1971, federal laws enacted by Congress prohibited cigarette advertising on broadcast television and radio. On January 11, 1978, the 14th anniversary of the first *Surgeon General's Report on Smoking and Health,* Secretary of Health, Education, and Welfare Joseph A. Califano, Jr. publicly declared a war on smoking.

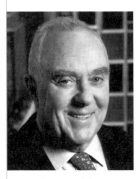

Joseph A. Califano, Jr.

Tobacco companies, consummate marketers of a product that depends on nicotine addiction for continued business, quickly found ways to combat the first Surgeon General's Report and a suddenly activist Congress. Since much of the work of creating smoke-free environments happens at the state and local levels, tobacco companies used their lobbying muscle and campaign donations to enlist the support of influential state legislators to keep anti-smoking legislation at bay. The preferred approach over the years has been to bottle up proposed legislation in committee, and tobacco companies have won those battles surprisingly often.

The terrain for anti-tobacco efforts changed significantly in 1999 with the Master Settlement Agreement (MSA) negotiated between the attorneys general of 46 states and five territories and the major tobacco companies. The attorneys general, led by Mississippi, signed a $206 billion agreement with tobacco companies to settle Medicaid lawsuits that had been filed to recover the high medical costs associated with treating terminal illnesses caused by smoking. Although $206 billion has now been completely distributed to the states, in varying amounts, the overall percentage of the settlement money dedicated to fighting tobacco addiction and, thus, helping reduce the associated Medicaid costs, has been surprisingly low. Instead, many states have chosen to balance their budgets with the windfall.

Recent developments in combating tobacco addiction include therapeutic agents, such as patches and gum, that are sold over the counter in drugstores. Therapeutics also include prescription antidepressants for patients with the co-morbidity of depression. ► Over the last decade, campaigns to reduce and prevent the prevalence of smoking among youth have mushroomed in states. Many of these programs take place in schools and in organizations serving youth such as Boys and Girls Clubs, led by local and state health departments. One such program is the Truth@ campaign, developed by the American Legacy Foundation. Truth@ is a hard-hitting advertising, grassroots and Internet program designed to prevent youth smoking; public health experts credit Truth@ for increasing anti-tobacco attitudes among young people, making it less likely that they will smoke.

The primary driver of the anti-smoking message comes through health education at the local level, assisted by a growing movement to eliminate smoking in the work-

▼

Over the last decade, campaigns to reduce and prevent the prevalence of smoking among youth have mushroomed in states.

place and other public facilities. These anti-smoking measures strengthen the message in campaigns aimed at youth.

► They also reinforce the message that environmental tobacco smoke (secondhand smoke) can be as deadly for innocent bystanders as for smokers themselves. While restaurant trade associations joined forces with tobacco companies to fight smoking restrictions at every turn, restaurants and bars have learned that smoking restrictions in fact help build business. In 2002, when New York City outlawed smoking in bars and taverns, tavern owners led a public outcry that helped contribute to a sharp drop in Mayor Michael Bloomberg's popularity. The mayor would not be swayed, however, stating that the decision was right and good for the public's health. With time, the outcry has dissipated and taverns have found that customers continue to sidle up to the bar. ◻

▼

They also reinforce the message that environmental tobacco smoke (secondhand smoke) can be as deadly for innocent bystanders as for smokers themselves.

Vignette

Mothers Against Drunk Driving (MADD)

Mothers Against Drunk Driving (MADD) was founded in 1980 at
a steak house in Sacramento, California, by a group of mothers who
were enraged that a repeat drunk-driving offender had killed Candace
Lightner's 13-year-old daughter, Cari. Two days before Cari's death,
the offender had been released on bail for a hit-and-run drunk-driving
crash, after having been convicted for two previous drunk-driving
crashes and a third that had been plea-bargained to "reckless accident."
When Cari died, the offender carried a valid California driver's
license, and the group of women rallying around Candace Lightner
vowed to organize to prevent drunk driving. MADD originally stood
for "Mothers Against Drunk Drivers," but in 1984 MADD changed
"Drivers" to "Driving."

Meanwhile, across the country in Maryland in 1979, Cindi Lamb's
five-and-a-half-month-old daughter Laura became one the world's
youngest quadriplegics when a repeat drunk driver traveling at 120
mph caused a head-on crash. Cindi Lamb and her friends began to
wage a war against drunk driving in Maryland. When the publicity
generated by Candace Lightner's group in California reached Cindi
Lamb the next year, the two groups joined forces. By 1981, MADD
had 11 chapters in four states.

What empowered MADD to grow? According to figures for 2000
from the National Highway Traffic Safety Administration (NHTSA),
three of every ten North Americans will be affected, at some point in
their lives, by an alcohol-related traffic crash. In 1999, roughly 17 percent of all drivers involved in fatal crashes were intoxicated at the time
of their crash. For every age from six through 33, traffic crashes are the
single greatest cause of death, and about 45 percent of these fatalities
are in alcohol-related crashes. In 2000, when 16,653 people were
killed in alcohol-related traffic crashes in the United States, these
fatalities reflected an increase for the first time in five years.

Examples of why MADD's mission resonates with people are legion.
One particularly horrific example was a bus crash in Carrollton,
Kentucky, on May 14, 1988. That day, a drunk driver in a pickup truck
drove the wrong way on I-71 and crashed head-on into a schoolbus
full of children, teens and chaperones who were heading home from
a church outing at an amusement park in Cincinnati. Flames killed 24
young people and three adults and injured 30 others. The driver of the
pickup, a repeat drunk-driving offender, survived. Just a few terrible

moments shattered the lives of 57 families and sent an entire community into shock.

In 1982, just two years after MADD organized at the steak house in Sacramento, President Ronald Reagan invited MADD to serve on the Presidential Task Force on drunk driving. By the end of that year, the organization had grown to 100 chapters. MADD's first national advocacy success, helping Congress enact a law that established the first National Drunk and Drugged Driving Awareness Week, came that December. In 1983, the organization opened national headquarters in Hurst, Texas, and became the subject of a made-for-television movie broadcast by NBC. The media attention helped open many more chapters. In 1984, with a strong push from MADD, Congress passed the federal "21" minimum legal drinking-age law, and MADD opened a chapter in Canada, the first of many international chapters.

Among the many services provided by MADD, victims' support and training are foremost. MADD chapters offer Victim Assistance Institutes to train volunteers to support victims of drunk driving and to serve as their advocates in the criminal justice system. In 1987, MADD established a national toll-free hotline to offer support to victims. After filing an amicus brief with the U.S. Supreme Court in 1987 defending the federal "21" law, which was upheld by the court,

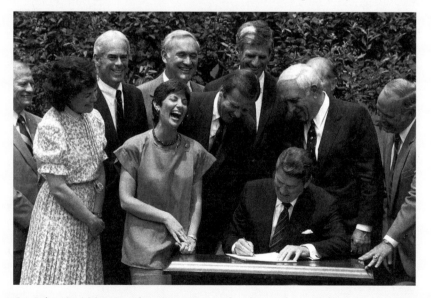

On July 17, 1984, President Reagan signs legislation that will force states to choose between a 21-year-old drinking age or a loss of federal aid. First row, left to right: Transportation Secretary Elizabeth Dole; Candy Lightner, founder of Mothers Against Drunk Driving (MADD). Second row, l. to r.: Rep. John Porter R-IL; Gov. Thomas Kean of NJ; Sen. Frank Lautenberg, D-NJ; and Rep. Norman Lent, R-NY. Third row, l. to r.: Rep. Gene Snyder, R-KY; and Sen. John Danforth (R-MO).

MADD pushed states to come on board with that law. By 1988, all states had passed laws establishing 21 as the legal minimum drinking age.

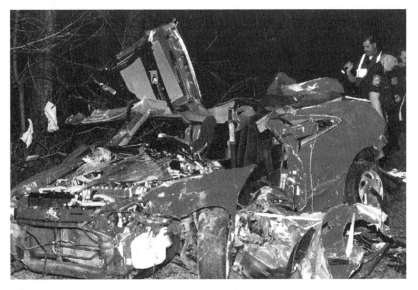

Wrecked car in which three teenagers died. All three had been drinking.

In 1990, MADD filed another amicus brief with the U.S. Supreme Court, this time defending the constitutionality of sobriety check-points. When the court ruled in favor of the checkpoints, MADD established the week of July Fourth as National Sobriety Checkpoint Week. Over the ensuing years, MADD worked with states to change sobriety laws to reflect a standard 0.08 blood alcohol content, down from 0.10 and a significant change. In 1994, NHTSA released figures showing that alcohol-related traffic deaths had dropped to a 30-year low during the previous year and credited MADD and tougher laws with making the difference. Unfortunately, that decline has not continued. In 1999, the MADD National Board of Directors voted unanimously to change the organization's mission statement to include the prevention of underage drinking. That same year, with the addition of two chapters in North Dakota, MADD was represented in all 50 states.

In becoming one of the most successful advocacy organizations in the world, Mothers Against Drunk Driving showed how a group of brokenhearted mothers, assembled loosely at first but fueled by outrage, could empower national change. With more than three million members and supporters, MADD today is the largest crime-victims' assistance organization in the world. ▫

Looking Ahead
Fighting Addiction in Young Women

Research shows that people who become addicted to any substance before the age of 21 have less of a chance of being able to break their addictive behavior. For reasons that are becoming clear through studies now under way, girls are more susceptible to addiction than boys.   ► Girls take up smoking, drugs and alcohol for different reasons than boys and become more vulnerable to long-lasting addiction. The challenge for the public health community, therefore, is to employ successful strategies aimed at youth, and especially girls, to prevent substance abuse in the first place. Effective

▼

Girls take up smoking, drugs and alcohol for different reasons than boys and become more vulnerable to long-lasting addiction.

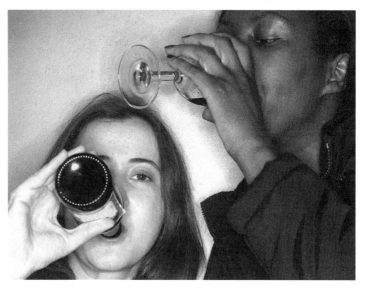

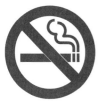

health education in the home, schools and community, supported by messages in the media, needs to reach children as early as possible in their preteens to prevent addictive behavior.

As Joseph Califano of the National Center on Addiction and Substance Abuse points out, "The issue of substance abuse and addiction – whether the substance is tobacco, alcohol, illicit or prescription drugs – is all about kids. A child who gets through age 21 without smoking, using drugs or abusing alcohol is virtually certain never to do so."

The National Center on Addiction and Substance Abuse at Columbia University in New York City, known as CASA, was founded in 1992. CASA calls for a nationwide overhaul in prevention and treatment programs serving youth, especially girls. Puberty is a time of higher risk for girls than boys, with girls who experience early puberty at significantly higher risk for using substances sooner, more often and in greater quantities than later-maturing peers. Girls are more likely than boys to be enticed into trying illicit substances in private settings by female acquaintances, female relatives or a boyfriend and are less likely to be asked for proof of age when buying cigarettes. Girls are also more likely than boys to be depressed, to have eating disorders, and to have a history of sexual or physical abuse, all of which increase the risk for substance abuse. Girls are more likely than boys to use alcohol and drugs to improve their mood, enhance sex and reduce inhibitions. As girls mature and become women, they are far less likely to beat their addictions than are men. They get hooked faster and suffer the consequences sooner than boys and young men.

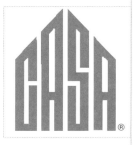

The National Center on Addiction and Substance Abuse logo.

Why should this be? It starts in the advertising and promotion of tobacco, with cigarette manufacturers knowingly targeting young girls. One-size-fits–all prevention efforts are partly to blame as well. Unisex approaches to prevention as well as treatment ignore the unique characteristics of substance abuse in young females and fail to influence millions. Physiological differences between the sexes also play a role. On average, the impact of one drink of alcohol for a woman has the impact of two drinks for a man.

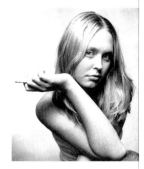

Advertising has promoted the "glamour" of smoking.

School-related transitions, from elementary to middle to high school and then to college, are risky times for girls. Parents, teachers and school counselors can make a difference in young girls' lives by encouraging them to talk about their anxieties and by validating their feelings of vulnerability. Furthermore, frequent changes in homes and neighborhoods increase the risk of substance abuse more for girls than for boys. Transitions unique to females, such as a girl's initial use of birth control or pregnancy, present key opportunities for intervention that are often missed. Because female substance use sinks more quickly and dangerously into abuse and addiction than does male substance use, timely and sensitive intervention is essential. Intervention should target all girls and young women who are going through key life transitions and also those known to be at high risk, either because of eating disorders, depression, or physical or sexual abuse. About 17 percent of high school girls report being abused physically, and 12 percent report being abused sexually, and these girls are at special risk for abusing substances earlier, more often and in greater quantities. Girls whose parents are known substance abusers are also at special risk.

In the United States today, more than 4.4 million women are alcoholics or abusers of alcohol, more than two million use illegal drugs, and more than 31 million smoke. In high schools, 27.7 percent of girls currently smoke, 45 percent drink alcohol, 26.4 percent binge drink, and 20 percent use marijuana. About 3.7 percent use cocaine and 4.2 percent use inhalants. Younger girls have been smoking and drinking as much as boys and are catching up in the use of illicit drugs. ▶ Girls initiate substance use nearly as early as boys but suffer consequences beyond those of boys.

▼

Girls initiate substance use nearly as early as boys but suffer consequences beyond those of boys.

About 34.5 percent of high school girls report regular feelings of sadness and hopelessness compared with 21.6 percent of boys. A strong link exists between feelings of depression and smoking, drinking or using drugs. Among high school girls who smoke and drink, those who report feeling depressed clearly outnumber those who have never smoked (47 percent vs. 25.3 percent) or drank alcohol (38.7 percent vs. 20 percent). Those who use marijuana are also likelier to report feeling sad or hopeless than those who have never used marijuana (42.9 percent vs. 29.7 percent). High school girls are more likely than boys to consider suicide (23.6 percent vs. 14.2 percent) and to attempt suicide (11.2 percent vs. 6.2 percent), and high school girls who smoke and drink are more than twice as likely to consider or attempt suicide than girls who have never smoked (37.7 percent vs. 14.4 percent) or drank (27.4 percent vs. 11.2 percent). The equivalent figures for marijuana are 34.5 percent vs. 19.5 percent.

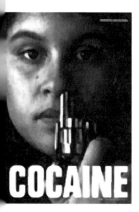

Poster from the Partnership for a Drug-Free America.

How can the public health community deal with these alarming statistics? Education, prevention, early diagnosis and treatment, the essential elements of any public health strategy, are increasingly being applied to substance abuse and addiction issues. Establishing awareness in the community can lead to the first line of defense, which are conversations that need to take place in the home. Most girls who have conversations with their parents about substance abuse say the conversations make them less likely to smoke, drink or use drugs. CASA research has consistently found that the more often children eat dinner with their parents, the less likely they are to smoke, drink or use drugs. As a result, CASA created an annual "Family Day" in 2001 to promote the idea that regular family time is a means to reduce substance abuse among children and teens. "Family Day" has since become a nationwide effort, held on the fourth Monday of September every year.

Health professionals must also be alert to signs of trouble. ▶ Pediatricians, family physicians, obstetricians/gynecologists, and dentists can all detect signs of substance abuse or eating disorders during routine checkups. They should screen young women for substance use and encourage treatment for those who seem to be in need. Clergy can also play a significant role. Since girls tend to be more religious than boys and hold more favorable opinions of religion, spirituality and religion can play protective roles with young women. The more frequently girls attend religious services, the less likely they are to smoke, drink, binge drink or use drugs.

▼

Pediatricians, family physicians, obstetricians/ gynecologists, and dentists can all detect signs of substance abuse or eating disorders during routine checkups.

As always in public health, messages about healthier outcomes must prompt individuals to change their behavior. Public health succeeds when individuals take responsibility for their own good health and encourage those around them to do the same. The cure for addiction comes when individuals change their behavior. Public health can recognize the extent of the problem, educate those at risk about the risks and provide assistance to those addicted, but it is the individual who, in the end, must rise to the challenge and overcome the addiction. While the public health community, friends and family members provide crucial support for changing behavior, it is the individual addict who must overcome the addiction. ▫

Photo credits

Page 191: Opium den, © CORBIS.

Page 192: Prohibitionist Carrie Nation, © Bettmann/CORBIS.

Page 193: Brain scan of cocaine user, courtesy The National Institute on Drug Abuse.

Page 194: Pavlov's dog illustration, courtesy www.Nobelprize.org, © 2005 The Nobel Foundation.

Page 196: Susan B. Anthony, © Bettmann/CORBIS.

Page 197: Prohibition ends, © Bettmann/CORBIS.

Page 197: Young man smoking marijuana, © Robert Essel NYC/CORBIS.

Page 201: Surgeon General's Report, © Bettmann/CORBIS.

Page 205: President Reagan signing drinking-age law, © Bettmann/CORBIS.

Page 206: Car wreck, courtesy of the CDC Public Health Image Library.

Page 207: Two women drinking, © Gary Houlder/CORBIS.

Page 208: Logo for CASA, courtesy The National Center on Addiction and Substance Abuse at Columbia University.

Page 208: Glamour shot of model smoking, © Chris Jones/CORBIS.

Page 209: Cocaine poster, public service announcements provided courtesy of the Partnership for Drug-Free America®.

Chapter 11

U.S. Public Health Infrastructure

Looking Back

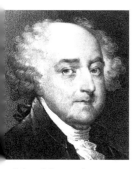

John Adams, the second president of the United States.

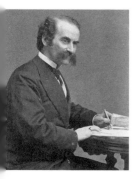

First supervising surgeon John Maynard Woodworth.

Public health has been an important concern in the United States dating back to the framers of the Constitution, who envisioned protection and promotion of public health among the federal government's responsibilities. On July 16, 1798, President John Adams signed a bill into law that provided for the care and relief of sick and injured merchant seamen in American ports. The earliest marine hospitals were located along the East Coast, with Boston as the site of the first such facility. They were established later along inland waterways, the Great Lakes, and the Gulf and Pacific Coasts. In 1870, reorganization converted the loose network of locally controlled hospitals into a centrally controlled Marine Hospital Service with its headquarters in Washington, D.C. The position of supervising surgeon (later known as the Surgeon General) was created to administer the service, and President Ulysses S. Grant appointed John Maynard Woodworth as the first supervising surgeon in 1871.

The scope of the Marine Hospital Service's responsibilities expanded beyond the care of merchant seamen in the closing decades of the 19th century, beginning with the control of infectious disease through better sanitation. As a result of its broadening responsibilities, the service's name was changed in 1902 to the Public Health and Marine Hospital Service. In 1912, the Marine Hospital Service became known officially as the Public Health Service.

As Elizabeth Fee and Theodore Brown describe in their article *The Unfulfilled Promise of Public Health: Déjà Vu All Over Again,* public health in the United States surged as a necessity-driven response to immediate local threats. The authors explain that these "threats" were closely tied in the popular imagination to epidemic disease, and as a consequence, public health was understood to be the set of measures undertaken to protect the local population from

epidemic disease. Based on this definition of public health,
it could be expected that the first local and state health
departments would arise during a yellow fever outbreak
that terrified the new nation between 1793 and 1806. In

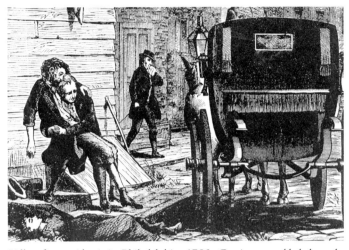

*Yellow fever epidemic in Philadelphia, 1793. Carriages rumbled through
the streets to pick up the dying and the dead.*

fact, the first Board of Health was established in Philadelphia in 1794, followed by Baltimore in 1797, Boston in
1799, Washington, D.C., in 1802, New Orleans in 1804,
and New York City in 1805.

► Once the yellow fever outbreak came under control,
public and budgetary support for these newly formed local
boards of health also diminished. Interest in public health
remained quiescent until 1830, when New York City
citizens formed a civilian group known as the "sanitary
reformers" in response to a cholera outbreak. The reformers pressured public officials to take their public health
responsibilities seriously and improve the city's living
conditions.

Fee and Brown further explain that from 1857 to 1860 the
sanitary reformers held "Sanitary Conventions." During the
Civil War, the group persuaded President Abraham Lincoln
to create a Sanitary Commission to investigate conditions
among the Union Forces and take measures to improve
sanitation and health interventions. One of the measures
taken by civilian and military authorities in response to the
Sanitary Commission's pressure was improved sanitation

▼

Once the yellow
fever outbreak
came under con-
trol, public and
budgetary support
for these newly
formed local
boards of health
also diminished.

among the troops. Another critical measure – educating officers and enlisted men – taught the closely confined troops about the spread of infectious diseases and the need for personal and public hygiene. After the war ended, Sanitary Commission measures continued in New York, Chicago and Massachusetts, creating a record of success for the first effective boards of health. ► By the 1870s, most major cities had instituted some form of public health organization.

▼

By the 1870s, most major cities had instituted some form of public health organization.

Advancing in history to the New Deal years in the 1930s and, again, visiting the Public Health Service, as it became known in 1912, Congress heeded President Franklin Roosevelt and, in response to the Great Depression, created the welfare state. The Public Health Service benefited from support in Congress and expanded greatly during the New Deal years. With the Social Security Act of 1935, Congress established social insurance and cash assistance programs that improved the public's health by ensuring income

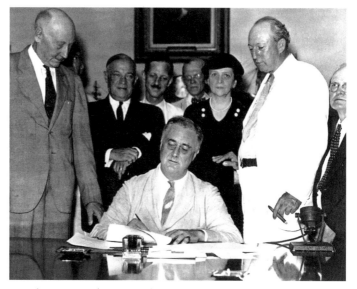

President Roosevelt signing the Social Security Act.

security for groups at greater risk of poverty and disease. Much later, in 1965, Congress enacted the Medicare and Medicaid programs, expanding social insurance. Medicare and Medicaid broadened significantly the role that the federal government plays in addressing health care issues for the needy.

The consolidation of the modern federal public health establishment came in the mid–20th century. In 1930, the Ransdell Act established the National Institutes of Health, which have evolved into the current well–funded engine for biomedical research and training throughout the United States. In 1946, the Centers for Disease Control (known as the CDC) was formed from the Office of Malaria Control in War Areas and became part of the Public Health Service, significantly expanding the federal government's public health responsibilities.

In 1953, the federal public health and social welfare functions were consolidated into one cabinet–level department, the Department of Health, Education and Welfare. This new department housed virtually all of the federal agencies with public health responsibilities that had evolved since the Civil War, including the Medicare and Medicaid programs. In 1979, when a new Department of Education was formed, the newly named Department of Health and Human Services (DHHS) became the home of federal health and social services programs.

Today the nation's public health system is a complex network of people, systems and organizations working at the local, state and national levels.   ►   The U.S. public health system is distinct from other parts of the health care system in two key respects: its primary emphasis is preventing disease and disability, and it focuses on population rather than individual health.

Both the public and private sectors play important roles in public health. The nation is served by more than 3,000 county and city health departments, 3,000 local boards of health, 59 state and territorial health departments, and more than 160,000 public and private laboratories. A series of federal health and environmental agencies set national standards and provide funding, training, scientific guidance and technical support.

Hospitals, clinics, managed care organizations, civic and volunteer groups, and national associations support the work of local, state and federal public health agencies. The associations include the National Association of County and City Health Officials (NACCHO), the Association of State and Territorial Health Officials (ASTHO), the Association of Public Health Laboratories (APHL), the

▼

The U.S. public health system is distinct from other parts of the health care system in two key respects: its primary emphasis is preventing disease and disability, and it focuses on population rather than individual health.

National Association of Local Boards of Health (NALBOH), the Council of State and Territorial Epidemiologists (CSTE) and the American Public Health Association (APHA).

Although these components are numerous, the public health infrastructure is but one piece of a larger public health system. The system depends on three interrelated components: the capacity and competency of the workforce, information and data systems, and organizational capacity. Deficiencies in one area can have a ripple effect throughout the entire public health system.

Workforce Capacity and Competency

Workforce capacity and competency refers to the expertise of professionals who work in federal, state and local public health agencies to protect the public's health. ► The governmental portion of the public health workforce includes 448,754 professionals deployed at the local, state and national levels. At the local level, public health workers are found in local health agencies and in private and non-profit organizations concerned with the public's health.

The most common professional disciplines within the U.S. public health workforce are nurses, physicians, environmental specialists, laboratorians, health educators, disease investigators, outreach workers and managers. Public health also includes dentists, social workers, nutritionists, anthropologists, psychologists, economists, political scientists, engineers, information technology specialists, public health informaticians, epidemiologists, biostatisticians and lawyers. Any professional whose primary function is to improve health can be considered part of the public health workforce. However, it is workers in official public health agencies who are on the front lines in tracking disease trends, implementing communitywide health promotion and disease-prevention programs, and responding to emerging threats and outbreaks.

The federal government has traditionally supported a variety of programs to enhance public health workforce capacity. For example, grant programs at the Health Resources and Services Administration (HRSA) are devoted to public health professional development and training. Over the last decade, CDC has also provided valuable training opportunities for state and local public health leaders and

▼

The governmental portion of the public health workforce includes 448,754 professionals deployed at the local, state and national levels.

professionals. In addition, state and local health departments are actively developing ways to strengthen their public health workforce. For example, New Jersey established credentials and competency-based training requirements for public health workers. In Pennsylvania, the Allegheny County Health Department joined the University of Pittsburgh Center for Public Health Practice to create a partnership for faculty and workforce development. Private foundations also help build workforce capacity by providing grants to schools of public health, funding education and training opportunities at the state and local level, supporting research and sponsoring national conferences.

Despite efforts to grow the workforce capacity of the nation, there is a gap between the increasing demands placed on the dedicated public health workforce and the growing complexity of disease patterns, interventions, partnerships, technology, tools and training necessary to meet the demands. There are 448,254 public health workers in the United States, according to U.S. Department of Labor statistics from 2004, compared with 490,000 lawyers, 532,740 bank tellers, and 2,026,000 fast food workers. In setting a public health goal to improve the public health workforce ► by the year 2010, the federal government calls for each community to be served by a "fully trained, culturally competent public health team, representing the optimal mix of professional disciplines."

▼

...by the year 2010, the federal government calls for each community to be served by a "fully trained, culturally competent public health team, representing the optimal mix of professional disciplines."

Surveillance and Information Systems

The delivery of effective public health services depends on timely and reliable information and data. Perhaps perceived as not as exciting as other public health disciplines, surveillance and information systems are nonetheless the heart of public health planning and interventions. These tools help to monitor disease and enable efficient communication among public and private health organizations, the media and the public. They also make it possible for health professionals to diagnose the health of populations, distribute resources to the right locations, and alert the public about public health issues and threats.

The ongoing systematic collection, analysis and interpretation of health-related data is called "surveillance." Surveillance systems provide data on illness, disability and death from acute and chronic conditions; on injuries; on personal environment and occupational risk factors; on preventive and treatment services; and on program costs. Data from these systems can assist prevention efforts by functioning as early-warning signals for new and emerging conditions. Data systems also facilitate planning, as public health agencies use data on disease prevalence to develop prevention programs.

► Although federal agencies take the lead in collecting national public health data, they represent only a fraction of the many necessary partners that collect, analyze and translate these data. Programs in each area collect information from local communities. Other data-collection systems depend upon the participation of private citizens nationwide. Still other systems rely on the administrative records and surveys of public and private health care organizations.

Despite advances in technology, many local health departments still lack access to basic information-system capabilities. Access is critical because state and local public health department staffs need the Internet and other electronic information systems to perform their job functions effectively. Similarly, it is essential that staff be trained to use these systems. In 1999, to address this issue, the CDC partnered with local and state health agencies, as well as national public health organizations, to develop the Health Alert Network (HAN), a nationwide, integrated information and communication system capable of distributing health alerts, prevention guidelines and other information. In 2000, the CDC launched another program, the National Electronic Disease Surveillance System, to provide national standards, specifications, and working prototypes so that information collected by local health departments can be used to detect and manage outbreaks that affect more than one area.

Organizational Capacity

Organizational capacity is the structure and mechanisms on which a functioning public health system relies – its facilities, laboratories and financing mechanisms. In order to perform activities and provide services that safeguard the health of a community, public health departments and laboratories must have modern facilities, adequate financing, successful partnerships with institutions in both the public and private sector, properly trained personnel and up-to-date information systems.

▼
Although federal agencies take the lead in collecting national public health data, they represent only a fraction of the many necessary partners that collect, analyze and translate these data.

In 1998 and 2000, studies performed by the University of North Carolina and the CDC's National Public Health Performance Standards Program measured health department performance. ► Both studies revealed that the state public health systems have half or less of the organizational capacity they need to optimally perform essential public health services. The average performance score for local public health departments was slightly higher than for state public health systems. In part, the cumulative result of budget cuts, lack of staff training and outmoded information systems and laboratories, these scores also reflect the growing demands on the public health system. The public health infrastructure has had trouble keeping pace with the demands for performance.

On two occasions, in 1988 and 2002, the Institute of Medicine (IOM) addressed public health infrastructure in two IOM reports. In the 1988 report, titled *The Future of Public Health*, IOM presented proposals for ensuring that public health service programs would be effective and efficient enough to deal not only with current challenges but future crises as well. The report identified the core functions of public health: assessment, policy development and assurance of essential health services. It also recommended the manner in which the performance of these core functions be divided among federal, state and local levels. The subsequent 2002 IOM report, titled *The Future of the Public's Health in the 21st Century*, reviewed the nation's public health capabilities and recommended a comprehensive framework for involving public health agencies with multiple partners in both the public and private sectors to create a more integrated public health system. Among the 2002 IOM report's recommendations for this integrated public health system were the following:

▼

...state public health systems have half or less of the organizational capacity they need to optimally perform essential public health services.

- ◆ Adopt a population health approach that considers multiple determinants of health.

- ◆ Strengthen government's public health functions, the backbone of the public health system.

- ◆ Develop new partners across sectors, requiring accountability in the process.

- ◆ Make decisions based on evidence.

◆ Enhance communication within this expanded public health system. ◻

Essential Public Health Functions*

1. Monitor health status to identify community health problems.

2. Diagnose and investigate health problems and health hazards in the community.

3. Inform, educate and empower people about health issues.

4. Mobilize community partnerships to identify and solve health problems.

5. Develop policies and plans that support individual and community health efforts.

6. Enforce laws and regulations that protect health and ensure safety.

7. Link people to needed personal health services and assure the provision of health care when it is otherwise unavailable.

8. Assure a competent public health and personal healthcare workforce.

9. Evaluate the effectiveness, accessibility, and quality of personal and population-based health services.

10. Research new insights and innovative solutions to health problems.

---

*From the Public Health Functions Project (1994-1999), directed by a Steering Committee chaired by the Assistant Secretary of Health and Surgeon General with the participation of CDC and a host of public health associations, foundations and organizations.

Case Study

The Creation of CDC

The Communicable Disease Center (CDC) opened in the old Office of Malaria Control in War Areas in Atlanta, Georgia, on July 1, 1946. As a part of the U.S. Public Health Service, the original CDC mission was to work with state and local health officials in the fight against malaria, then still prevalent in several Southern states, as well as typhus and other communicable diseases. Its founder, Joseph W. Mountin, MD, a visionary public

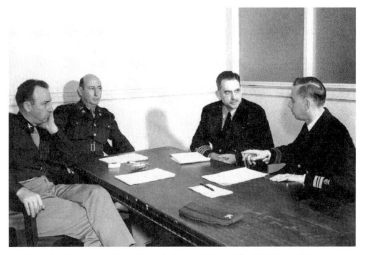

Dr. Joseph Mountin, third from left, meeting with CDC staffers.

health leader, had high hopes for this small and comparatively insignificant branch of the Public Health Service. Dr. Mountin received his medical degree from Marquette University in Milwaukee, Wisconsin, in 1914. He began his career with the Public Health Service during World War I working in sanitation in the temporary living quarters specially built by the U.S. Army for soldiers in military areas throughout the United States. In his distinguished career with the Public Health Service, Mountin became widely known as the father of many service programs. In late November 1951, he was appointed to the post of bureau chief with the rank of Assistant Surgeon General. Mountin died unexpectedly the following year at the Naval Medical Center in Bethesda.

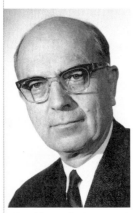

Dr. Alexander Langmuir

During the first years of CDC, medical epidemiologists were scarce. It was not until 1949 that Dr. Alexander Langmuir, now known as the father of infectious disease epidemiology, arrived to head the epidemiology branch. He launched the first-ever disease surveillance program and confirmed his suspicions that malaria control, the largest part of the CDC budget, had long since become unnecessary. Subsequently, disease surveillance became the cornerstone of CDC's mission of service and, in time, changed the practice of public health. Langmuir was CDC's chief epidemiologist from 1949 to 1970. He spent the rest of his life teaching at Harvard Medical School and at Johns Hopkins, where he had earned his degree in public health. In 1993, he died of kidney cancer at the age of 83.

World events also had an impact on CDC's mission. In 1950, the start of the Korean War gave impetus to creating the Epidemic Intelligence Service (EIS). With the threat of biological warfare looming, Langmuir wanted to train epidemiologists to detect new emerging agents and at the same time guard against common threats to public health. In 1955, CDC broadened its focus to include poliomyelitis (polio) and established the Polio Surveillance Unit.

Two major health crises in the mid-1950s cemented CDC's credibility and long-term survival. In 1955, after polio appeared in children who had received the Salk

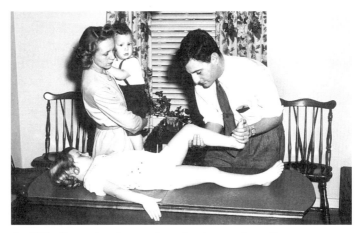

An EIS officer using the muscle evaluation test for polio.

vaccine, only recently approved, CDC stopped the national inoculation program. The cases were traced to contaminated vaccine from a laboratory in California;

once the problem was corrected, the inoculation program resumed, at least for first- and second-graders. Two years later, surveillance traced the course of a massive influenza epidemic. From data gathered in 1957 and subsequent years, national guidelines for influenza vaccine were developed.

In the 1950s and 1960s, CDC grew by acquisition. The venereal disease program came to Atlanta in 1957 and with it, the first Public Health Advisors. The tuberculosis and immunization programs were moved under CDC's "umbrella" in 1960; and in 1961, CDC took over publication of the *Morbidity and Mortality Weekly Report* (MMWR). The MMWR, which lists important data on deaths and certain diseases from every state every week, is still published every week and is considered an essential public health tool. The Foreign Quarantine Service, one of the oldest and most prestigious units of PHS, became part of CDC in 1967, followed by the long-established nutrition program and the National Institute for Occupational Safety and Health.

One of CDC's greatest accomplishments, the worldwide eradication of smallpox, was launched in 1966. The Smallpox Eradication Program aimed to eradicate smallpox and control measles in 20 African countries and support the worldwide efforts of the World Health Organization's smallpox crusade. The disease had killed millions of people over the centuries. By the late 1970s, just over a decade later, CDC efforts helped eradicate smallpox from the world. CDC also achieved notable success at home tracking new emerging infections such as Legionnaire's disease, toxic-shock syndrome and hantavirus. More importantly, the MMWR published the first report of a new and fatal disease, acquired immunodeficiency syndrome (AIDS), in the June 5, 1981, issue. During the 1990s and early 2000s, CDC broadened its focus to address chronic disease prevention and obesity.

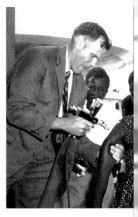

Dr. Stan Foster, EIS officer, administering smallpox vaccine to a Nigerian woman in 1967.

As CDC's activities expanded in scope far beyond communicable diseases to include chronic disease control and health promotion, its name had to be changed to reflect a broader mission. In 1970, the name became the Center for Disease Control. In 1981, after extensive reorganization, "Center" became "Centers." In 1992, the words "and Prevention" were added, but by law, CDC retained its well-known three-letter abbreviation. ◻

Vignette

Surgeon General's Report of 1964

More than 40 years ago on January 11, 1964, Luther L. Terry, MD, Surgeon General of the U.S. Public Health Service, released the report of the Surgeon General's Advisory Committee on Smoking and Health. This landmark document, now referred to as the first *Surgeon General's Report on Smoking and Health*, had a tremendous impact on public attitudes and policy for three important reasons. First, an official U.S. agency recognized for the first time that cigarette smoking caused cancer and other serious diseases. Second, it prompted a series of public health actions reflecting changes in societal attitudes toward the health hazards of tobacco use. Third, the Surgeon General's report was the first to receive widespread media and public attention. Although evidence that smoking caused harm had accumulated since the 1930s, official sources did not recognize the ill effects at the time. Epidemiologists used statistics and large-scale, long-term case control surveys to link the increase in lung cancer mortality to smoking. Pathologists and laboratory scientists confirmed the statistical relationship of smoking to lung cancer as well as to other serious diseases, such as bronchitis, emphysema and coronary heart disease. In 1957, then-Surgeon General Leroy E. Burney declared as the official position of the U.S. Public Health Service that smoking caused lung cancer.

The impulse for an official report on smoking and health did not come until 1961, however, pushed by an alliance of prominent private health organizations. The American Cancer Society, the American Heart Association, the National Tuberculosis Association, and the American Public Health Association called for a national commission on smoking in a letter addressed to President John F. Kennedy. The letter sought a commission dedicated to "seeking a solution to this health problem that would interfere least with the freedom of industry or the happiness of individuals."

The Kennedy administration responded the following year. In 1962, recently appointed Surgeon General Luther L. Terry announced that he would convene a committee of experts to conduct a comprehensive review of the scientific literature on the smoking question. Terry invited representatives of the four voluntary medical organizations who had first proposed the commission, as well as the Food and Drug Administration, the Federal Trade Commission, the American Medical Association, and the Tobacco Institute (the lobbying arm of the tobacco industry) to nominate ten commission members.

From November 1962 through January 1964, the committee reviewed more than 7,000 scientific articles with the help of more than 150 consultants. The advisory committee concluded that cigarette smoking caused both lung cancer and chronic bronchitis. The committee recognized for the first time, officially, that "cigarette smoking is a health hazard of sufficient importance in the United States to warrant appropriate remedial action."

The 1964 Surgeon General's report became the first of a series of steps to reduce the impact of tobacco use on the health of the American people. The circumstances surrounding the release of the first report in 1964 were peculiar. Surgeon General Terry issued the commission's report on a Saturday, a strategy meant to minimize the effect on the stock market and maximize coverage in the Sunday papers. "This strategy succeeded," Terry remembered two decades later, "because the report hit the country like a bombshell. It was front-page news and a lead story on every radio and television station in the United States and many abroad."

Among the steps that followed the report were banning tobacco advertising on broadcast media, placing mandatory health warnings on cigarette packages and developing effective treatments for tobacco dependence. The Office of the Surgeon General has issued 27 subsequent reports on tobacco use, covering such topics as environmental (i.e., secondhand) tobacco smoke. These reports helped lead the way to smoke-free public places, restaurants and bars.

The widespread media and public attention led to significant changes in public attitudes toward smoking. A Gallup survey conducted in 1958 found that only 44 percent of Americans believed smoking caused cancer; that figure grew to 78 percent by 1968. Between 1965 and 2002, adult smoking rates have been cut from 42.4 percent to 22.5 percent, nearly in half, and per-capita consumption of tobacco products has fallen from 4,345 cigarettes in 1963 to 1,979 cigarettes in 2002, more than half.

The 1964 Surgeon General's report was significant because it marked the first of a series of authoritative scientific statements by the Surgeon General that helped shape the debate on the responsibility of government, physicians and individual citizens for the nation's health. Indeed, Surgeon General's reports since 1964 have addressed a broad range of health issues. These include secondhand smoke, maternal and child health, nutrition and physical exercise, mental health, and issues that lie outside medicine, such as suicide and gun violence, that are studied for how they affect public health. ◘

Looking Ahead

Public Health – A 21st Century Perspective

The 21st century presents a new set of challenges to the nation's health. Whether confronting bioterrorism attacks, emerging infections, lifestyle behaviors, disparities in health status, or increases in chronic disease and injury rates, the public health community now more than ever needs a strengthened infrastructure. ► Public health needs to gain capacity as it prepares to respond to acute and chronic threats to the nation's health, not all now known. Only a public health system supported by political will, public and private partnerships, and other financial resources can meet ongoing and new health challenges.

As Dr. William Keck of the Department of Community Health Sciences at the Northeastern Ohio Universities College of Medicine points out, "A continually expanding public health agenda in an era of shrinking governmental resources diminishes the ability of many local health departments to meet basic community health needs, let alone lift their communities to the highest levels of health possible. The successful public health department of the future will develop multiple funding sources, advocate effectively for resources to meet community needs, and build strong collaborative linkages with other community health agencies and the illness care system. It will otherwise be impossible to ensure that each citizen has access to a seamless web of services that promote health, prevent illness and injury, diagnose disease early and provide disease treatment that is efficient and effective."

Bioterrorism

Bioterrorism is defined as the unlawful release of biologic agents or toxins to kill or sicken people, animals or plants with the intent to intimidate or coerce a government or civilian population. A bioterrorism attack would represent a major public health threat in the United States. CDC, the government agency in charge of responding to public health emergencies for decades, must now prepare for bioterrorism attacks.

▼

Public health needs to gain capacity as it prepares to respond to acute and chronic threats to the nation's health....

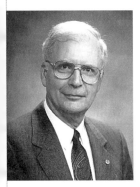

Dr. William Keck of Northeastern Ohio Universities College of Medicine.

CDC and public health authorities became aware of the threat of domestic bioterrorism after several small acts of focused bacteriologic criminal assault in the United States. These acts included the intentional contamination of salad bars with *Salmonella* organisms in 1984 in Oregon and of muffins and pastries with *Shigella* organisms in Texas in 1996. As a result, the United States government decided to revisit and update a national plan for bioterrorism preparedness and response. In 1999, as part of this strategy, CDC collaborated with the Association of Public Health Laboratories and the Federal Bureau of Investigation to establish the Laboratory Response Network. This network develops local, state and federal public health laboratory capacity to respond to bioterrorism events.

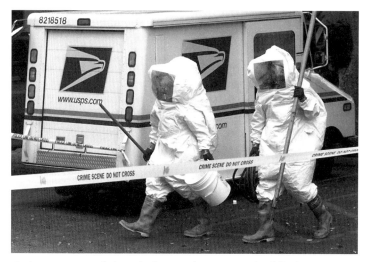

Anthrax was spread through the postal system in the fall of 2001.

Only in the fall of 2001 were CDC's bioterrorism plans put into action, in response to an anthrax attack in the U.S. At a time of heightened tension due to the events of September 11, letters containing anthrax powder spread this infectious disease deliberately through the postal system; 22 people were infected and five people died.

Lifestyle and Behavior Change

While this century's medical advances and public health efforts have dramatically reduced the threat of infectious disease in the U.S., poor health due to lifestyle behaviors remains a threat to public health. Poor lifestyle behaviors are linked to chronic diseases, the heaviest burden on the health care system today. These behaviors involve tobacco use, alcohol and drug abuse, lack of healthy diet and exercise, and risky sexual practices. In particular, poor nutrition and a sedentary lifestyle are considered by some experts to be "the 21st century plague" as they lead to obesity and diabetes, now considered national epidemics. They also contribute to a host of other serious medical problems, such as heart disease and cancer – the two leading causes of death in the U.S.

Public health professionals know that promoting healthy behaviors is one of the best ways to prevent disease and disability. Consequently, many public health activities are designed to help individuals and communities achieve and maintain a healthy lifestyle at any age. For example, CDC launched a campaign called VERB (to connote action) in 2002 to fight childhood obesity, encouraging young people ages nine to 13 to be physically active every day. The campaign combines paid advertising, marketing strategies and partnership efforts to reach the distinct audiences of tweens and adults/influencers. As CDC Director Dr. Julie L. Gerberding said, "The VERB campaign has surpassed expectations and is responsible for improving physical activity levels among youth." In February 2004, CDC released the results of a telephone survey that indicate that physical activity among the nation's youth is increasing as a result of the VERB campaign.

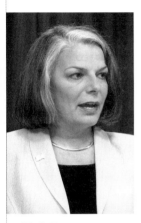

CDC Director
Julie L. Gerberding

Chronic–Disease Prevention and Control

Chronic diseases, such as heart disease, stroke, diabetes and cancer, cause 70 percent of all deaths in the United States each year. A large number of these deaths are preventable. People with chronic conditions are the largest, most costly and fastest-growing group in health care, and their numbers are expected to swell in the 21st century.

From specific laboratory measures to more complex studies of behaviors and risk factors, CDC's efforts are designed to understand the causes and consequences of chronic diseases and to place the powerful tools of prevention within reach of more people every day. Moreover, CDC works to ensure that advances in basic scientific and behavioral research are put into practice to benefit all Americans. As part of its mission, CDC works with states to develop comprehensive, sustainable prevention programs that target the leading causes of death and disability in our society and their risk factors. In addition, numerous efforts to manage chronic disease, along with social marketing campaigns, changes in food (such as removal of trans fats) and a new food pyramid have gained an increasing role in chronic-disease prevention. New approaches to prevention are crucial to fight chronic diseases in this century.

Infectious Diseases and Emerging Threats

Despite incredible gains in combating infectious diseases, they remain a public health concern in the 21st century. Infectious diseases are the third leading cause of death in the United States and still predominate worldwide, with acute lower respiratory tract infections, HIV/AIDS, diarrheal diseases, tuberculosis and malaria as the major threats.

Although the combination of improved hygiene and sanitation, vaccinations and antibiotics has helped turn the tide against infectious diseases in this country, new diseases and the resurgence of old ones make infectious diseases a constant concern. Emerging infections are those that have not been previously recognized. ► The AIDS pandemic is an example of a truly new and emerging infectious disease whose public health impact had not been previously experienced. On the other hand, infections that have been experienced previously reappear in a more virulent form or in a new epidemiological setting. The influenza type A pandemics of 1918, 1957 and 1968 are examples of this.

Global air travel, now widely available and affordable, introduces infected travelers to the U.S. with diseases that once might have stayed overseas. For example, severe acute respiratory syndrome (SARS) was first reported in Asia in February 2003. Over the next few months, due to global air travel, the illness spread to more than two dozen countries in North America, South America, Europe and Asia. According to the World Health Organization (WHO), a total of 8,098 people worldwide became sick with SARS during the 2003 outbreak. Of these, 774 died. In the United States, only eight people had laboratory evidence of SARS infection and all of them had been traveling in other countries where SARS had been identified. Fortunately, CDC worked closely with the WHO and other partners in a global effort to address the

▼

The AIDS pandemic is an example of a truly new and emerging infectious disease whose public health impact had not been previously experienced.

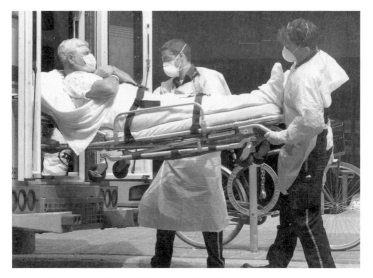

Paramedics during the SARS outbreak in Toronto.

SARS outbreak of 2003, preventing SARS from spreading more widely in the United States.

► CDC continues its work of increasing the capacity of laboratories and surveillance systems here and abroad to detect and monitor changes in disease patterns and to serve as an early-warning system. For example, surveillance centers in both the U.S. and Asia monitor the ever-present threat of influenza pandemics. CDC also continues to work with public and private partners to change the way antibiotics are prescribed and used in hospitals and other settings. CDC helps form working teams that link epidemiology, partnerships, education of health care providers and patients, and vector control to counter the spread of specific infectious disease threats. These threats range from sexually transmitted diseases, like syphilis and chlamydia, to bloodborne threats, like hepatitis C. The teams help control existing infectious disease threats and prepare the nation for new ones.

Meeting the challenges of infectious diseases in the 21st century means that the scientific and technological advances that form the foundation of a public health response must evolve quickly and continually. As former CDC director Dr. Jeffrey Koplan observed in the 2002 IOM Report, "We are only as prepared as the least prepared among us." ◻

▼

CDC continues its work of increasing the capacity of laboratories and surveillance systems here and abroad to detect and monitor changes in disease patterns and to serve as an early-warning system.

Epilogue

Santayana's admonition, "Those who forget the past are doomed to repeat it," should never happen to the public health community. In celebrating ten milestones of public health in the United States during the 20th century, this book outlines potential challenges that, if addressed based on lessons learned from the past, will create the next generation of milestones in public health. Although we cannot be certain what the 21st century milestones will be, we can be certain that the public health community will face challenges in achieving them and, in the process, will improve the health and well-being of the nation. As always with public health, success redefines the challenge.

Certain common denominators – technological advances, sound public policies and legislation, adoption of individual healthier behaviors and corporate responsibility – have helped the public health community meet the challenges of the 20th century and produce solutions. Public health's biggest challenge has been gaining traction in these areas simultaneously. As the problems faced by the public health community grow more complex, so do the solutions.

Fortunately, public health is a diverse field that engages a wide spectrum of expertise. The population's health depends on the collective work of attorneys, environmentalists, journalists, legislators, social workers and teachers, as well as administrators, laboratory scientists and researchers. The population's health advances when workers from many different fields collaborate to implement educational programs, develop public policies and legislation, administer services and conduct research. If the next set of milestones is to be achieved, this diverse workforce will need to work in a synchronized manner that captures the public's attention and changes behavior.

Public health seeks to protect the health of entire populations, and future public health milestones will be so far-reaching that they will affect every aspect of society. To accomplish its goals, the public health community will need to protect individual rights and privacy, prompt the public to respond to messages that point the way to healthier lifestyles and to persuade corporations to tap their resources to assist in reaching the goals. Lessons learned in the 20th century must be assessed with open minds as society searches for new ways to improve the public's health. Society must learn from the milestones outlined in this book and build on their success.

Could a newly enacted federal law dramatically reduce death rates on our highways due to drunk driving by repeat offenders? Preliminary figures for 2004 from the National Highway Traffic Safety Administration show a slight decline in highway deaths but also show that three categories of drivers – repeat offenders, those with very high blood alcohol levels, and those who continue to drive with suspended licenses despite convictions for drunk driving – account for nearly 40 percent of fatal crashes, unchanged for many years. For the milestone of reducing death rates due to repeat offenders to be possible, drivers themselves would have to abstain from excessive drinking. Improvements in automobile and highway design, such as an ignition interlock that would prevent a car from starting if a sensor detects that the driver's blood alcohol level is too high, would also play a role. Finally, Congress would play its role by nationalizing standards for stricter enforcement of drunk driving.

Could public health messages about eating healthy diets and exercising regularly reduce dramatically the rate of obesity in our youth? Public health experts continue to be alarmed by obesity statistics that lead to unacceptably high rates of diabetes and incipient cardiovascular disease. The public health response has been to promote a combination of healthy diets, regular physical activity and early screening for warning signs of metabolic syndrome. To conquer this challenge and build a healthier society, individuals, food corporations, government and communities will have to rally together.

Could the silent epidemic of tooth decay be conquered? Proven public health interventions – water fluoridation and sealant programs – would need to be far more universal than they are today; access to dentists, far more prevalent. These measures are part of the solution. For the milestone to be achieved, responsible individuals would need to eat healthy diets and practice good personal hygiene. Public health messages highlighting healthy outcomes, employed by public health experts to change behavior, can succeed only when individuals and society as a whole respond. New laws, improvements in technology and refinements of public health techniques are never enough.

Sentinel public health milestones occur when society's attitude and behavior change so significantly that the preventive or screening measure is adopted routinely. For example, seat belts are a proven means to reduce mortality in car crashes, and laws requiring them are effective only when individuals voluntarily comply. Most people now don't think twice about buckling up – especially their children, in safety-tested car seats – and this compliance has saved countless lives. Public health messages offered proof of improved mortality, so manufacturers installed seat belts. Legal requirements, coupled with public campaigns designed to educate about seat belts, changed society's attitude, and this led to changes in behavior.

Who would have thought that regulations promoting smoke-free indoor environments could effectively eliminate environmental smoke as a threat to the public's health? People no longer light up on airplanes and in schools and, in many states, in workplaces and other public spaces. Labels on cigarette packages warn pregnant women that smoking is dangerous to the health of their unborn children. Laws enacted to restrict smoking in public spaces and the warnings about its health hazards have been factors in changing attitudes and behavior toward smoking. Similar changes in behavior have occurred with drinking and driving, drinking alcohol during pregnancy, and the use of bicycle helmets.

Advances in public health in the 21st century could surprise us. In 50 years, a new edition of *Milestones in Public Health* might highlight 10 advances that can hardly be contemplated today. Even then, the public health community will have moved on to new challenges, and the story will repeat itself. This is the appeal of public health, a dynamic field that builds on past successes but strives always to find new ways to improve the nation's health. The public health community, in marshalling all available resources, will engage workers across a wide variety of fields to persuade a reluctant public to change behavior, reluctant legislatures to pass laws that protect and promote health, and reluctant scientists to develop and test technologies that can prevent illnesses or detect and cure them. New generations will demonstrate the value of public health, a field that refuses to accept things as they are. Scientists will be rewarded, public officials won over, legislatures persuaded, and new laws and regulations passed that protect and promote better health outcomes.

The milestones of this new century depend on the best of our nation's youth enlisting in the field to seek new ways to improve the public's health. The work of a new generation, inspired by the successes of earlier generations, is sure to bring about the next milestones in public health.

Barbara A. DeBuono, MD, MPH
November 2005

References

Chapter 1. *Vaccines*

Looking Back

1. BBC Homepage History. Edward Jenner (1749-1823). www.bbc.co.uk./history/historic_figures/jenner_edward.shtml.
2. BBC Homepage History. Donald Ainslie Henderson (1928 -). www.bbc.co.uk./history/historic_figures/henderson_donald_ainslie.shtml.
3. Bennett, Joslyn Tobin. History of Vaccines. *Grinnell College.* December 2001.
4. CDC. Smallpox Vaccination and Adverse Reactions. *Supplement to MMWR.* February 21, 2003.
5. Fox, Maggie. More U.S. Children Vaccinated Than Ever – Report. *Reuters Health.* July 31, 2003.
6. Maybury Okonek, Bonnie A. and Peters, Pamela M., Ph.D. Vaccines – How and Why? *The National Health Museum's Access Excellence.* www.accessexcellence.org/AE/AEC/CC/vaccines_how_why.html.
7. The Medical Letter on Drugs and Therapeutics. Smallpox Vaccine. *The Medical Letter, Inc.*, Vol. 45 (Issue 1147), January 6, 2003.
8. Nobel Museum. Emil von Behring – Biography. www.nobel.se/medicine/laureates/1901/behring.cio.html.
9. Ross, Emma. Childhood Vaccine-Autism Study Retracted. *Associated Press.* March 3, 2003.
10. World Health Organization. The History of Vaccination. www.who.int/vaccines-diseases/history/history.shtml.

Case Study: Eradication of Smallpox

1. Fenner, Frank. The Eradication of Smallpox. *Progress in Medical Virology* 23, 1-21, 1977.
2. Fenner, Frank. The Eradication of Smallpox. *Impact of Science on Society* 150, 147-158, 1988.
3. Fenner, Frank. A successful eradication campaign. Global eradication of smallpox. *Reviews of Infectious Diseases* 4, 916-922, 1982.
4. Fenner, Frank. The global eradication of smallpox. *Medical Journal of Australia* 1, 455-457, 1980.
5. Fenner, Frank. Eradicating smallpox: Lessons for the future. *Radius,* 15, 9-14, 2002.
6. Fenner, Frank. History of smallpox. In *Microbes Hunters – Then and Now* (H. Koprowski and M.B.A. Oldstone, eds.), pp. 25-37. Med-Ed Press, Bloomington, Ill., 1996.
7. Fenner, Frank, Chairman of Global Commission. The Global Eradication of Smallpox. Final Report of the Global Commission for the Certification of the Eradication of Smallpox. World Health Organization, Geneva. History of International Public Health, No. 4, 122 pages, 1980.
8. Fenner, Frank. Lessons from the smallpox eradication campaign. In *Vaccines 85,* (R.A. Lerner, R.M. Chanock and F. Brown, eds.), pp. 143-146, Cold Spring Harbor Laboratory, New York.
9. Fenner, Frank, Henderson, DA, et al. Smallpox and Its Eradication, Chapter 31, Lessons and Benefits (pp. 1345-1370). World Health Organization, 1988.
10. Feuerstein-Kadgien, Bernadette, MD, and Korn, Klaus, MD. Cowpox infection. *New England Journal of Medicine.* January 30, 2003, Vol. 348, No. 5:415-425.
11. Fewell, Heather. The History of Smallpox; The Rise and Fall of a Disease. *What You Need to Know About Dermatology.* http://dermatology.about.com/library/blsmallpoxhistory.htm.
12. Flight, Colette. Smallpox: eradicating the scourge. www.bbc.co.uk/history/discover/medicine/smallpox_01.shtml.
13. Henderson, D. A. and Fenner, F. Smallpox and vaccinia. In "Vaccines" Second Edition. (S.A. Plotkin and E.A. Mortimer, Jr., eds), pp. 13-40. W.B. Saunders Company, Philadelphia, 1994.
14. Mack, Thomas, MD, MPH. A different view of smallpox and vaccination (Sounding Boards). *New England Journal of Medicine.* January 30, 2003, Vol. 348, No. 5:460-463.

Vignette: Hib Vaccine

1. BMJ. Vaccination and type 1 diabetes mellitus. www.bmj.com. May 1999.
2. CDC. *Haemophilus influenzae* Serotype b (Hib) Disease. *Division of Bacterial and Mycotic Diseases, Disease Information.* www.cdc.gov/ncidod/dbmd/diseaseinfo/haeminflueserob_t.htm.
3. CDC. Impact of Vaccines Universally Recommended for Children – United States, 1990-1999. www.cdc.gov/mmwr/preview/mmwrhtml/00056803.htm. April 2, 1999; 48(12); 243-248.
4. CDC. Progress Toward Elimination of *Haemophilus influenzae* Type b Invasive Disease Among Infants and Children – United States, 1998-2000. *MMWR Weekly.* March 22, 2002.
5. Doctor's Guide. New Combination Vaccine May Reduce Number of Childhood Shots Needed. www.docguide.com. January 20, 1997.
6. Gilbert, Lyn. Emerging Infectious Diseases. INOCULUM, Centre for Infectious Diseases and Microbiology, University of Sydney. Published in the *Canberra Times.* August 24, 2000.
7. Health Canada. Impact of Vaccines Universally Recommended for Children United States, 1990-1999. *CCDR,* Volume 25-14, July 15, 1999.
8. Steinberg, Jennifer. New Vaccine Hits Hib Hard. *Snapshots of Science & Medicine, Stories of Discovery.* http://science-education.nih.gov/snapshots.nsf. Posted April 23, 1999.

9. University of Rochester. FDA approves CHS-researched vaccine. *Currents.* March 20, 2000.

10. Wise, Jacqui. UK introduces new meningitis C vaccine. *BMJ,* Volume 319, July 31, 1999.

Looking Ahead: Preparedness and the Development of New Vaccines

1. 2003 Cancer Vaccines – 2nd Annual Conference on Advances in Designing. www.knowledgepress.com/events/10311228.htm. Boston, April 23-25, 2003.

2. A study forecasts unprecedented Market Opportunity for vaccine development. www.biotechwithitaly.com. October 15, 2001.

3. Altman, Lawrence K. Pocket of Opposition to Vaccine Threatens Polio Eradication. *New York Times.* December 9, 2003.

4. Altman, Lawrence K. World Health Organization Seeks Eradication of Polio by 2005. *New York Times.* July 29, 2003.

5. Antex Biologics. Preclinical Studies on Antex's Traveler's Diarrhea Vaccine Show 100 Percent Effectiveness in Animals. *Press Release.* April 4, 2001.

6. Associated Press. Hospital Patients Face Risks from Smallpox-Vaccine Use. From *WSJ Online.* March 25, 2003.

7. Associated Press. Study Says Insurers Should Pay for Vaccinations. *New York Times.* August 4, 2003.

8. Australian Centre for International & Tropical Health & Nutrition. Vaccine Development at ACITHN. *The University of Queensland.* Modified February 3, 2003.

9. Blendon, Robert J., ScD, et al. The public and the smallpox threat. *New England Journal of Medicine.* January 30, 2003, Vol. 348, No. 5:426-432.

10. BMJ.com. Vaccination in utero may cut vertical transmission. *BMJ,* Volume 321, August 5, 2000.

11. BMJ.com. Vaccine protects against Ebola virus. *BMJ,* Volume 321, December 9, 2000.

12. BMJ.com news roundup. Scientists isolate HIV blocker in placenta. *BMJ,* Volume 322, December 9, 2000.

13. BMJ.com news roundup. End to rubella in US thwarted by unvaccinated, foreign-born population. *BMJ,* Volume 324, February 2, 2002.

14. Bmj.com news roundup. Doubts raised over cancer vaccine study. *BMJ,* Volume 323, July 28, 2001.

15. Bozzette, Samuel A., MD, PhD., et al. A model for a smallpox-vaccination policy. *New England Journal of Medicine.* January 30, 2003, Vol. 348, No. 5:416-425.

16. Bremer, Joel G., MD, DTPH, Arita, Isao, MD, and Fenner, Frank, MD. Preventing the return of smallpox. *New England Journal of Medicine.* January 30, 2003, Vol. 348, No. 5:463-466.

17. CDC. Development of Immunization Registries. *Program in Brief.* February 2002.

18. CDC. Infectious Diseases. *Program in Brief.* February 2002.

19. CDC. Tracking Vaccine-Preventable Diseases. *Program in Brief.* February 2002.

20. Chase, Marilyn. NIH Study Points to Vaccine for Smallpox That's Safer. *Wall Street Journal.* July 15, 2003.

21. Ciment, James. US drug companies announce vaccine initiative. *BMJ,* Volume 320, March 18, 2000.

22. Connolly, Ceci. Focus on Smallpox Threat Revived: Experts Say Immunization Program is Crucial to Homeland Security. *Washington Post.* July 17, 2003.

23. Connolly, Ceci. Smallpox Campaign Taxing Health Resources: Program Siphons Funds, Staffing from Other Projects, State and Local Officials Say. *Washington Post.* March 10, 2003.

24. Folkers, Gregory K. and Fauci, Anthony S., NIAID. The Role of U.S. Government Agencies in Vaccine Research and Development. *Nature Medicine Vaccine Supplement.* May 1998.

25. Friedman, Jonathan. Smallpox Strategy: Waiting won't work. *National Review.* 2003.

26. Friedman, Stephen, MD, MPH. 2003 Health Alert #11 – Smallpox Vaccination in People with a History of Cardiac Disease. *City of New York Department of Health and Mental Hygiene.* March 26, 2003.

27. Global Alliance for Vaccines and Immunization. Seminar in PowerPoint format.

28. Goldhammer, Alan, Ph.D. Cost of Smallpox Vaccinations. *PhRMA.* April 3, 2003.

29. Gottlieb, Scott. Vaccine could give protection against cervical cancer. *BMJ,* Vol. 325:1259 November 30, 2002.

30. Gorman, James. Looking for a vaccine to defang the Lyme tick. *New York Times.* May 20, 2003.

31. Grabenstein, John D., EdM, MS Pharm, FASHP and Wilson, James P., PharmD, Ph.D. Are Vaccines Safe? Risk Communication Applied to Vaccination. *Hospital Pharmacy* 1999; Vol. 34, No. 6, pp 713-729.

32. Grady, Denise, and Altman, Lawrence K. Beyond cute: Exotic pets come bearing exotic germs. *New York Times.* June 17, 2003.

33. Grantmakers Health. Victims of Our Own Success: Will Immunization Remain the Paradigm of Effective Prevention? Based on a Grantmakers in Health Roundtable, Washington, D.C. Issue, Brief No. 4.

34. Healy, Bernadine, MD. Time for a pause. *U.S. News and World Report.* April 21, 2003.

35. Herper, Matthew. Help IBM Take On Smallpox. *Forbes.* February 5, 2003.

36. Jackson, Trevor. Public less worried about MMR vaccine than many other issues. *BMJ,* Volume 324, March 16, 2002.

37. Langreth, Robert. Biotechs See Dollar Signs in War. *Forbes.* February 27, 2003.

38. Longbottom, Helen. Emerging infectious diseases. *CDI,* Volume 21, No 7, April 3, 1997.

39. Marwick, Charles. Improved anthrax vaccine is needed, claims report. *BMJ*, Volume 324, March 16, 2002.

40. McNeil, Donald G., Jr. African strain of polio virus hits Indonesia. *New York Times*. May 3, 2005.

41. McNeil, Donald G., Jr. Many Balking at Vaccination for Smallpox. *New York Times*. February 7, 2003.

42. McNeil, Donald G., Jr. National Programs to Vaccinate for Smallpox Come to a Halt. *New York Times*. June 19, 2003.

43. Moukheiber, Zina. Seeking a Safer Smallpox Vaccine. *Forbes*. March 14, 2003.

44. National Institute of Allergy and Infectious Diseases. Minority Health Research Initiatives: Microbiology and Infectious Diseases. www.aiaid.nih.gove/facts/mwhhp2.htm.

45. Nossal, Sir Gustav. Protecting Our Progeny: The Future of Vaccines. *Perspectives in Health Magazine,* the magazine of the Pan American Health Organization. Volume 7, No. 1, 2002.

46. Oakeshott, Isabel. Vaccine "cure" for cancer. *This is London*. September 22, 2003.

47. Payne, Doug. Ireland's measles outbreak kills two. *BMJ*, Volume 321, July 22, 2000.

48. Poland, Gregory A., Murray, Dennis, Bonilla-Guerrero, Ruben. New Vaccine Development. Clinical review in *BMJ*, Volume 324, June 1, 2002.

49. Pollack, Andrew. F.D.A. Backs Flu Vaccine Given by Mist, Not a Needle. *New York Times*. June 18, 2003.

50. Reuters Top Science and Health News. British scientists are developing vaccines.

51. Review & Outlook. The Politics of Autism: Lawsuits and emotion vs. science and childhood vaccines. *Wall Street Journal*. December 29, 2003.

52. Schmid, Randolph E. Panel recommends against smallpox shots. *Salon.com*. August 12, 2003.

53. Schoeberl, Joshua. U.S. vaccination rates up; Iowa ranks seventh. *Iowa Health Focus,* Iowa Department of Public Health. September 2000.

54. Schraeder, Terry L., MD, and Campion, Edward W., MD. Smallpox vaccination – The call to arms (Perspective). *New England Journal of Medicine*. January 30, 2003, Vol. 348, No. 5:381-382.

55. Sepkowitz, Kent A., MD. How contagious is vaccinia? (Current Concepts). *New England Journal of Medicine*. January 30, 2003, Vol. 348, No. 5:439-446.

56. Srivastava, Indresh K., PhD, and Liu, Margaret A., MD. Gene vaccines (Review). *Annals of Internal Medicine*. April 1, 2003, Vol, 138, No. 7:550-559.

57. U.S. Department of Health and Human Services. Shaping the Future of Breast Cancer Awareness, Research, Diagnosis and Treatment. *HHS Fact Sheet*. October 12, 2000.

58. Vaccines in the 21st Century. www.studentbmj.com/back_issues/1299/new_tech/new_tech5.html.

59. World Health Organization. Vaccines, Immunization and Biologicals. www.who.int/vaccines/en/rotavirus.shtml. Updated May 2002.

60. Wysocki, Bernard, Jr. Lack of Vaccines Goes Beyond Flu Inoculations. *Wall Street Journal*. December 8, 2003.

Chapter 2. *Automotive Safety*

Looking Back

1. Alliance of Automobile Manufacturers. The facts on SUV safety. www.autoalliance.org. American Legislative Exchange Council. Cellular phones and driving/Drunk drivers/Highway Funding. www.alec.org.

2. American Medical Association. Traffic death toll may be declining, but experts not ready to celebrate (and ensuing articles). *JAMA Medical News & Perspectives*. July 15, 1992, Vol. 268, No. 3:301-318.

3. Associated Press. Slowly, more motorists accepting cell phone ban. *Governors Highway Safety Association/ AP via eWatch Web Pubs*. August 24, 2003.

4. CDC. Achievements in public health, 1900-1999 motor-vehicle safety: A 20th century public health achievement. *MMWR*. May 14, 1999. 48(19);369-374.

5. CDC. Motor vehicle safety quick facts. National *Center for Injury Prevention and Control*. www.cdc.gov/ncipc/duip/factsmv.htm.

6. Durbin, Dee-Ann. Traffic deaths increase, injuries fall. *Governors Highway Safety Association*. www.statehigh-waysafety.org. July 17, 2003.

7. Ford Motor Company. Clue into safety/ Mobility: Our position/Safety: Our position. www.ford.com.

8. General Motors. A family affair: GM's crash test dummies have been making an impact on automotive safety for 25 years. *Safety/Protecting Occupants/Dummies*. www.gm.com. January 7, 2002.

9. General Motors. Congressman Dale Kildee joins greater Flint Safe Kids for Safety Seat checkup. *Safety/Protecting Occupants/Child Passenger Safety*. www.gm.com. October 22, 2003.

10. General Motors. History timelines: 1900 to 1930/1930 to 1940/1940 to 1960/1960 to 1970/1970 to 1980/1980 to 1990/1990 to 2000/2000 to 2002. www.gm.com.

11. Governors Highway Safety Association. What is GHSA? www.statehighwaysafety.org. Hakim, Danny. Once world leader in traffic safety, U.S. drops to No. 9. *New York Times*. November 27, 2003.

12. Hingson, Ralph, ScD, Heeren, Timothy, PhD, and Winter, Michael, MPH. Lowering state legal blood alcohol limits to 0.08%: The effect on fatal motor vehicle crashes. *American Journal of Public Health*. September 1996, Vol. 86, No. 9:1297-1299.

13. Insurance Institute for Highway Safety. DUI/DWI laws as of October 2003. www.iihs.org.

14. Insurance Institute for Highway Safety. Fatality facts: General 2002/Children 2002/State by State 2002/Gender 2002/Alcohol 2002/Older people 2002/Pedestrians 2002/Roadside hazards 2002/Teenagers 2002. www.iihs.org.

15. Insurance Institute for Highway Safety. Q&A: Alcohol: General/Administrative license suspension/Deterrence & enforcement. www.iihs.org. As of June 2003.

16. Insurance Institute for Highway Safety. Q&A: Pedestrians/Red light running/Speed and speed limits/Speed: Law enforcement/Urban crashes. www.iihs.org. As of June 2003.

17. Insurance Institute for Highway Safety. Q&A: Teenagers: General/Graduated driver licensing. www.iihs.org. As of June 2003.

18. Insurance Institute for Highway Safety. Status Report. *Vol. 38, No. 3.* March 15, 2003.

19. Johnson, Malcolm. Lawmakers go slow on cell phone bill: Measure to curb drivers' use lacks solid data in state. *Governors Highway Safety Administration/AP.* July 14, 2003.

20. Kafka, Joe. South Dakotans examine cell phone use: Legislators might tackle issue during upcoming session. *Governors Highway Safety Association/AP.* November 17, 2003.

21. Kristof, Nicholas D. 117 deaths each day. *New York Times.* March 13, 2004.

22. Lange, Robert C. Welcome from Bob Lange, Executive Director of Vehicle Safety, General Motors. www.gm.com.

23. Lundegaard, Karen, et al. New world goal: Halting rise in traffic deaths. *Wall Street Journal.* April 7, 2004.

24. Madigan, Erin. New Jersey cracks down on drowsy driving. *Governors Highway Safety Association/Stateline.org.* November 18, 2003.

25. McCartt, Anne T., PhD, Braver, Elisa R., PhD, and Geary, Lori L., MPH. Drivers' use of hand-held cell phones before and after New York State's cell phone law. *Preventive Medicine.* 36 (2003) 629-635.

26. Miami Herald. Car Safety Devices Hailed as Life-Savers. January 19, 2005.

27. Miami Herald. Death rate in accidents high among Hispanic children. *Road Safety/AP.* October 7, 2003.

28. National Center for Statistics and Analysis. Motor vehicle traffic crashes as a leading cause of death in the United States for 2000, by age group. www.nrd.nhtsa.dot.gov.

29. National Safety Council. Dr. William Haddon, Jr., Class of 1987/Dr. John Lane, Class of 1987/James Economos, Class of 1988/Nils Bohlin, Class of 1989/Dr. Richard Bishop, Class of 1989/Hugh DeHaven, Class of 1990/Louis Morony, Class of 1990/William Franey, Class of 1991/Dr. Thomas Seals, Class of 1992/Elizabeth Dole, Class of 1993/Don Buck, Class of 1997. *Safety & Health Hall of Fame International.* www.shhofi.org.

30. New York City Department of Transportation. Safety City: A program for NYC school children/Safety information/Safety Programs/Traffic safety educational materials. www.nyc.gov.

31. Pickler, Nedra. Alcohol-related traffic death rate drops. *Governors Highway Safety Association/AP.* December 18, 2002.

32. Porter, A. First fatal car crash in Britain occurred in 1898. Letter to Editor, *BMJ,* Vol. 317, July 18, 1998.

33. Robertson, Leon S., PhD. Reducing death on the road: The effects of minimum safety standards, publicized crash tests, seat belts, and alcohol. *American Journal of Public Health.* January 1996, Vol. 86, No. 1:31-34.

34. Subramanian, Rajesh. Motor vehicle traffic crashes as a leading cause of death in the United States, 2000. *National Center for Statistics and Analysis/Traffic Safety Facts Research Note.* October 2003.

35. What You Need to Know About Inventors. The history of crash test dummies, Parts 1 and 2. http://inventors.about.com. 2003.

36. White, Joseph B. Latest highway deaths report paints a discouraging picture. *Wall Street Journal/*"Eyes on the Road." April 28, 2003.

37. Williams, Leslie. Cell phones get bad rap, experts say/Study: Driver gawking worse than talking. *Governors Highway Safety Association, Times Picayune.* August 26, 2003.

Case Study: Development of Seat Belts

1. Associated Press. More Americans buckling up than ever. *Governors Highway Safety Association/AP.* August 25, 2003.

2. Associated Press. Seat belt usage increases in 40 states, NHTSA says. AP. November 17, 2003.

3. Durbin, Dee-Ann. Nationwide seat belt campaign starts this week. *Governors Highway Safety Association/AP.* May 12, 2003.

4. Durbin, Dee-Ann. Study blames deaths on slack seat-belt laws. *Governors Highway Safety Association/AP.* November 17, 2003.

5. Ford Motor Company. Safety Belts: Belt-Minder/Booster Seats. www.ford.com.

6. General Motors. GM studies safety belt reminders that click with drivers. *Safety/News & Issues/News.* www.gm.com. November 24, 2003.

7. General Motors. Safety belt & child restrain use. *Public Policy Issues.* www.gm.com.

8. Golden, Al, MPH, and Hatcher, Barbara J., PhD, MPH, RN. Buckling up America: Making a difference at the local level. *American Journal of Public Health.* November 2001, Vol. 91, No. 11:1795-1796.

9. Insurance Institute for Highway Safety. Child restraint, belt laws as of October 2003. www.iihs.org.

10. Osberg, J. Scott, MA, and Di Scala, Carla, PhD. Morbidity among pediatric motor vehicle crash victims: The effectiveness of seat belts. *American Journal of Public Health.* March 1992, Vol. 82, No. 3:422-425.

11. Ritter, Karl. Nils Bohlin, inventor of three-point seat belt, dies in Sweden at 82. *Detroit News.* September 26, 2002.

12. School Transportation News. Occupant Restraint: Seat belt history. www.stnonline.com.

13. Sequi-Gomez, Maria, MD, ScD, et al. Where children sit in cars: The impact of Rhode Island's new legislation. *American Journal of Public Health.* February 2001, Vol. 91, No. 2:311-313.

14. U.S. Department of Transportation. New DOT data show rising safety belt use rates in most states. *NHTSA 49-03 News.* November 17, 2003.

15. U.S. Department of Transportation. Safety belt use in 2003. *NHTSA/NCSA.* DOT HS 809 646. September 2003.

16. Wald, Matthew L. TV ad campaign for seat belts to focus on high-risk drivers. *New York Times.* May 12, 2003.

17. White, Joseph B. Eyes on the Road: Regulators want tough push on enforcing seat-belt laws. *Wall Street Journal Online.* August 4, 2003.

Vignette: Air Bags

1. Bellis, Mary. Air Bags – Allen Breed. *What You Need to Know About Inventors.*

2. Cooper, Josephine S. Letter addressed to the Honorable Rosalyn G. Millman, Deputy Administrator, NHTSA, RE: Side air bag test procedure and evaluation protocol; alliance member commitment. *Alliance of Automobile Manufacturers.* August 8, 2000.

3. Ford Motor Company. Air bags. www.ford.com/en/innovation/safety/airbags.htm.

4. General Motor. Air bags. *Public Policy Issues.* www.gm.com.

5. Insurance Institute for Highway Safety. Q&A: air bags. www.iihs.org/safety_facts/qanda/airbags.htm. June 2003.

6. Massachusetts Institute of Technology. Allen K. Breed: Automotive air bags. *Inventor of the Week Archive, Lemelson-MIT Program.* http://web.mit.due/invent/iow/breed.html.

7. National Center for Statistics and Analysis. Special crash investigations: Adult drivers seriously injured by DAB normalized by vehicle registrations. October 1, 2003.

8. U.S. Department of Transportation. Counts for air bag-related fatalities and seriously injured persons: Counts for confirmed air bag-related fatalities through 10/1/2003. www.nrd.nhtsa.dot.gov.

9. Wald, Matthew L. Fear of air bag sends children to back seat, saving many. *New York Times.* August 27, 2003.

Looking Ahead: Advances in Automobile Manufacturing

1. Alliance of Automobile Manufacturers. Fast facts: Advanced technology, auto safety enhancements, clean vehicle facts/Cleaner fuels make cleaner cars. www.autoalliance.org.

2. Alliance of Automobile Manufactuerer. Automaker back nationwide safety belt enforcement campaign focusing on teens. *Press Release.* May 19, 2003.

3. Alliance of Automobile Manufacturers. Automakers demonstrate clean diesel vehicles. *Press Release.* October 16, 20003.

4. American Legislative Exchange Council. Air pollution and automobile emissions reductions, automobile insurance. www.alec.org.

5. Augenstein, David M. The race to the 21st century. *Fleet Equipment.* April 1995.

6. Bayles, Fred. States trying to shift the decline in driver's education. *Governors Highway Safety Assocation/USA Today.* September 22, 2003.

7. Coleman, Kate. Aging drivers can reassess their changing abilities. *Governors Highway Safety Association/Herald-Mail.* October 11, 2003.

8. Costales, Troy. Statement for NTSB symposium on driver education and training. *Governors Highway Safety Association.* October 28-29, 2003.

9. Evans, Leonard, D.Phil. A new traffic safety vision for the United States (Editorial). *American Journal of Public Health.* September 2003, Vol. 93, No. 9.

10. Ewing, Reid, PhD, Schieber, Richard A., MD, MPH, and Zegeer, Charles V., MS. Urban sprawl as a risk factor in motor vehicle occupant and pedestrial fatalities. *American Journal of Public Health.* September 2003, Vol. 93, No. 9:1541-1545.

11. Ferguson, Susan A., PhD, et al. Daylight Saving Time and motor vehicle crashes: The reduction in pedestrian and vehicle occupant fatalities. *American Journal of Public Health.* January 1995, Vol. 85, No. 1:92-95.

12. Ford Motor Company. Advanced vehicle technology/Rollover protection/Family safety/Telematics for safety/Intelligent architecture. *Public Policy.* www.ford.com.

13. Ford Motor Company. Air quality and vehicle emissions, driver distraction lab, global climate change, green materials, teen driver study. www.ford.com.

14. General Motors. Safety: Daytime running lamps (DRLs)/Driver distraction & workload/Light Trucks/Tire safety/Traffic safety. *Public Policy Issues.* www.gm.com.

15. General Motors. GM responds to new NHTSA dynamic rollover NCAP test program/OnStar helps police locate stolen vehicles quickly. *Safety/News & Issues/News.* www.gm.com. June 18, 2003.

16. General Motors. New GM study shows daytime running lamps continue to reduce crashes. *Safety/Helping You Avoid a Crash/New Features.* www.gm.com. October 28, 2003.

17. General Motors. GMC Savana and Chevrolet Express 15-passenger vans with vehicle stability enhancement system hit the market. *Safety/News & Issues/News.* www.gm.com. October 21, 2003.

18. General Motors. OnStar, GM help spearhead effort to improve emergency services response/OnStar Fact Sheet. *Safety/Security/OnStar.* www.gm.com. 2003.

19. Governors Highway Safety Association. Public Health and safety groups urge members of Congress to oppose H.R. 1305. www.statehighwaysafety.org. April 15, 2002.

20. Insurance Institute for Highway Safety. Q&A: Antilock brakes: Cars, truck, motorcycles/Q&A: Bumpers/Q&A: Daytime running lights. www.iihs.org. As of June 2003.

21. Lavizzo-Mourey, Risa, MD, MBA and McGinnis, J. Michael, MD, MPP. Making the case for active living communities (Editorial). *American Journal of Public Health.* September 2003, Vol. 93, No. 9.

22. McMahon, Patrick. Orlando tops list of danger zones for pedestrians: Road design puts speed over safety, report says; worst areas all in South. *Governors Highway Safety Association/USA Today.* November 21, 2002.

23. Retting, Richard A., MS, Ferguson, Susan A., PhD, and McCartt, Anne T., PhD. A review of evidence-based traffic engineering measure designed to reduce pedestrian-motor vehicle crashes. *American Journal of Public Health.* September 2003, Vol. 93, No. 9:1456-1463.3.

24. Retting, Richard A., MS, et al. Crash and injury reduction following installation of roundabouts in the United States. *American Journal of Public Health.* April 2001, Vol. 91, No. 4:628-631.

25. Retting, Richard A., MS, and Kyrychenko, Sergey Y., MS. Reductions in injury crashes associated with red light camera enforcement in Oxnard, California. *American Journal of Public Health.* November 2002, Vol. 92, No. 11:1822-1825.

26. Roberts, Ian. Reducing road traffic would improve quality of life as well as preventing injury. *Editorial, BMJ.* Vol. 316, January 24, 1998.

27. Scarborough, Senta. "In your face" ads make roads safer. *Governors Highway Safety Association/Arizona Republic.* August 30, 2003.

28. Strassburger, Robert. Letter to the Honorable Sue Bailey, Administrator, NHTSA, RE: Statement of principles on human machine interface (HMI) for in-vehicle information and communication systems. *Alliance of Automobile Manufacturers.* December 21, 2000.

29. Vartabedian, Ralph. Drunk-driving reforms stir safety debates. *Governors Highway Safety Association/LA Times.* October 2, 2003.

30. White, Joseph B. The danger of drowsy driving: States work to wake up motorists to hazards of driving while sleepy. *Wall Street Journal/*"Eyes on the Road." November 24, 2003.

31. White, Joseph B. The next frontier in automotive safety: Systems that stop driver's own mistakes. *Wall Street Journal/*"Eyes on the Road." October 18, 2004.

Chapter 3. *Environmental Health*

Looking Back

1. American Journal of Public Health. Built Environment and Health (entire issue). September 2003.

2. American Lung Association. Milestones in air pollution history. www.californialung.org/spotlight/clearnair03-milestones.html.

3. Bailey, Ronald. Silent Spring at 40: Rachel Carson's classic is not aging well. *ReasonOnline.* June 12, 2002.

4. Baker, Randall. Rachel Carson's Silent Spring and the beginning of the environmental movement in the United States. www.spea.indiana.edu/bakerr/v600/rachel_carson_and_silent_spring.htm.

5. Global Lead Network. Timeline: 8,500 years of lead, 79 years of leaded gasoline. www.globalleadnet.org/advocacy/initiatives/TIMEnation.cfm.

6. History of selected public health events in Chicago, 1834-1999. From *Public Health: What It Is and How It Works,* 2nd Edition (Aspen Publishers). www.aspenpublishers.com/books.

7. Jackson, Richard J., MD, MPH. The impact of the built environment on health: An emerging field (Editorial). *American Journal of Public Health.* September 2003, Vol. 93, No. 9:1382-1383.

8. Markowitz, Gerald, and Rosner, David. *Deceit and Denial: The Deadly Politics of Industrial Pollution.* The Milbank Memorial Fund, University of California Press (Berkeley and Los Angeles, CA). 2002.

9. National Resources Defense Council. The story of Silent Spring. Toxic Chemicals & Health: Pesticides: In Brief: History. www.nrdc.org/health/pesticides/hcarson.asp.

10. Rogers, Paul G. The Clean Air Act of 1970. *EPA Journal.* U.S. Environmental Protection Agency. January/February 1990.

11. Ramazzini Institute for Occupational and Environmental Health Research. The Selikoff Fund for Environmental and Occupational Cancer Research. Genes, Ethics & Environment. www.ramazziniusa.org.

12. Rosner, David, and Markowitz, Gerald. Lead: The relevance of history. Mealey's Litigation Report: Lead. www.mealeys.com/ledcom.html. November 1, 2001; Vol. 11, Issue 3.

13. Samet, Jonathan M., MD, MS, and Spengler, John D., PhD. Indoor environments and health: Moving into the 21st century. *American Journal of Public Health.* September 2003, Vol. 93, No. 9:1489-1493.

14. U.S. Environmental Protection Agency. www.epa.gov/history/org/orginins/reorg.htm.

15. U.S. Environmental Protection Agency. www.epa.gov/history/topics/caa70/11.htm.

16. Warren, Christian. *Brush with Death: A Social History of Lead Poisoning.* The Johns Hopkins University Press (Baltimore, MD). 2000.

Case Study: Lead Poisoning

1. American Academy of Pediatrics. Screening for elevated blood lead levels (RE9815). *Pediatrics/Policy Statement.* June 1998, Vol. 101, No. 6:1072-1078.

2. Brody, Jane E. Even low lead levels pose perils for children. *New York Times.* August 5, 2003.

3. CDC. Blood lead levels in young children − United States and selected states, 1996-1999. *MMWR.* December 22, 2000. 49(50);1133-7.

4. CDC. CDC's Lead Poisoning Prevention Program. *National Center for Environment Health.* www.cdc.gov/nceh/lead/factsheets/leadfcts.htm.

5. CDC. Childhood Lead Poisoning. *National Center for Environmental Health.* www.cdc.gov/nceh/lead.

6. CDC. Fatal pediatric lead poisoning − New Hampshire, 2000. *MMWR.* June 8, 2001. 50(22);457-9.

7. CDC. Managing elevated blood lead levels among young children: Recommendations from the Advisory Committee on Childhood Lead Poisoning Prevention. National *Center for Environmental Health.* www.cdc.gov/nceh/lead/CaseManagement/QA_CM.htm.

8. CDC. Trends in blood lead levels among children − Boston, Massachusetts, 1994-1999. *MMWR.* May 4, 2001. 50(17);337-9.

9. Healthy People 2010. Objectives 8-11. Eliminate elevated blood lead levels in children. *Toxics and Waste.*

10. Heinz Awards. Environment: Herbert Needleman, 2nd Annual Heinz Award Recipient. www.heinzawards.net.

11. Johnson, Gordon S., Jr. Testimony of Don Ryan, Executive Director, Alliance to End Childhood Lead Poisoning, on Policy Driven Lawsuits. *To Senate Judiciary Committee.* November 2, 1999.

12. Kitman, Jamie Lincoln. The secret history of lead. *The Nation.* March 20, 2000.

13. Kovarick, William and Hermes, Matthew E. Fuels and society C: 4. Phase out of lead (TEL). *Kennesaw State University.* http://chemcases.com.

14. Lead Advisory Service Australia. The importance of the availability of "spot tests" for lead in paint. *A factsheet for hardware & paint trade store manager.* www.lead.org.au/fs/fst14.html.

15. LEAD Group, Inc. Australian world first with ban on candles that can cause lead poisoning. *LEAD Action News Fact Sheet.* Vol. 7, No. 4.

16. MECA. MECA advocates the banning of lead in gasoline worldwide. *Press Release.* November 16, 1998.

17. Nash, Denis, PhD, MPH, et al. Blood lead, blood pressure, and hypertension in perimenopausal and post-menopausal women. JAMA. March 26, 2003, Vol. 289, No. 12:1523-1532.

18. National Safety Council. Lead Poisoning. *Fact Sheet Library.* www.nsc.org/library/facts/lead.htm.

19. New York State Department of Health. Physician's Handbook on Childhood Lead Poisoning Prevention. *Info for Providers.* www.health.state.ny.us/nysdoh/lead/handbook/phc1.htm.

20. Parkins, Patricia. Lead Poisoning Awareness Day 2000: Have we really resolved the lead issue? *Lead Advisory Serviced Australia.* www.lead.org.au/fs/fst13.html. Last updated March 27, 2003.

21. Pertowski, Carol. A., MD. Lead Poisoning: Public Health Importance in "From Data to Action: CDC's Public Health Surveillance for Women, Infants, and Children." *Child Health.*

22. Reyes, Jessica Wolpaw. The impact of prenatal lead exposure on infant health. *Department of Economics, Amherst College/University of Texas Austin.* 2003.

23. Rhode Island Department of Health. Rhode Island Lead Screening Plan. *RIDOH Childhood Lead Poisoning Prevention Program.* October 2000.

24. Romano, Jay. Lead paint regulation is in limbo. *New York Times.* July 13, 2003.

25. SecurityWorld.com. The dangers of lead poisoning. *The Education Station.* www.securityworld.com/library/health/leadpoisoning.html.

26. University of North Carolina Chapel Hill School of Public Health. Working together: Community-based approaches to prevent childhood lead poisoning. *Environmental Resource Program.*

27. U.S. Department of Health and Human Services, Centers for Disease Control and Prevention. Recommendations for blood lead screening of young children enrolled in Medicaid: Targeting a group at high risk. Atlanta, Georgia. *Advisory Committee on Childhood Lead Poisoning Prevention (ACCLPP)/MMWR Recommendations and Reports.* December 8, 2000, Vol. 49, No. RR-14.

28. U.S. Department of Housing and Urban Development. Martinez announces $6.5 million to protect children from lead hazards at home. *Press Release.* www.hud.gov/news. February 5, 2003.

29. U.S. Department of Justice. U.S. settles cases against Chicago, N.Y. and L.A. landlords: More than 16,000 apartments to become lead safe. *Press Release.* www.usdoj.gov. October 2, 2001.

30. U.S. Environmental Protection Agency. EPA's efforts to reduce lead. *Air Quality Where You Live.* www.epa.gov/air/urbanair/lead/effrt.html. Last updated October 16, 2002.

31. U.S. Environmental Protection Agency. Lead Awareness Program: Protect your child from lead poisoning. *Lead in Paint, Dust, and Soil.* www.epa.gov/opptintr/lead/index.html.

32. U.S. Senate Committee on Banking, Housing, and Urban Affairs. Hearing on "Lead-based paint poisoning: Federal responses"; Prepared statement of Mr. Adam Sharp, Assistant Associate Administrator, Office of Prevention, Pesticides and Toxic Substances, Environmental Protection Agency. *Subcommittee on Housing and Transportation.* June 5, 2002.

33. World Bank Group. Removal of lead from gasoline. *Pollution Prevention and Abatement Handbook.* Effective July 1998.

34. World Health Organization. Asia: Experts call on governments to remove lead from gasoline. *Press Release WHO/15.* March 7, 2002.

Vignette: Asbestos

1. Agency for Toxic Substances and Disease Registry. Proposed public health response plan for Libby, Montana and other sites with exposure to tremolite asbestos in vermiculite ore. *ATSDR Resources & Studies on Asbestos.* May 31, 2000.

2. Agency for Toxic Substances and Disease Registry. Year 2000 medical testing of individuals potentially exposed to asbestoform minerals associated with vermiculite in Libby, Montana: A report to the community. *ATSDR Resources & Studies on Asbestos.* August 23, 2001.

3. American Insurance Association. The asbestos litigation crisis by the numbers. *AIA Advocate.* January 3, 2003.

4. Asbestos Victims' Compensation Act of 2003. H.R. 1737. *108th Congress, 1st Session.* April 10, 2003.

5. Beck, Darlene. Libby's future defeat is not a community trait. www.folkways.org.

6. CDC. Current trends use of death certificates for surveillance of work-related illnesses – New Hampshire. MMWR. August 29, 1986. 35(34);537-40.

7. Early, Ludwick, Sweeney and Strauss, LLC. What is mesothelioma? *Asbestos Diseases/Mesothelioma.* www.mesothelioma.com.

8. Egilman, David, MD, MPH. WebMD live chat transcript: The hazards of asbestos with David Egilman, MD. October 7, 1999. www.mesotheliomaweb.org.

9. Falk, Henry, MD, MPH. Statement on ATSDR's public health response plan in Libby, MT before the Senate Committee on Environment and Public Works Subcommittee on Superfund, Toxics, Risk, and Waste Management. *Department of Health & Human Services/Assistant Secretary for Legislation.* www.hhs.gov/asl/testify. June 20, 2002.

10. Gee, David, and Greenberg, Morris. Chapter 5. Asbestos: from "magic" to malevolent mineral (from "late lessons from early warnings: the precautionary principle 1896-2000). *European Environmental Agency/EEA Reports.* Environmental Issue Report No. 22. 2002.

11. Global Environment & Technology Foundation. Asbestos strategies: GETF releases recommendations report on asbestos use and management. www.getf.org. May 16, 2003.

12. Harvard Medical School. Malignant mesothelioma. www.intelihealth.com. Last reviewed March 27, 2001.

13. Kazan-Allen, Laurie. New research confirms hazards of asbestos-cement. March 16, 2003. www.btinternet.com.

14. KazanLaw. The firm's role in asbestos litigation. www.kazanlaw.com.

15. KazanLaw. What is asbestos? www.mesothelioma-facts.com

16. KazanLaw. What are asbestos diseases?/Asbestosis/Benign pleural diseases. www.mesothelioma-facts.com. 2003.

17. Legal Information Institute. Sec. 4011. – Findings and purpose. *US Code Collection.* Title 20, Chapter 52 and Title 15, Chapter 53.

18. Martin, Lawrence, MD, FACP, FCCP. Runaway asbestos litigation – why it's a medical problem. www.mtsinai.org/pulmonary/Asbestos/AsbestosEditorial.htm. Revised November 18, 2002.

19. Mesothelioma Facts and Information Newsletter. Asbestos in the home. www.mesothelioma-facts.com.

20. Mesothelioma Facts and Information Newsletter. What is mesothelioma? www.mesothelioma-facts.com. August 4, 2003.

21. Molloy, Laurence B. Background on asbestos. www.nyenvirolaw.org. February 7, 2002.

22. Ravenesi, Bill. Gallery I Breath Taken: The Landscape & Biography of Asbestos, An Exhibition. *Boston University School of Public Health, Department of Environmental Health.* www.bumc.bu.edu/SPH/Gallery. 1990.

23. Renner, Rebecca. Asbestos in the air. *ScientificAmerican.com.* February 21, 2000.

24. Rowley Ashworth, Solicitors. Asbestos-related disease – still a serious problem. *RA Briefing.* www.asbestosadvice.co.uk.

25. *Sacramento Bee.* "The Asbestos Danger." www.sacbee.com/static/archive.news/projects/asbestos/harm.html.

26. Schneider, Andrew and Smith, Carol. Asbestos industry pays Crayola's expert millions. *Seattle Post-Intelligencer.* May 30, 2000.

27. Schneider, Andrew and Smith, Carol. Certified lab finds crayon asbestos, ABC reports. *Seattle Post-Intelligencer.* May 27, 2000.

28. Schneider, Andrew and Smith, Carol. Major brands of kids' crayons contain asbestos, tests show. *Seattle Post-Intelligencer.* May 23, 2000.

29. Schneider, Andrew and Smith, Carol. Old dispute rekindled over content of mine's talc. *Seattle Post-Intelligencer.* May 30, 2000.

30. Sebok, Anthony J. The new asbestos bill, Part One: Why it is imperative that it pass. *Asbestos Claims Trust/LitigationDataSource.com.* July 22, 2003.

31. U.S. Environmental Protection Agency. Asbestos in your home. www.epa.gov/asbestos/ashome.html. Updated January 15, 2003.

32. U.S. Environmental Protection Agency. Asbestos Ban and Phase Out. www.epa.gov/asbestos/ban.html. Updated January 15, 2003.

33. U.S. Environmental Protection Agency. Common questions on the Asbestos NESHAP. www.epa.gov/region04/air/asbestos/asbqa.htm.

34. U.S. Environmental Protection Agency. EPA Asbestos Materials Bans: Clarification. May 18, 1999.

35. U.S. Environmental Protection Agency. Lead Contamination Control and Asbestos Information Acts of 1988. *History/Press Release.* www.epa.gov. November 1, 1988.

36. U.S. Geological Survey. Some facts about asbestos. *USGS Fact Sheet FS-01201.* March 2001.

37. Work Safe. What kinds of building materials may contain asbestos? www.worksafe.org. 2003.

38. Work Safe. Where might I find asbestos in my home? www.worksafe.org. 2003.

39. Zumwalt, James G. II, Lt. Col. USMCR (Ret.). Statement to Senate Hearing. June 17, 2002. www.mesothel.com

Looking Ahead: Asthma

1. AAAAI. Tips to remember: Asthma & Allergy Medications. *American Academy of Allergy, Asthma and Immunology.* www.aaaai.org/patients.

2. American Thoracic Society. Two differing pathologies in severe asthma. *Press Release Archives.* www.thoracic.org/news. September 1999.

3. Asthma and Allergy Foundation of America. Asthma: What is Asthma? www.aafa.org.

4. Ball, Thomas M., MD, MPH, et al. Siblings, day-care attendance, and the risk of asthma and wheezing during childhood. *New England Journal of Medicine.* August 24, 2000, Vol. 343, No. 8:538-543.

5. BlackHealthCare.com. Asthma: A concern for minority populations. *Asthma – Description.* www.blackhealthcare.com/BHC/Asthma/Description.asp.

6. Braun-Fahrlaender, Charlotte, MD, et al. Environmental exposure to endotoxin and its relation to asthma in school-age children. *New England Journal of Medicine.* September 19, 2002, Vol. 437, No. 12:869-877.

7. Brody, Jane E. Even low lead levels pose perils for children. *New York Times.* August 5, 2003.

8. Brody, Jane E. Families grab an asthma lifeline that keeps children well and active. *New York Times.* October 28, 2003.

9. Busse, William W., MD, and Lemanske, Robert F., MD. Asthma. *New England Journal of Medicine.* February 1, 2001, Vol. 344, No. 5:350-362.

10. Cardwell, Diane. 1 in 3 children in Brooklyn area exposed to dangerous lead levels, a study finds. *New York Times.* June 9, 2003.

11. CDC. CDC study links improved air quality with decreased emergency visits for asthma. *Press Release, Media Relations.* February 21, 2001.

12. Clean School Bus. Whitman announces new partnership to reduce children's exposure to emissions from diesel school buses. www.epa.gov/cleanschoolbus. April 7, 2003.

13. Coyle, Yvonne Marie, MD, et al. Effectiveness of acute asthma care among inner-city adults. *Archives of Internal Medicine.* July 14, 2003, Vol. 163, No. 13.

14. D'Amato, G. Environmental urban factors (air pollution and allergens) and the rising trends in allergic respiratory diseases. *Allergy/Blackwell Synergy.* August 2002, Vol. 57, Issue s72, Page 30.

15. Edozien, Frankie. Kids breathe easier as asthma plummets. *New York Post.* January 14, 2004.

16. Fang, Kezhong et al. S-nitrosoglutathione breakdown prevents airway smooth muscle relaxation in the guinea pig. *American Journal of Physiology – Lung Cellular and Molecular Physiology.* October 2000, Vol. 279, Issue 4, L716-721.

17. Fidler, Eric. School health centers benefit asthmatics. *Associated Press.* February 10, 2003.

18. Frisch, Dana. Asthma symptoms go untreated in many teens. *Yahoo News/Reuters Health.* June 13, 2003.

19. Fujimoto, Keisaku, et al. Sputum eosinophilia and bronchial responsiveness in patients with chronic non-productive cough responsive to anti-asthma therapy. *Blackwell Synergy.* June 2003, Vol. 8, Issue 2, Page 168.

20. Geraghty, Jim. The Cairo street. *National Review Online.* June 4, 2003.

21. Health News. Study looks at asthma risk, indoor pools. *Occupational & Environmental Medicine.* May 25, 2003; 60L385-394.

22. Hoppe, Carrie. Advances in treating asthma and allergic diseases. *Discover.* March 2000. JHMI. Race plus roaches: A breathtaking link. www.hopkinsmedicine.org/press. June 11, 1996.

23. LaurusHealth.com. Breathing easier: New advances help doctors understand and treat asthma effectively. *Future of Medicine.* C.2003 VHA.

24. LaurusHealth.com. FDA expected to OK first biotech asthma drug. *Today's Headlines.* June 6, 2003.

25. LaurusHealth.com. In some, throat clearing first sign of asthma. *Today's Headlines/Reuters Health.* April 4, 2003.

26. LaurusHealth.com. Study gives more proof of "thunderstorm asthma." *Today's Headlines/Reuters Health.* March 13, 2003.

27. LaurusHealth.com. Traffic pollution linked to severe asthma attacks. *Today's Headlines/Reuters.* June 6, 2003.

28. Lindqvist, Ari, MD, et al. Salmeterol resolves airway obstruction but does not possess anti-eosinophil efficacy in newly diagnosed asthma: A randomized, double-blind, parallel group biopsy study comparing the effects of salmeterol, fluticasone propionate, and disodium cromoglycate. *Journal of Allergy and Clinical Immunology.* July 2003, Vol. 112, No. 1.

29. Masoli, Matthew, MBBS, MRCP, Holt, Shaun, BPharm, MBChB, and Beasley, Richard, MBChB, FRACP, DM. Editorial: What to do at step 3 of the asthma guidelines – increase the dose of inhaled corticosteroids or add a long-acting beta-agonist drug? *Journal of Allergy and Clinical Immunology.* 2003;112:10-1.

30. Murphy, Kate. Fight for Breath. *UTMB Quarterly.* Winter 2000.

31. National Institutes of Health. Grants awarded to implement inner-city asthma intervention. *NIH Press Release.* February 5, 2001.

32. Nelson, BV, et al. Expired nitric oxide as a marker for childhood asthma (Abstract). *Journal of Pediatrics.* March 1997, 130(3).

33. Neumeister, Larry. Study: 1 in 4 Harlem children has asthma. *Associated Press.* April 21, 2003.

34. NIAID. Asthma and allergy statistics. *Fact Sheet.* www.medhelp.org/NIHlib/DG-489.html.

35. NIAID. NIAID inner-city asthma study finds multiple factors lead to increased asthma morbidity. *NIAID-NEWS Press Release.* February 19, 1997.

36. NIAID. Significant items in House and Senate Appropriations Committee Reports, FY2002. http://biodefense.niaid.nih.gov/director/congress/2002/cj/sigitems.htm.

37. NIAID. NIAID Study: Cockroaches important cause of asthma morbidity among inner-city children. www.hhs.gov/news/press/1997pres/970507b.html. May 7, 1997.

38. Perez-Pena, Richard. Asthma project reaches out in Harlem. *New York Times.* May 1, 2003.

39. Picado, C. et al. Dietary micronutrients/antioxidants and their relationship with bronchial asthma severity. *Allergy/Blackwell Synergy.* January 2001, Vol. 56, Issue 1, Page 43.

40. Ricks, Delthia. Assessing the scope of WTC ailments: Experts study how lung ills may worsen. *Newsday.* October 1, 2002.

41. Rosenstreich, David L., MD, et al. The role of cockroach allergy and exposure to cockroach allergen in causing morbidity among inner-city children with asthma. *New England Journal of Medicine.* May 8, 1997, Vol. 336, No. 19:1356-1363.

42. Schmid, Randolph E. Compound may improve treatment for asthma. www.salon.com (Associated Press). January 11, 2004.

43. Szczeklik, A., Nizankowska, E., and Duplaga, M. Natural history of aspirin-induced asthma (Abstract). *European Respiratory Journal/Blackwell Synergy.* September 2000, Vol. 16, Issue 3, Page 432.

44. University of Virginia Health System. Helping millions to breathe normally. *Report from the Dean, 2000-2001.*

45. Weiss, Scott T., MD. Eat dirt – the hygiene hypothesis and allergic diseases (Editorial). *New England Journal of Medicine.* September 19, 2002, Vol. 347, No. 12:930-931.

46. Wijga, AH, et al. Association of consumption of products containing milk fat with reduced asthma risk in pre-school children: The PIAMA birth cohort study. *Thorax.* 2003;58:567-572.

Chapter 4. *Infectious Disease Control*

Looking Back

1. Altman, Lawrence K., MD. The search for SARS's past may help predict its future. *New York Times.* May 20, 2003.

2. Bakalar, Nicholas. More diseases pinned on old culprit: Germs. *New York Times.* May 17, 2005.

3. Baker, Jeffrey P. and Katz, Samuel L. Childhood vaccine development: An overview. *Pediatric Research.* Vol. 55, No. 2, 2004.

4. Berlinguer, Giovanni. The interchange of disease and health between the old and new worlds. *International Journal of Health Services.* 1993, Vol. 93, No. 4:703-715.

5. Campos-Outcalt, Doug, MD, MPA, and Aickin, Mikel, PhD. Incidence of infectious disease and the licen-sure of immunobiologics in the United States. *American Journal of Preventive Medicine.* Vol. 13, No. 2, 1997.

6. CDC. Achievements in Public Health, 1900-1999: Control of Infectious Diseases. *MMWR.* July 30, 1999, Vol. 48, No. 29.

7. CDC. Centers for Disease Control (CDC) in the United States: 50 years. From *Epidemiological Bulletin/PAHO.* Vol. 17, No. 3 (1996).

8. CDC. Control of infectious diseases, 1900-1999. *MMWR.* 1999;48:621-629.

9. CDC. Notifiable disease surveillance and notifiable disease statistics – United States, June 1946 and June 1996. *MMWR.* June 28, 1996, Vol. 45, No. 25.

10. CDC. Part 3: Historical summaries of notifiable diseases in the United States, 1970-2001. *MMWR.* May 2, 2003, Vol. 50, No. 53.

11. CDC. Questions and answers about TB. *National Center for HIV, STD, and TB Prevention/Division of Tuberculosis Elimination.* www.cdc.gov/nchstp/tb.

12. CDC. Summary of notifiable diseases, United States 1990. *MMWR.* October 4, 1991, Vol. 39, No. 53.

13. Cohen, Mitchell L. Changing patterns of infectious disease. *Nature.* August 17, 2000, Vol. 406.

14. Cunha, Burke A., MD, Guest Editor. Historical aspects of infectous diseases, part I (Preface). *Infectious Disease Clinics of North America.* 18 (2004) xi-xv.

15. Curtis, Valerie, and Biran, Adam. Dirt, disgust, and disease: Is hygiene in our genes? *Perspectives in Biology and Medicine.* Winter 2001, Vol. 44, No. 1:17-31.

16. Denny, Floyd W., Jr. Infectious diseases and the last 100 years in the American Pediatric Society. *Pediatric Research.* Vol. 27, No. 6 (Suppl), 1990.

17. Donoghue, Helen D. et al. Tuberculosis: From prehistory to Robert Koch, as revealed by ancient DNA. *The Lancet.* September 2004, Vol, 4.

18. Dowling, Harry F., MD. Human experimentation in infectious diseases. *JAMA.* November 28, 1966, Vol. 198, No. 9.

19. Drotman, D. Peter. Emerging infectious diseases: A brief biolographical heritage. *Emerging Infectious Diseases.* July-September 1998, Vol. 4, No. 3.

20. Evans, Alfred S. Ruminations on infectious disease epidemiology: Retrospective, curspective, and prospective, with discussion by Phil Brachman and R.H. Morrow. *International Journal of Epidemiology.* 1985, Vol. 14, No. 2.

21. Ewald, Paul W., PhD. Evolution of virulence. *Infectious Disease Clinics of North America.* 18 (2004) 1-15.

22. Fauci, Anthony S. Fifty years: Advancing knowledge, improving health (Scientific Address). *Journal of Human Virology.* January/February 1999, Vol. 2, No. 1.

23. Finland, Maxwell. Gaps in therapy for infectious diseases: A historical perspective (with a Conference Summary). *Journal of Infectious Diseases.* Vol. 145, No. 3, March 1982.

24. Grady, Denise, and Altman, Lawrence K. Beyond cute: Exotic pets come bearing exotic germs. *New York Times.* June 17, 2003.

25. Gibbs, Ronald S., MD. After Office Hours: Impact of infectious diseases on women's health, 1776-2026. *Obstetrics & Gynecology.* Vol. 97, No. 5, June 2001.

26. Greenwood, David. Reflections at the end of the millennium (Editorial). *Journal of Medical Microbiology.* Vol. 48 (1999), 1051-1053.

27. Imperato, Pascal James. Historical precedent and the obligation to treat AIDS patients. *Journal of Community Health.* Winter 1989, Vol. 14, No. 4.

28. Jarcho, Saul, MD. Transatlantic transmission of infectious diseases: The applicability of paleopathology. *Bulletin of the New York Academy of Medicine.* Vol. 66, No. 6, November-December, 1990.

29. Kass, Edward H., MD, PhD. A brief perspective on the early history of American infectious disease epidemiology. *Yale Journal of Biology and Medicine.* 60 (1987), 341-348.

30. Kass, Edward H., MD, PhD. History of the specialty of infectious diseases in the United States. *Annals of Internal Medicine.* May, 1987, Vol. 106, No. 5:745-756.

31. King, Nicholas B. The scale politics of emerging diseases. *Osiris.* 2004, 19: 062-076.

32. Kinkead, Gwen. To study disease, Britain plans a genetic census. *New York Times.* December 31, 2002.

33. Landsberger, Max, MD. Communicable diseases across the oceans. *New York State Journal of Medicine.* August 1975.

34. Lederberg, Joshua. Pathways of Discovery/Infectious History. *Science.* Vol. 288, April 14, 2000.

35. Mechnikov, Il'ia Il'ich. Classics in infectious diseases: Immunity in infective diseases. *Reviews of Infectious Diseases.* Vol. 10, No. 1, January-February, 1988.

36. Melosi, Martin V. Cleaning up our act: Germ consciousness in America. *Reviews in American History.* 27 (1999) 259-266.

37. Mortimer, Edward A., Jr. Immunization against infectious disease. *Science.* Vol. 200, May 26, 1978.

38. Nathanson, Neal, and Alexander, E. Russell. Infectious disease epidemiology. *American Journal of Epidemiology.* Vol. 144, No. 8 (Suppl), 1996.

39. National Institutes of Health. Teacher's Guide: Understanding emerging and re-emerging infectious diseases. http://science.education.nih.gov.

40. Petersen, Eskild A., MD, and Mandel, Richard M., MD. Infectious diseases: Old diseases return and new agents emerge (Editorial). Archives of Internal Medicine. August 7/21, 1995, Vol. 155.

41. Ramsay, A. Melvin, MA, MD. Infectious diseases. *The Practitioner.* May 1980, Vol. 224.

42. Risse, Guenter B. Epidemics and medicine: The influence of disease on medical thought and practice. *Bulletin of the History of Medicine.* Vol. 53, 1979.

43. Robbins, Jim. Montana lab tries to identify tick-borne disease. *New York Times.* May 20, 2003.

44. Rosati, Louis A., MD. The microbe, creator of the pathologist: An inter-related history of pathology, microbiology, and infectious disease. *Annals of Diagnostic Pathology.* Vol. 5, No. 3 (June), 2001: pp. 184-189.

45. Satcher, David, MD, PhD. Emerging infections: Getting ahead of the curve. *Emerging Infectious Diseases.* Vol. 1, No. 1, January-March 1995.

46. Schwartz, David A. and Herman, Chester J. Editorial response: The importance of the autopsy in emerging and re-emerging infectious disease. *Clinical Infectious Diseases.* 1996;23:248-54.

47. Sink, Mindy. West Nile virus is still a threat as fall nears. *New York Times.* September 16, 2003.

48. Thomson, Daniel, CB, MD. The ebb and flow of infection. *JAMA.* January 19, 1976, Vol. 235, No. 3.

49. Tomes, Nancy, PhD. The making of a germ panic, then and now. *American Journal of Public Health.* February 2000, Vol. 90, No. 2.

50. Weinstein, Louis. Infectious diseases (Editorial). *Hospital Practice.* October 1976.

51. Weksler, Marc E. Immunology and the elderly: An historical perspective for future international action. *Mechanisms of Aging and Development (Elsevier).* 93 (1997) 1-6.

52. Wilson, Mary E., MD. Travel and the emergence of infectious diseases. *Emerging Infectious Diseases.* Vol. 1, No. 2, April-June 1995.

53. Winkelstein, Warren, Jr. Epidemiologic highlights of the past with look towards the future. Journal of Public Health Policy. Vol. 22, No. I.

54. Yoshikawa, Thomas T. Perspective: Aging and infectious Diseases: Past, present, and future. *Journal of Infectious Diseases.* 1997;176:1053-7.

Case Study: HIV/AIDS

1. AIDS Education Global Information System. So little time…An AIDS history. www.aegis.com/topics/timeline.

2. Altman, Lawrence K., MD. AIDS expert helps doctors learn from the dead to help the living. *New York Times.* February 18, 2003.

3. Altman, Lawrence K. Officials Push Use of a 20-Minute H.I.V. Test. *New York Times.* February 12, 2003.

4. CDC. A glance at the HIV epidemic. *HIV/AIDS Update.*

5. CDC. Basic statistics. *National Center for HIV, STD and TB Prevention, Divisions of HIV/AIDS Prevention.* www.cdc.gov/hiv/stats.htm. July 6, 2004.

6. CDC. CDC-HIV vaccine unit: The world needs a vaccine. *National Center for HIV, STD and TB Prevention/Divisions of HIV/AIDS Prevention.* www.cdc.gov/hiv/vaccine. April 12, 1999.

7. CDC. CDC-funded study to examine critical questions in HIV vaccine research. *Update.* April 2001.

8. CDC. Diagnoses of HIV/AIDS – 32 States, 2000-2003. *MMWR.* December 3, 2004, Vol. 53, No. 47:1106-1110.

9. CDC. Fact Sheets: HIV and its transmission//HIV/AIDS among African Americans//HIV/AIDS among Hispanics//HIV/AIDS among women/Human Immunodifficiency Virus Type 2/Young people at risk: HIV/AIDS among America's youth. *National Center for HIV, STD and TB Prevention/Divisions of HIV/AIDS Prevention.* www.cdc.gov/hiv/pubs/facts. Updates from March 11, 2002 through December 2, 2004.

10. CDC. Frequently asked questions: What is AIDS?/What is HIV?/Where did HIV come from? *National Center for HIV, STD and TB Prevention/Divisions of HIV/AIDS Prevention.* www.cdc.gov.hiv/pubs/faq.

11. CDC. HIV/AIDS surveillance report: Cases of HIV infection and AIDS in the United States, 2003. www.cdc.gov/hiv/stats/hasrlink.htm. 2004, Vol. 15:1-46.

12. CDC. HIV prevalence trends in selected populations in the United States: Results from National Serosurveillance, 1993-1997. *National Center for HIV, STD and TB Prevention/Divisions of HIV/AIDS Prevention.* www.cdc.gov/hiv/pubs/hivprevalence. November 14, 2001.

13. Dreifus, Claudia. Agency seeks a virus-killer for women to help control the spread of AIDS; A conversation with Zeda Rosenberg. *New York Times.* July 29, 2003.

14. Hughes, Walter T., MD. Prologue to AIDS: The recognition of infectious opportunists. *Medicine.* Williams & Wilkins, Baltimore. 1998, Vol. 77, No. 4:227-32.

15. Johnston, Margaret I. and Flores, Jorge. Progress in HIV vaccine development. *Current Opinion in Pharmacology.* Elsevier Science, Ltd. 2001, Vol. 1:504-510.

16. Lerner, Sharon. Making new efforts to convince youths they're not invulnerable to H.I.V. *New York Times.* August 5, 2003.

17. LGBT Health Channel. HIV & AIDS. www.gayhealthchannel.com/hivaids/history.shtml. March 9, 2004.

18. McNeil, Donald G., Jr. From Eli Lilly to front line in AIDS war. *New York Times.* July 29, 2003.

19. Rojcewicz, Stephen J., Jr., MD. AIDS controversies in the mirror of history (Letters to the Editor). *American Journal of Psychiatry.* July 1988, Vol. 145, No. 7:898.

20. Sartorius, Norman. Paths of Medicine: The puzzle of AIDS. *Croatian Medical Journal.* 2004, Vol. 45, No. 2:230-231.

21. Sternberg, Steve. AIDS fight hits racial divide: Vaccine's effects on black patients ignites social and scientific storm. *USA Today.* April 1, 2003.

22. The NIAID Division of AIDS. General Info: Challenges in developing AIDS vaccines/Developing a safe and effective AIDS vaccine. www.niaid.nih.gov/daids/vaccine.

23. Vaughan, Marvin A., MD, and Li, James T.C., MD, PhD. Prevention of AIDS: Lessons from Osler (To the Editor). *New England Journal of Medicine.* June 12, 1986, Vol. 314, No. 24:1578-79.

24. U.S. Department of Health and Human Services. Health information for patients: HIV and its treatment: What you should know (Fact Sheets)/About the HIV treatment guidelines/Approved medications to treat HIV infection/HIV treatment regimen failure/Recommended HIV treatment regimens/Understanding HIV prevention. *AIDSinfo, National Institutes of Health.* http://aidsinfo.nih.gov. May-October 2004.

25. U.S. Department of Health and Human Services. HIV preventive vaccine fact sheet, March 2003/HIV preventive vaccine. *AIDSinfo/National Institutes of Health.* http://aidsinfo.nih.gov/other.

26. U.S. Department of Health and Human Services. HIV vaccines explained (brochure). *Division of AIDS, National Institute of Allergy and Infectious Diseases, National Institutes of Health.* February 2004.

27. Villarosa, Linda. Despite need for H.I.V. vaccines, fear mutes call for volunteers. *New York Times.* May 27, 2003.

28. Witte, M.H., and Witte, C.L. Lymphspiration: Ignorance of infectious diseases: The case of AIDS, Kaposi sarcoma, and lymphology. *Lymphology.* 2000, Vol. 33:95-121.

Vignette: Development of Penicillin

1. Diggins, Francis W.E. The discovery of penicillin: So many get it wrong. *Biologist.* 2000, Vol. 47, No. 3:115-119.

2. Hayes, G.W., MD, Keating, C.L., MD, and Newman, J.S., MD. The golden anniversary of the silver bullet (Essay). *JAMA.* October 6, 1993, Vol. 270, No. 13:1610-11.

3. Henderson, John Warren, MD. The yellow brick road to penicillin: A story of serendipity. *Mayo Clinic Proceedings.* July 1997, Vol. 72:683-687.

4. Lerner, Phillip I., MD. Producing penicillin. *New England Journal of Medicine.* August 5, 2004, Vol. 351, No. 6:524.

5. Ligon, B. Lee, PhD. Penicillin: Its discovery and early development. *Seminars in Pediatric Infectious Diseases.* January 2004, Vol. 15, No. 1:52-57.

6. Markowitz, Milton, MD. Long-acting penicillins: Historical perspectives. *Pediatric Infectious Disease* (Williams & Wilkins Co.) September 1985, Vol. 4, No. 5:570-573.

7. Microbial World. Penicillin: The story of an antibiotic. *Penicillin and Other Antibiotics.* http://helios.bto.ed.ac.uk/bto/microbes/penicill.htm.

8. Nobel Prize. The discovery of penicillin. http://nobelprize.org.

9. Radetsky, Michael, MD, CM. The discovery of penicillin. *Pediatric Infectious Disease Journal* (Williams & Wilkins). September 1996, Vol. 15, No. 9:811-818.

10. Sartin, Jeffrey S., MD, and Perry, Harold O., MD. From mercury to malaria to penicillin: The history of the treatment of syphilis at the Mayo Clinic – 1916-1955 *Journal of the American Academy of Dermatology.* February 1995, Vol. 32, No. 2, Part 1:255-261.

11. Sternbach, George, MD, FACEP, and Varon, Joseph, MD. Alexander Fleming: The spectrum of penicillin. *Journal of Emergency Medicine* (Pergamon Press). 1992, Vol. 10, pp. 89-92.

12. Stollerman, Gene H., MD. The global impact of penicillin: Then and now. *Mount Sinai Journal of Medicine.* March 1993, Vol. 60, No. 2:112-119.

13. Wainwright, Milton. The history of the therapeutic use of crude penicillin. *Medical History.* 1987, Vol. 31, pp. 41-50.

14. Weisse, Allen B. The long pause: The discovery and rediscovery of penicillin. *Hospital Practice.* August 15, 1991. pp. 93-118.

Looking Ahead: Antibiotic Resistance

1. Altman, Lawrence K., MD. To Contain Ailment, A Test Heads the Wish List. *New York Times.* April 18, 2003.

2. American College of Physicians. Legislative update. www.acponline.org/ear/legislative.htm.

3. American College of Physicians. What you can do to reduce the threat of antibiotic resistance. www.acponline.org/ear/whatyou.htm.

4. Barlam, Tamar, MD. Antibiotics in jeopardy. *Center for Science in the Public Interest, Antibiotic Resistance Project.* http://cspinet.org/ar/antibiotics_jeopardy.html.

5. Bren, Linda. Antibiotic resistance from down on the chicken farm. *U.S. Food and Drug Administration/FDA Consumer Magazine.* January-February 2001.

6. Bren, Linda. Battle of the bugs: Fighting antibiotic resistance. *U.S. Food and Drug Administration, FDA Consumer Magazine.* July-August 2002.

7. Besser, Richard E., MD. Antimicrobial prescribing in the United States: Good news, bad news. Annals of Internal Medicine. April 1, 2003, Vol. 138, No. 7:605-606.

8. CDC. Antimicrobial resistance: Prevention tips. *National Center for Infectious Diseases.* www.cdc.gov/drugresistance/general/prevention_tips.htm. June 5, 2001.

9. CDC. Campaign to prevent antimicrobial resistance in healthcare settings: Campaign goals and methods/ Overview of the campaign/Partnerships/Why a campaign? www.cdc.gov/drugresistance/health care.

10. CDC. Get smart: Know when antibiotics work: Background on antibiotic resistance/General information about antibiotic resistance. www.cdc.gov/drugresistance/community. February 10-December 1, 2004.

11. CDC. Issues in healthcare settings: Antimicrobial resistance: A growing threat to public health. *Division of Healthcare Quality Promotion.* www.cdc.gov/ndidod/hip/Aresist/am_res.htm. June 1999.

12. Center for Science in the Public Interest. Consumer tips for using antibiotics. http://cspinet.org/ar/ar_tips.html.

13. Center for Science in the Public Interest. House bill introduced to preserve effectiveness of antibiotics. *CSPI Newsroom.* November 10, 1999.

14. CNN.com. Antibiotic resistance a growing threat, WHO reports. *CNN.com.health, from staff reports.* June 12, 2000.

15. Davis, Jeanie Lerche. Antibiotic resistance in healthy adults. *WebMD Medical News.* October 9, 2003.

16. Dowell, Scott F., et al. Principles of judicious use of antimicrobial agents for pediatric upper respiratory tract infections. *Pediatrics.* January 1998, Vol. 101, No. 1 (Suppl):163-165.

17. Eng, Jodi Vanden, et al. Consumer attitudes and use of antibiotics. *Emerging Infectious Diseases.* September 2003, Vol. 9, No. 9:1128-1135.

18. Federal Interagency Task Force on Antimicrobial Resistance. Second annual progress report: Implementaton of "A Public Health Action Plan to Combat Antimicrobial Resistance, Part I: Domestic Issues" (Draft). July 2, 2004.

19. Gonzales, Ralph, MD, MSPH, et al. Principles of appropriate antibiotic use for treatment of acute respiratory tract infections in adults: Background, specific aims, and methods. *Annals of Internal Medicine.* March 20, 2001, Vol. 134, Issue 6:479-486.

20. Kampmeier, Rudolph H., MD. In Retrospect: From watchful waiting to antibiotics. *JAMA.* November 3, 1989, Vol, 262, No. 17:2433-2436.

21. Lewis, Ricki, PhD. The rise of antibiotic-resistant infections. *U.S. Food and Drug Administration/FDA Consumer Magazine.* www.fda.gov/fdac/features/795_antibio.html. September 1995.

22. Lieberman, Patricia B., PhD, and Wootan, Margo G., DSc. Protecting the crown jewels of medicine: A strategic plan to preserve the effectiveness of antibiotics. *Center for Science in the Public Interest.* http://cspinet.org/reports/abiotic.htm. 1998.

23. Manning, Anita. Antibiotic resistance on the rise. *USA Today.* September 29, 2002.

24. McKay, Betsy. U.S. Agency Urging Doctors, Patients to Use Treatments in Moderation. *Wall Street Journal Online.* September 17, 2003.

25. Nordenberg, Tamar. Miracle drugs vs. superbugs: Preserving the usefulness of antibiotics/Animal use: Medicine and more. *U.S. Food and Drug Administration/FDA Consumer Magazine.* www.fda.gov/fdac/features/1998/698_bugs.html. November-December 1998.

26. Pollack, Andrew. With SARS, antivirus arms race heats up. *New York Times.* May 27, 2003.

27. Reuters. Children Receive Fewer Antibiotics: Study Shows a Five-Year Drop. *Washington Post.* September 2, 2003.

28. Rosenstein, Nancy, et al. The common cold – Principles of judicious use of antimicrobial agents. *Pediatrics.* January 1998, Vol. 101, No. 1 (Suppl):181-184.

29. Tuller, David. If SARS Hits U.S., Quarantine Could Too. *New York Times.* December 9, 2003.

30. Tuller, David. Mystery Surrounds a Virulent Skin Infection. *New York Times.* February 4, 2003.

31. Union of Concerned Scientists. Food and environment: Myths and realities about antibiotic resistance (FAQs). *FEED.* www.ucusa.org. December 6, 2003.

32. U.S. Department of Health and Human Services. Exploring: The problem of antibiotic resistance. *National Institute of Allergy and Infectious Diseases.* www.niaid.nih.gov/factsheets/antimicro.htm. April 6, 2004.

33. U.S. Department of Health and Human Services. HHS, public health partners unveil new campaign to promote awareness of proper antibiotic use. *News Release.* September 17, 2003.

34. U.S. Food and Drug Administration. FDA issues guidance on evaluating the safety of antimicrobial new animal drugs to help prevent creating new resistant bacteria. *FDA News.* October 23, 2003.

35. U.S. Food and Drug Administration. FDA publishes final rule to require labeling about antibiotic resistance. *FDA News.* February 5, 2003.

36. Washington State Department of Health. Do you really need an antibiotic? www.doh.wa.gov/Topics/antibiotics.htm. December 15, 2004.

Chapter 5. *Cancer*

Looking Back

1. American Cancer Society. Cancer reference information. www.cancer.org.

2. DeLisa, Joel A, MD, MS. Cancer rehabilitation in the New Millennium: Opportunities and challenges. New York, New York. June 4-5, 1999.

3. DeVita, Jr., Vincent T, MD. A perspective on the War on Cancer. New Haven, CT. Page 352.

4. Evaluation Review. *SAGE Publications.* 1999, Vol. 23, No. 3:259-280.

5. Freireich, Emil J. A perspective on cancer therapy. *Clinical Cancer Research.* September 2002, Vol. 8:2764-2765.

6. Gerber LH, and Vargo, M. Rehabilitation for patients with cancer diagnoses. In Rehabilitation medicine: Principles and Practice, 3rd Ed. (DeLisa, J.A., and Gans, B.M., editors). Lippincott-Raven (Philadelphia, PA). 1998:1293-1317.

7. Hamilton, Lee. National Cancer Act. *The Center on Congress at Indiana University, Congressional Moment Radio Series.* http://congress.indiana.edu/radio_series/national_cancer_act.php.

8. Jemal, Ahmedin, PhD, and Clegg, Limin X., PhD. Annual Report to the Nation on the Status of Cancer, 1975-2001. July 1, 2004, Vol. 101, Issue 1.

9. Kardinal, Carl G., and Yarbro, John W. A conceptual history of cancer. *Seminar in Oncology.* December 1979, Vol. 6, No. 4:396-406.

10. Lasker Foundation. www.laskerfoundation.org/about/albertmary.html.

11. Li, MC, Hertz, R., and Spencer, D.B. Effects of methotrexate therapy upon choriocarcinoma and chorioadenoma. *Proceedings of the Society for Experimental Biological Medicine.* 1956, Vol. 93:361.

12. Nash, J.M. The enemy within. *Time Magazine.* 1996, Fall Special Issue:15-23.

13. National Cancer Institute. By-Pass Budget Requests. www3.cancer.gov/public/factbk/bypass.htm.

14. National Cancer Institute. Executive Summary:1999 By-Pass Budget Request. http://plan1999.cancer.gov/executive/index.html.

15. National Cancer Institute 2003;95:1681–91.

16. Schlessel Harper, Wendy, guest editor, with Donna Hoel. Postgraduate medicine: Raising the curtain on cancer: Is the puzzle finally becoming clear? *Cancer.* September 1997, Vol. 102, No. 3.

17. Skolnick, Andrew A. Leader in War on Cancer looks ahead: Talking with Vincent T. DeVita, Jr., MD. *JAMA.* February 15, 1995, Vol. 273, No.7.

18. Sporn, Michael B. The war on cancer. *The Lancet.* May 18, 1996, Vol. 347.

19. Stillman, Frances A. Evaluation of the American Stop Smoking Intervention Study (ASSIST): A Report of Outcomes. *Journal of the National Cancer Institute.* November 19, 2003, Vol. 95, No. 22:1.

20. Watson, J.D., and Crick, F.H.C. A structure for deoxyribose nucleic acid. 1953, Vol. 171:737.

Case Study: Screening Tools for Cancer Detection

1. American Cancer Society. American Cancer Society issues new guidelines for cancer screening. *Primary Care & Cancer.* April 2000, Vol. 20, No 4.

2. American Cancer Society. Breast cancer facts and figures, 2001.

3. American Cancer Society. Cancer facts and figures 2003.

4. American Cancer Society. Cancer facts and figures 2004. November 15, 2004.

5. American Cancer Society. Colorectal cancer PDQ screening. www.cancer.gov/cancertopics/pdq/screening/colorectal.

6. *American Journal of Preventive Medicine.* September/October 1996, Vol. 12, No. 5:340-41.

7. Barton, Claudia L., DVM. The historical background of cytology. Department of Small Animal Medicine and Surgery, College of Veterinary Medicine, Texas A&M University. www.cvm.tamu.edu/cancer/professional/Cytology/asp/A_History.asp.

8. Brody, Jane E. Questions outnumber answers on P.S.A. test. *New York Times.* February 18, 2003.

9. CDC. Colorectal cancer prevention and control initiatives. *Cancer Prevention and Control.* www.cdc.gov/cancer/colorctl.

10. CDC. National Center for Chronic Disease Prevention and Health Promotion. http://cdc.gov/cancer/prostate/index.htm.

11. Cervical cancer trends and the Pap smear. *Primary Care & Cancer.* June 1997, Vol. 17, No 6.

12. Collins, Patricia M. Tumor markers and screening tools in cancer detection. *Nursing Clinics of North America.* June 1990, Vol. 25, No. 2.

13. Dolinsky, Christopher, MD. Breast cancer: The basics. Oncolink. www.oncolink.org/types/article.cfm. May 29, 2003.

14. Ford K, Marcus E, and Lum B. Breast cancer screening, diagnosis, and treatment. *Disease of a Month.* September 1999, Vol. 45, No. 9.

15. Greenwald, P. Colon cancer overview. *Cancer.* 1992, Vol. 70:1260-1271.

16. Health Encyclopedia. Diseases and conditions. www.healthscout.com/ency/68/329/main.html.

17. *Health Scout News.* Those at highest risk miss head and neck cancer screens. April 9, 2003.

18. History of Mammography. GE Healthcare. www.gehealthcare.com/rad/whc/mswhhis.html.

19. Ismail, Jatoi. Screening clinical breast examination. *Surgical Clinics of North America.* 2003, Vol. 83:790-1.

20. Kim, Hyon Ju, MD. Genetic predisposition to cancer, an overview. *Spring Symposium 1997, Laboratory of Medical Genetics, Ajou University Institute for Medical Sciences.* Ajou University School of Medicine, Suwon, Korea. 1997.

21. Lee, Nancy C., MD. Testimony on screening programs for breast and cervical cancer before the U.S. House of Representatives Committee on Commerce, Subcommittee on Health and Environment. www.hhs.gov/asl/testify/t990721a.html. July 21, 1999.

22. MedTerms Online Medical Dictionary. www.medterms.com.

23. Mellors, Robert C., MD, PhD. Neoplasia. Pathology Lecture Notes, Weill Medical College of Cornell University (New York City). http://edcenter.med.cornell.edu/CUMC_PathNotes/Neoplasia.

24. Mohandas, K. M. Genetic predisposition to cancer (Special section: cancer). *Current Science.* September 10, 2001, Vol. 81, No. 5:482.

25. National Cancer Institute. Cancer facts. http://cis.nci.nih.gov/fact/5_28.htm.

26. National Cancer Institute. Colorectal cancer PDQ screening. www.cancer.gov/cancertopics/pdq/screening/colorectal.

27. National Cancer Institute. Prostate cancer PDQ screening. www.cancer.gov.

28. Pignone M, et al. Screening for colorectal cancer in adults at average risk: Summary of the evidence for the U.S. Preventive Services Task Force. *Annals of Internal Medicine.* 2002, Vol. 137:132-41.

29. Rauscher, Megan. Americans confused about cancer prevention: Survey. *Reuters Health.* June 4, 2003.

30. Ries LA, Wingo PA, Miller DS, et al. The annual report to the nation on the status of cancer, 1973-1997, with special section on colorectal cancer. *Cancer.* 2000;88:2398-2424.

31. Smith, Robert A., PhD, et al. American Cancer Society guidelines for the early detection of cancer. *Cancer J Clin.* January-February 2000, Vol. 50, No. 1:34-49.

32. Study findings advise tests for colon cancer. *Managed Care & Cancer.* November/December 2000, Vol. 2, No. 6.

33. Susan G. Komen Breast Cancer Foundation. Former U.S. First Lady Betty Ford congratulates the Komen Foundation on its 20th Anniversary. www.komenswmichigan.org/bfordletter.htm.

34. Thompson, Ian M., MD, and Optenberg, Scott A., PhD. An overview cost-utility analysis of prostate cancer screening. *Oncology.* November 1995, Vol 9, No. 11.

35. Tuller, David. Some urge type of Pap test to find cancer in gay men. *New York Times.* February 18, 2003.

36. Wolff, W.I. Colonoscopy: History and development. *American Journal of Gastroenterology.* September 1989, Vol. 84, No. 9:1017-25.

37. Wright, Thomas C., Jr., MD, and Schiffman, Mark, MD. Adding a test for human papillomavirus DNA to cervical-cancer screening. *New England Journal of Medicine.* February 6, 2003, Vol. 348, No. 6:489-490.

Vignette: Skin Cancer and Sunblock/SPF Products

1. American Cancer Society. Cancer facts and figures 2004. www.cancer.org.

2. Brody, Jane E. A second opinion on sunshine: It can be good medicine after all. *New York Times.* June 17, 2003.

3. CDC. Cancer prevention and control: Facts and statistics about skin cancer. www.cdc.gov/chooseyourcover/skin.htm. Last reviewed November 1, 2004.

4. CDC. Skin cancer tools, resources, and projects. www.cdc.gov/cancer/nscpep.

5. Moloney, Fergal J, Collins, Sinead, and Murphy, Gillian M. Sunscreens: Safety, efficacy and appropriate use. *American Journal of Clinical Dermatology.* 2002, Vol. 3:185-191.

6. Nicol, Noreen, and Schlepp Susan L. Sunscreen use: An overview. *Plastic Surgical Nursing.* Fall 1999, Vol. 19, No. 3.

7. Rudavsky, Shari. Dark side of the sun. *Miami Herald.* May 1, 2003.

8. Schneider, LS, et al. "Block the sun, not the fun": Evaluation of a skin cancer prevention program for child care centers. *American Journal of Preventive Medicine.* 1998, Vol.17, Issue 1:31-37.

9. Schering-Plough HealthCare Products, Inc. Coppertone. www.coppertone.com.

10. Skin Cancer Foundation. The Skin Cancer Foundation sunproofs America! www.skincancer.org/news/040207-sunproof.php. February 7, 2004.

11. United States Preventive Services Task Force. Counseling to prevent skin cancer: Recommendations and rationale. *Internet Journal of Oncology.* 2004, Vol. 2, No. 1.

Looking Ahead: Genomic Research and Medicine

1. Alliance for Cancer Gene Therapy. Genes and their relationship to cancer. www.acgtfoundation.org/whatis.html.

2. American Society of Gene Therapy. www.asgt.org/media.shtml.

3. Cancer Consultants. Gene therapy appears effective for recurrent head and neck cancer. *Oncology Resource Center.* http://patient.cancerconsultants.com/gene_cancer_news.aspx.

4. Chung, Daniel C., MD, and Rustgi, Anil K., MD. The hereditary nonpolyposis colorectal cancer syndrome: Genetics and clinical implications (Review). *Annals of Internal Medicine.* April 1, 2003, Vol. 138, No. 7:560-570.

5. Collins, Francis S. MD, PhD. Appearance before U.S. House of Representatives Subcommittee on Health and Committee on Energy and Commerce. May 22, 2003.

6. Cooper, Richard S., MD, and Psaty, Bruce M., MD, PhD. Genomics and medicine: Distraction, incremental progress, or the dawn of a new age? (Perspective). *Annals of Internal Medicine.* April 1, 2003, Vol. 138, No. 7:576-580.

7. Durkin, Walter James, MD. Cancer Drug Therapy. *Primary Care.* December 1992, Vol. 19, No. 4:759-760.

8. Ensenauer, Regina E, MD, et al. Primer on Medical Genomics: Part VIII: Essentials of Medical Genetics for the Practicing Physician. *Mayo Clinic Proceedings.* 2003;78:846-857.

9. Evans, William E., PharmD., and McLeod, Howard L., PharmD. Pharmacogenomics – Drug disposition, drug targets, and side effects. *New England Journal of Medicine.* February 6, 2003, Vol. 348, No. 6:538-549.

10. Goldstein, David B., PhD. Pharmacogenetics in the laboratory and the clinic. *New England Journal of Medicine.* February 6, 2003, Vol. 348, No. 6:553-556.

11. Green, Michael J., MD, MS, and Botkin, Jeffrey R., MD, MPH. "Genetic Exceptionalism" in medicine: Clarifying the differences between genetic and nongenetic tests (Perspective). *Annals of Internal Medicine.* April 1, 2003, Vol. 138, No. 7:571-575.

12. Grosse, Scott and Teutsch, Steven. Genetics and Prevention Effectiveness. Part IV: Developing, implementing, and evaluating population interventions. In Genetics and Public Health in the 21st Century. Using Genetic Information to Improve Health and Prevent Disease (Ed) by Muin J. Khoury, Wylie Burke and Elizabeth J. Thomson. New York: Oxford University Press, 2000.

13. Jacobs, Paul. Biotech start-up takes step toward personalized cancer treatment. *San Jose Mercury News.* June 3, 2003.

14. Kelly, William N., MD. From the double helix to genomic medicine (Editorial). *Annals of Internal Medicine.* April 1, 2003, Vol. 138, No. 7:603-604.

15. Khoury MJ, Burke W, Thomsen EJ (Editors). Genetics and public health: a framework for the integration of human genetics into public health practice. In Genetics and Public Health in the 21st Century. New York: Oxford University Press, 2000.

16. Kim, Hyon Ju, MD. Genetic Predisposition to Cancer, an overview. 1997 Spring Symposium, Laboratory of Medical Genetics, Ajou University Institute for Medical Sciences. Ajou University School of Medicine, Suwon, Korea.

17. Krasner, Jeffrey. Marketing of cancer-gene test raises ethical, medical concerns. *Boston Globe.* March 26, 2003.

18. Kristof, Nicholas D. Staying alive, staying human. *New York Times.* February 11, 2003.

19. Mariani, Sara M., MD, PhD. Functional genomics: Improving cancer prognosis and drug development (Conference Report, Highlights from Keystone Meeting on Functional Genomics: Global Analysis of Complex Biological Systems, February 20-25, 2003, Santa Fe, NM). *Medscape General Medicine.* March 14, 2003, Vol. 5, No. 1.

20. Masood, Shahla MD. Breast cancer risk assessment and genetic testing: FCAP, MIAC. *Jacksonville Medicine.* March 1998. www.dcmsonline.org/jaxmedicine/1998journals/march98/riskassessment.pdf.

21. Michener, Chad M, MD, et al. Cancer detection and prevention. *International Society of Preventive Oncology* (Elsevier). 2002, Vol. 26:249-255.

22. National Cancer Institute. Herceptin (trastuzumab): Questions and answers. http://cis.nci.nih.gov/fact/7_45.htm. Reviewed February 14, 2002.

23. National Institutes of Health. National Human Genome Research Institute. www.genome.gov/10001772.

24. Neergaard, Lauran. Study: Tamoxifen could benefit 2 million women. Associated Press. April 1, 2003.

25. Pollack, Andrew. New cancer test stirs hope and concern. *New York Times.* February 3, 2004.

26. U.S. Department of Energy. Office of Science: Human Genome Project Information. www.ornl.gov/sci/techresources/Human_Genome/project/50yr.shtml.

27. Wade, Nicholas. Watson and Crick, both aligned and apart, reinvented biology. *New York Times.* February 25, 2003.

28. Wessel, David. Wanted: Public policies to help genetic testing fulfill its promise. *Wall Street Journal.* June 19, 2003.

29. Weinshilboum, Richard, MD. Genomic medicine: Inheritance and drug response. *New England Journal of Medicine.* February 6, 2003, Vol. 348, No. 6:529-537.

30. World Health Organization. Genomics section. www.who.int/genomics/elsi/en.

Chapter 6. *Cardiovascular Disease*

Looking Back

1. ALLHAT. Facts About ALLHAT: New Findings About Drugs to Lower High Blood Pressure and Cholesterol. www.nhlbi.hih.gov/health/allhat/facts.htm.

2. Audio-Digest Foundation. Cardiovascular Issues – Highlights of the American Academy of Physicians' 52nd Annual Scientific Assembly. September 20-24, 2000, Dallas. *Audio-Digest Family Practice.* Volume 48, Issue 44, November 28, 2000.

3. Bailar, John, MD, PhD. Hormone-Replacement Therapy and Cardiovascular Diseases. *New England Journal of Medicine.* August 7, 2003, 6; 349: 521-522.

4. BMJ Journals – http://bmj.bmjjournals.com/cgi/content/full/312/7047/1680.

5. Bussey, Henry, PharmD, and Fagan, Susan, PharmD. Antiplatelet Therapy and Stroke Prevention. *American Society of Consultant Pharmacists' 31st Annual Meeting,* Boston, 2000.

6. Diabetes Care. Aspirin Prophylaxis against Cardiovascular Disease in Diabetes. www.abcdiabetescare.org.uk/aspirin_prophylaxis_against_card.htm.

7. HealingWithNutrition.com. Cardiovascular Disease Facts, Disease Prevention and Treatment Strategies.

8. Landers, Susan J. Aspirin, the wonder drug: It's not just for headaches anymore. *amednews.com.* July 22, 2002. www.ama-assn.org/sci-pubs/amnews/pick_02/hlsa0722.htm.

9. Majorowicz, Karen, RN, ARNP. Management of Coronary Heart Disease. Continuing Education Course from *Continuing Education Online.* Released February 20, 2001. www.netce.com.

10. Rowland, Rhonda. Aspirin can cut heart risk for the healthy. *CNN.com.* January 14, 2002.

11. Schulman, Sam, MD. Care of Patients Receiving Long-Term Anticoagulant Therapy. *New England Journal of Medicine.* August 14, 2003. Number 7, Volume 349:675-683.

12. United Kingdom Philately. www.ukphilately.org.uk/nps/article1/heart.htm.

13. University of Iowa Hospitals and Clinics. www.uihealthcare.com/depts/medmuseum/galleryexhibits/beat-goesonhistory/02bloodpressure.html.

14. WebDesk.com. Aspirin and Heart Health – Role of Aspirin in Preventing Heart Attacks and Stroke. www.webdesk.com/asprin-heart-health. February 5, 2002.

15. Weill Medical College of Cornell University. In the Development of Heart Disease, LDL Cholesterol Isn't the Only Villain – Weill Cornell Dean and Cardiovascular Expert Stresses 'Metabolic Syndrome' at New York City International Heart Conference. *Press Release.* June 9, 2003.

16. Your Family's Health. Aspirin and Heart Disease. www.yourfamilyshealth.com/cardiology/aspirin.

17. Your Family's Health. What You Should Know About Diabetes and Heart Disease. www.yourfamily'health.com/cardiology/diabetes.

Case Study: Risk Assessment

1. Ahern, Cathy, R.N. What's Now and What's Next in Heart Disease Management. Presentation at *Mayo Health System Regional Food Day*. October 29, 2002.

2. American Heart Association. Tests to Diagnose Heart Disease. www.americanheart.org.

3. American Heart Association. Men with 3 of 5 metabolic abnormalities risk diabetes, heart disease. *Journal Report*. July 15, 2003. www.americanheart.org/presenter.jhtml?identifier=3013637.

4. Boyles, Salynn. Simple Blood Test Predicts Heart Disease: CRP Better Than Cholesterol at Predicting Risk. *WebMDHealth*. November 13, 2002.

5. Breast Cancer Source. Troponin T can be used to detect missed heart attacks. *AstraZeneca* website.

6. Brigham and Women's Hospital. CRP shown to predict heart disease among patients with metabolic syndrome. *Press Release*. January 27, 2003. www.brighamandwomens.org/publicaffairs/new/crp_and_metabolic_sydrome.asp.

7. Bueller, Harry R., MD, and Prins, Martin H., MD. Secondary Prophylaxis with Warfarin for Venous Thromboembolism. *New England Journal of Medicine*. August 14, 2003. Number 7, Volume 349:702-704.

8. Children's Hospital Boston. New tool fights heart disease. *Children's News Online*. c.2003.

9. Chobanian, Abram V., MD, et al. The Seventh Report of the Joint National Committee on Prevention, Detection, Evaluation, and Treatment of High Blood Pressure – The JNC 7 Report. *JAMA*. 2003;289:2560-2571.

10. Clancy, Mike. Chest pain units: Evidence of their usefulness is limited by encouraging. *BMJ Publishing Company*. 2002;325:116-117 (20 July).

11. Collinson, PO, Premachandram, S, Hashemi, K. Prospective audit of incidence of prognostically important myocardial damage in patients discharged from emergency department. *BMJ Publishing Group, Ltd.* 2000;320:1702-1705 (24 June). http://bmj.com/cgi/content/full/320/7251/1702.

12. Grady, Denise. High Blood Sugar Also Poses Risk to Heart. *New York Times*. September 21, 2004.

13. Grant, Ross. Women Unhappy With Care for Heart Disease. *HealthScoutNews*. January 29, 2003.

14. Griffith, Robert W., MD. The Metabolic Syndrome: Time for Action! *Health and Age, A Novartis Foundation*. August 10, 2001. http://www.healthandage.ch/PHome/gm=20!gid2=1237.

15. Hajjar, Ihab, MD, MS, Kotchen, Theodore A., MD. Trends in Prevalence, Awareness, Treatment, and Control of Hypertension in the United States, 1988-2000. *JAMA*. 2003;290:199-206 (July 9).

16. Health and Age, A Novartis Foundation. Metabolic Syndrome Boosts Cardiovascular Disease Risk. Tufts University. January 17, 2003.

17. Hellmich, Nanci. Belly full of danger: That gut is called visceral fat, and it's the deadliest kind. *USA Today*. February 26, 2003.

18. Kearon, Clive, M.B., Ph.D. et al. Comparison of Low-Intensity Warfarin Therapy with Conventional-Intensity Warfarin Therapy for Long-Term Prevention of Recurrent Venous Thromboembolism. *New England Journal of Medicine*. August 14, 2003. Number 7, Volume 349:631-639.

19. McCook, Alison. Pre-Diabetic Syndrome Ups Risk of Death in Men. *LifeScan Diabetes News*. August 18, 2003. www.lifescan.com/care/news/dn120302-1.html.

20. National Institutes of Health. NHLBI Issues New High Blood Pressure Clinical Practice Guidelines. *NIH News Release*. May 14, 2003.

21. Pearson, Thomas A., MD, PhD, MPH. New Tools for Coronary Risk Assessment: What Are Their Advantages and Limitations? *Circulation*. 2002;105:886-892.

22. Pearson, Thomas A., MD, MPH, PhD, et al. American Heart Association Guide for Improving Cardiovascular Health at the Community Level – A Statement for Public Health Practitioners, Healthcare Providers, and Health Policy Makers From the American Heart Association Expert Panel on Population and Prevention Science. *Circulation*. 2003;107:645-651.

23. Pearson, Thomas A., MD, PhD, et al. AHA Guidelines for Primary Prevention of Cardiovascular Disease and Stroke: 2002 Update – Consensus Panel Guide to Comprehensive Risk Reduction for Adult Patients Without Coronary or Other Atherosclerotic Vascular Diseases. *Circulation*. 2002;106:388-391.

24. Pearson, Thomas A., MD, PhD (Co-Chair) et al. Markers of Inflammation and Cardiovascular Disease; Application to Clinical and Public Health Practice – A Statement for Healthcare Professionals from the Centers for Disease Control and Prevention and the American Heart Association. *Circulation*. 2003;107:499-511.

25. Science Blog. CRP improves cardiovascular risk prediction in metabolic syndrome. *American Heart Association*. January 28, 2003. www.scienceblog.com/community/article876.html.

26. Tanne, Janice Hopkins. US guidelines say blood pressure of 120/80 mm Hg is not 'normal.' *BMJ Publishing Company*. 2003;326:1104 (24 May).

27. Tanzi, Maria G., Pharm.D. Cardiovascular Disease in Women. *Clinical Trends in Pharmacy Practice*, Fujisawa Healthcare, Inc. 2003.

28. Tarkan, Laurie. Low Cholesterol? Don't Brag Quite Yet. *New York Times*. May 10, 2005.

29. Taylor, C, Forrest-Hay, A, Meek, S. ROMEO: a rapid rule out strategy for low risk chest pain. Does it work in UK emergency department? *Emergency Medicine Journal*. 2002;19:395-399.

Vignette: Statins

1. Altman, Lawrence K., MD. Heart-Health Lessons from the Clinton Case. *New York Times.* September 21, 2004.

2. American Heart Association. Cholesterol-Lowering Drugs. http://www.americanheart.org/presenter.jhtml?identifier=4510

3. Fallon, Sally and Enig, Mary G., PhD. The Dangers of Statin Drugs: What You Haven't Been Told About Cholesterol-Lowering Medication, Part I. www.mercola.com/2004/jul/21/statin_drugs.htm.

4. Gotto, Jr., Antonio M., MD, DPhil. Statins: Powerful Drugs for Lowering Cholesterol, Advice for Patients. *Cardiology Patient Page, Circulation.* 2002;105:1514-1516.

5. Manning, Anita. Statins can lower diabetics' heart risk. *USA Today.* June 7, 2004.

6. http://nhlbisupport.com/chd1/meds1.htm. Statins.

7. Mercola.com. Half the Population Will be Taking Statins. http://www.mercola.com/fcgi.

8. O'Neil, John. Treatments: Statins and Diabetes: New Advice. *New York Times.* April 20, 2004.

Looking Ahead: Obesity in Young Populations

1. Altman, Lawrence K. Clinton joins fight against child obesity. *New York Times.* May 4, 2005.

2. American Diabetes Association. Management of Dyslipidemia in Children and Adolescents with Diabetes. *Diabetes Care.* 26:2194-2197, 2003.

3. American Heart Association. Heart health should be the front line of diabetes care. *Charity Wire.* May 7, 2002.

4. Briefings in Education. Public Schools and Junk Food. *New York Times.* May 29, 2005.

5. Brody, Jane. Exercise is a habit; here's why to pick it up. *New York Times.* September 16, 2003.

6. Brody, Jane. With Fruits and Vegetables, More Can Be Less. *New York Times.* October 5, 2004.

7. Dotinga, Randy. Obese Kids as Unhappy as Those With Cancer. *HealthScoutNews.* April 8, 2004.

8. Foody, JoAnne M., MD. Guidelines: Hypertension Prevention and Management – JNC 7. *Journal Watch Cardiology.* June 13, 2003.

9. Fox, Maggie. Obesity Top Health Problem in U.S., Agency Head Says. *Washington Post.* October 28, 2003.

10. Goode, Erica. The Gorge-Yourself Environment. *New York Times.* July 22, 2003.

11. Goodnough, Abby. New York City Schools Cut Down on Fat and Sweets in Menus. *New York Times.* June 25, 2003.

12. Grundy, Scott M. Early Detection of High Cholesterol Levels in Young Adults. *JAMA.* July 19, 2000; 284: 365-67.

13. Hambrecht, Ranier et al. Effect of Exercise Training on Left Ventricular Function and Peripheral Resistance in Patients with Chronic Heart Failure. *JAMA.* June 21, 2000; 283: 3095-3101.

14. Haney, Daniel Q. Doctors see ominous rise in adult form of diabetes in children. *Associated Press.* April 9, 2003.

15. Kirchheimer, Sid. Breakfast Reduces Diabetes, Heart Disease; Morning Meal May Reduce Obesity, Other Health Risks by 50%. *WebMD Medical News.* March 6, 2003.

16. Kolata, Gina. Two studies suggest a protein has a big role in heart disease. *New York Times.* January 6, 2005.

17. Kottke, Thomas E., MD, MSPH, Stroebel, Robert J., MD, Hoffman, Rebecca S., BA. JNC 7 – It's More Than High Blood Pressure. *JAMA.* 2003;289:2573-2575.

18. Matthews, Karen A. Youthful hostility linked to adult heart disease. *Health Psychology.* 2003;22:279-286.

19. Meckler, Laura. Obesity Reported to Cost U.S. $93B a Year. *Associated Press.* May 14, 2003. http://www.healthaffairs.org.

20. Mercola.com. Modest Weight Loss May Cut Heart Risks of Obesity. www.mercola.com/fcgi. January 15, 2002.

21. Mozes, Alan. Youthful hostility linked to adult heart disease. *CYC-NET.* 28 May 2003.

22. Niaura, Raymond et al. Hostility, the Metabolic Syndrome, and Incident Coronary Heart Disease. *Health Psychology.* 2002, Vol. 21, No. 6, 588-593.

23. Orr, Andrea. CDC: Obesity Fastest Growing Health Threat in U.S. *Reuters.* June 5, 2003.

24. Perez-Pena, Richard. Obesity on Rise in New York City Public Schools. *New York Times.* July 9, 2003.

25. Science Blog. Obese People Experience Delay in Feeling Full, UF Researchers Find. www.scienceblog.com/community/article1110.html. February 26, 2003.

26. Scott, Janny. Life at the top in America isn't just better, it's longer. *New York Times.* May 16, 2005.

27. Stamler, Jeremiah et al. Relationships of Baseline Serum Cholesterol Levels in 3 Large Cohorts of Younger Men to Long-Term Coronary, Cardiovascular and All-Cause Mortality and Longevity. *JAMA.* July 19, 2000; 284; 311-18.

28. Stampfer, Meir J. et al. Primary Prevention of Coronary Heart Disease in Women Through Diet and Lifestyle. *New England Journal of Medicine.* July 6, 2000; 343: 16-22.

29. Stein, Rob. Risk Syndrome Found in Overweight Teens: Early Diabetes, Heart Diseases Likelier. *Washington Post.* August 12, 2003.

30. Thomas RJ et al. Attempts at changing dietary and exercise habits to reduce risk of cardiovascular disease: who's doing what in the community? www.ncbi.nlm.hih.gov. 2002.

31. U.S. Department of Health and Human Services. Overweight and Obesity Threaten U.S. Health Gains – Communities Can Help Address the Problem, Surgeon General Says. *Press Release.* December 13, 2001.

32. U.S. Pharmacist. Patient Consult: Metabolic Syndrome. www.uspharmacist.com. No. 27:11.November 15, 2002.

33. Wade, Nicholas. Drug in test acts on gene tied to heart. *New York Times.* May 11, 2005.

34. Ware, James H., PhD. Interpreting Incomplete Data in Studies of Diet and Weight Loss. *New England Journal of Medicine.* Volume 348:2136-2137, May 22, 2003.

35. Warner, Melanie. Striking back at the food police. *New York Times.* June 12, 2005.

36. Williams, Christine L., MD, MPH, Chairman, et al. Cardiovascular Health in Childhood – A Statement for Health Professionals From the Committee on Atherosclerosis, Hypertension, and Obesity in the Young (AHOY) of the Council on Cardiovascular Disease in the Young, American Heart Association. *Circulation.* 2002;106:143.

37. Winslow, Ron. Heart-Disease Warning Signs Begin as Early as Childhood. *Wall Street Journal.* March 18, 2003.

Chapter 7. *Safer and Healthier Foods*

Looking Back

1. Backstrand, Jeffrey R., PhD. The history and future of food fortification in the United States: A public helath perspective. *Nutrition Reviews.* January 2002, Vol. 60, No. 1:15-26.

2. Barkan, Ilyse D., JD. Industry invites regulation: The passage of the Pure Food and Drug Act of 1906. *American Journal of Public Health.* January 1985, Vol. 75, No. 1:18-26.

3. Begley, Timothy H. Methods and approaches used by FDA to evaluate the safety of food packaging materials. *Food Additives and Contaminants.* 1997, Vol. 14, No. 6-7:545-553.

4. Binkley, JK, Eales, J, and Jekanowski, M. The relation between dietary change and rising US obesity. *International Journal of Obesity.* 2000, Vol. 24:1032-1039.

5. Briefel, Ronette R., and Johnson, Clifford L. Secular trends in dietary intake in the United States. *Annual Review of Nutrition.* 2004, Vol. 24:401-31.

6. Burditt, George M., Esq. The history of food law. *Food and Drug Law Journal.* 1995, Vol. 50, 50th Anniversary Special Issue.

7. Burdock, George A., and Carabin, Ioana G. Generally recognized as safe (GRAS): History and description. *Toxicology Letters* (Elsevier). 2004, Vol. 150:3-18.

8. Carlson, Andrea, PhD, et al. Revision of USDA's low-cost, moderate-cost, and liberal food plans. *Family Economics and Nutrition Review.* 2003, Vol. 15, No. 2:43-51.

9. Carpenter, Kenneth J. The relationship of pellagra to corn and the low availability of niacin in cereals. *University of California, Department of Nutritional Sciences, Berkeley, CA.*

10. CDC. Nutrition & Physical Activity: Overweight and Obesity: Defining overweight and obesity/Economic consequences/Health consequences/U.S. obesity trends, 1985-2002. *National Center for Chronic Disease Prevention and Health Promotion.* www.cdc.gov/nccdphp/dnpa/obesity. Last updated June 2004.

11. Champagne, Catherine M., Bogle, Margaret L., and Karge III, William H. Part 1. Evaluation of aggregated food consumption patterns at the national, provincial and community level: Using national dietary data to measure dietary changes. *Public Health Nutrition.* 2002, Vol. 5, No. 6A:985-989.

12. Cordle, Frank, PhD, MPH, and Kolbye, Albert C., MD, MPH. Food safety and public health: Interaction of science and law in the federal regulatory process. *Cancer.* 1979, Vol. 43, No. 5, May Supplement:2143-2150.

13. Darby, William J., MD, PhD. A perspective on food legislation. *Special Report, Nutrition Reviews.* November 1981, Vol. 39, No. 11:413-416.

14. Daynard, Richard A., JD, PhD, Hash, Lauren E., Robbins, Anthony, MD, MPA. Food litigation: Lessons from the tobacco wars. *JAMA.* 2002; 288:2179.

15. Dirks, Robert. Diet and nutrition in poor and minority communities in the United States 100 years ago. *Annual Review of Nutrition.* 2003, Vol. 23:81-100.

16. Drexler, Madeline. Modern Meat: Cultivating resistance. An excerpt from "Secret Agents: The Menace of Emerging Infections" (Joseph Henry Press, 2002). *PBS, Frontline.* www.pbs.org/wgbh. 2002.

17. Dunkelberger, Edward, Esq. The statutory basis for the FDA's food safety assurance programs: From GMP, to Emergency Permit Control, to HACCP. *Food and Drug Law Journal.* 1995, Vol. 50, Issue 3:357-383.

18. Fennema, Owen R., PhD. Food additives – an unending controversy. *American Journal of Clinical Nutrition.* 1987, Vol. 46:201-3.

19. Field, AE, et al. Association between fruit and vegetable intake and change in body mass index among a large sample of children and adolescents in the United States. *International Journal of Obesity.* 2003, Vol. 27:821-826.

20. Fortin, Neal D. The hang-up with HACCP: The resistance to translating science into food safety law. *Food and Drug Law Journal.* 2003, Vol. 58, Issue 4:565-593.

21. French, Simone A. Pricing effects on food choices (presented at the Symposium: Sugar and Fat – From Genes to Culture, New Orleans). *Experimental Biology '02 Meeting, American Society for Nutritional Sciences.* April 23, 2002.

22. Goldsmith, Grace A., MD. Niacin: Antipellagra factor, hypocholesterolemic agent. *JAMA.* October 11, 1965, Vol. 194, No. 2:147-153.

23. Hayes, Jr., Arthur Hull, MD. Food and drug regulation after 75 years. *JAMA.* September 11, 1981, Vol. 246, No. 11:1223-1226.

24. Heckman, Jerome H. United States of America and European regulation of food packaging: Finding common ground to reach a common goal. *Food Additives and Contaminants.* 1994, Vol. 11, No. 2:271-283.

25. Hegsted, D. Mark, PhD. Food and nutrition policy: Probability and practicality. *Journal of The American Dietetic Association.* May 1979, Vol. 74:534-538.

26. Hutt, Peter Barton. Government regulation of the integrity of the food supply. *Annual Review of Nutrition.* 1984, Vol. 4:1-20.

27. Kay, Gwen. Health public relations: FDA's 1930s legislative campaign. *Bulletin of Historical Medicine.* 2001, Vol. 75, 446-487.

28. Kessler, David A. The evolution of national nutrition policy. *Annual Review of Nutrition.* 1995, Vol. 15:xiii-xxvi.

29. King, Charles Glen, PhD, FAPHA. Fifty years of experience in nutrition and a look to the future. *American Journal of Public Health.* November 1968, Vol. 58, No. 11:2015-2020.

30. Lewis, Carol. The "Poison Squad" and the advent of food and drug regulation. *FDA Consumer, U.S. Food and Drug Adminstration.* November-December 2002.

31. Miller, Sanford A. Science, law and society: The pursuit of food safety. *Journal of Nutrition* (American Institute of Nutrition). 1993, Vol. 123:279-284.

32. Morris, Jr., J. Glenn. The color of hamburger: Slow steps toward the development of a science-based food safety system in the United States. *Transactions of the American Clinical and Climatological Association.* 2003, Vol. 114:191-202.

33. Mrak, Emil M. Some of the developments in food production and their impact on nutrition. *Journal of Nutrition.* 1967, Vol. 91, Supplement 1:55-61.

34. Nestle, Marion, PhD, MPH. Increasing portion sizes in American diets: More calories, more obesity. *Journal of The American Dietetic Association.* January 2003, Vol. 103, No. 1:39-40.

35. Nielsen, Samara Joy, and Popkin, Barry M., PhD. Patterns and trends in food portion sizes, 1977-1998. *JAMA.* January 22/29, 2003, Vol. 289, No. 4:450-453.

36. Nielsen, Samara Joy, Siega-Riz, Anna Maria, and Popkin, Barry M. Trends in energy intake in U.S. between 1977 and 1996: Similar shifts seen across age groups. *Obesity Research.* May 2002, Vol.. 10, No. 5:370-378.

37. Park, Youngmee K., PhD, et al. Effectiveness of food fortification in the United States: The case of pellagra. *American Journal of Public Health.* May 2000, Vol. 90, No. 5:727-738.

38. Pennington, Jean A.T., et al. History of the Food and Drug Administration's Total Diet Study (Part II), 1987-1993. *Journal of AOAC International.* 1996, Vol. 79, No. 1:163-170.

39. Pollan, Michael. The (agri)cultural contradictions of obesity. *New York Times Magazine.* October 12, 2003.

40. Popkin, Barry M. and Nielsen, Samara Joy. The sweetening of the world's diet. *Obesity Research.* November 2003, Vol. 11, No. 11:1325-1332.

41. Popkin, Barry M., PhD, Zizza, Claire, PhD, and Siega-Riz, Anna Maria, PhD. Who is leading the change? U.S. dietary quality comparison between 1965 and 1996. *American Journal of Preventive Medicine.* 2003, Vol. 25, No. 1:1-8.

42. Rados, Carol. GRAS: Time-tested, and trusted, food ingredients. *FDA Consumer Magazine, U.S. Food and Drug Administration.* March-April 2004.

43. Smiciklas-Wright, Helen, PhD., et al. Foods commonly eaten in the United States, 1989-1991 and 1994-1996: Are portion sizes changing? *Journal of The American Dietetic Association.* January 2003, Vol. 103, No. 1:41-47.

44. Steele, James H., DVM, MPH. History, trends, and extent of pasteurization. Commentary, *JAVMA.* July 15, 2000, Vol. 217, No. 2:175-178.

45. Thom, Susan, RD, CDE, and Kulkarni, Karmeen, RD, MS, CDE. Labeling lingo: History and trends. *The Diabetes Educator.* November-December 1990, Vol. 16, No. 6:489-496.

46. U.S. Department of Agriculture. Nutrient content of the U.S. food supply, 1909-99: A summary report (Home Economics Research Report No. 55). *Center for Nutrition Policy and Promotion.* June 2002.

47. U.S. Department of Agriculture. The Thrifty Food Plan, 1999 (Executive Summary). *Center for Nutrition Policy and Promotion.* August 1999.

48. U.S. Department of Agriculture. USDA releases studies of new thrifty food plan, nutritional status of WIC participants. *Press Release.* August 19, 1999, No. 0341.99.

49. U.S. Department of Agriculture. United States Food Safety System. *U.S. Food and Drug Administration.* www.foodsafety.org. March 3, 2000.

50. U.S. Department of Health and Human Services. HHS unveils FDA strategy to help reduce obesity: New "Calories Count" approach builds on HHS' education, research efforts. *Press Release.* March 12, 2004.

51. U.S. Department of Health and Human Services. Overweight and Obesity: At a Glance/A Vision for the Future/Health consequences. www.surgeongeneral.gov/topics/obesity/calltoaction/fact_glance.htm.

52. U.S. Department of Health and Human Services. Surgeon General's healthy weight advice for consumers. www.surgeongeneral.gov/topics/obesity/calltoaction/fact_advice.htm.

53. U.S. Food and Drug Administration. Report of the working group on obesity. *Backgrounder.* www.fda.gov/oc/initiatives/obesity/backgrounder.html. March 12, 2004.

54. Weisburger, John H. The 37 year history of the Delaney Clause. *Experimental Toxic Pathology* (Gustav Fischer Verlag, Jena). 1996, Vol. 48, Nos. 2-3:183-188.

55. Welsh, Susan O., PhD, RD, and Marston, Ruth M. Review of trends in food use in the United States, 1909 to 1980. *Journal of the American Dietetic Association.* August 1982, Vol. 81:120-128.

56. Wiser, Vivian. Part I: Healthy Livestock – Wholesome Meat: A short history. From "100 Years of Animal Health, 1884-1984," *The Associates of the National Agricultural Library, Inc.* (Beltsville, MD). 1987.

57. Wiser, Vivian. Part V: Meat and poultry meat inspection in the United States Department of Agriculture. From "100 Years of Animal Health 1884-1984." *The Associates of the National Agricultural Library, Inc.* (Beltsville, MD). 1987.

58. Wood, Donna J. The strategic use of public policy: Business support for the 1906 Food and Drug Act. *Business History Review* (Harvard College). Autumn 1985, Vol. 59:403-432.

59. Young, James Harvey. From oysters to after-dinner mints: The role of the early Food and Drug inspector. *Journal of the History of Medicine and Allied Sciences.* January 1987, Vol. 42:30-53.

60. Young, James Harvey. The pig that fell into the privy: Upton Sinclair's The Jungle and the Meat Inspection Amendments of 1906. *Bulletin of Historical Medicine.* 1985, Vol. 59:467-480.

61. Young, Lisa R., PhD, RD, and Nestle, Marion, PhD, MPH. Expanding portion sizes in the US marketplace: Implications for nutrition counseling. *Journal of The American Dietetic Association.* February 2003, Vol. 103, No. 2:231-234.

62. Young, Lisa R., MS, and Nestle, Marion, PhD, MPH. Portion sizes in dietary assessment: Issues and policy implications. *Nutrition Reviews.* June 1995, Vol. 53, No. 6:149-158.

63. Young, Lisa R., PhD, RD, and Nestle, Marion, PhD, MPH. The contribution of expanding portion sizes to the US obesity epidemic. *American Journal of Public Health.* February 2002, Vol. 92, No. 2:246-249.

64. Yuhas, Joan A., PhD, RD, LD, Bolland, Janet E., MS, RD, LD, and Bolland, Thomas W., PhD. The impact of training, food type, gender, and container size on the estimation of food portion sizes. *The Journal of the American Dietetic Association.* October 1989, Vol. 89, No. 10:1473-1477.

65. Ziporyn, Terra, PhD. The Food and Drug Administration: How "those regulations" came to be. *JAMA.* October 18, 1985, Vol. 254, No. 15:2037-2046.

Case Study: Jack in the Box *E. coli* Outbreak

1. American Medical Association. Foodborne Illnesses Table: Bacterial Agents. www.ama-assn.org. January 2001.

2. Bender, Jeffrey B., DVM, MS, et al. Food-borne disease in the 21st century: What challenges await us? *Postgraduate Medicine.* August 1999, Vol. 106, No. 2:109-119.

3. CDC. Escherichia coli O157:H7: General information/Technical information. *Division of Bacterial and Mycotic Diseases, Disease Information.* www.cdc.gov/ncidod/dbmd/diseaseinfo.

4. CDC. Preliminary FoodNet data on the incidence of infection with pathogens transmitted commonly through food – selected sites, United States, 2003. *MMWR.* April 30, 2004, Vol. 53, No. 16:338-343.

5. Cohen, Elizabeth (correspondent). Study: Browned ground beef no safeguard against E. coli. *Health Story Page, CNN Interactive.* www.cnn.com/HEALTH/9705/19/brown.burgers. May 19, 1997.

6. Dargatz, David A. DVM, PhD. Food safety pathogens on the farm. From "Pathogen Reduction Dialogue, Panel 1." *USDA Centers for Epidemiology and Animal Health* (Ft. Collins, CO). May 6, 2002.

7. Deliganis, Chryssa V. Death by apple juice: The problem of foodborne illness, the regulatory response, and further suggestions for reform. *Food and Drug Law Journal.* 1998, Vol. 53:681-728.

8. Drexler, Madeline. Modern Meat: Secret Agent O157: The evolution of a killer. An excerpt from "Secret Agents: The Menace of Emerging Infections" (Joseph Henry Press, 2002). *PBS, Frontline.* www.pbs.org/wgbh. 2002.

9. Entine, Jon. How "Jack" turned crisis into opportunity. *Business Digest.* November/December 1999.

10. Eskin, Sandra B., et al. Ten years after the Jack-in-the-Box outbreak: Why are people still dying from contaminated food? S.T.O.P. looks at the state of foodborne illness and the U.S. public health response. Centers for Disease Control and Prevention (Atlanta). February 2003.

11. Jack in the Box. About our company/History. www.jackinthebox.com.

12. Jack in the Box. Food Safety: CPSI recognizes Jack in the Box restaurants for food safety leadership. *News Release.* www.jackinthebox.com. November 15, 1996.

13. Johnson, Steve. Modern Meat: The politics of meat. *Public Broadcasting System, Frontline.* 2002. www.pbs.org/wgbh/pages/frontline/shows/meat/politics.

14. Kent, Rosann. Grilling the suspect in food-related illness. *University of Georgia Research Magazine.* www.ovpr.uga.edu/researchnews. Fall 1993.

15. McKee, Garry L. Statement by Administrator, FSIS. *News and Information, Food Safety and Inspection Service, USDA.* February 7, 2003.

16. Parham, Delila R., DVM. HACCP impacts on contamination levels in meat and poultry products: FSIS perspective. From "Pathogen Reduction Dialogue, Panel 2." *USDA Food Safety and Inspection Service, Office of Public Health and Science.* May 6, 2002.

17. Pollan, Michael. Power Steer. *New York Times Magazine*. March 31, 2002.

18. Public Broadcasting System. Modern Meat: Food-borne Illnesses. *Frontline*. www.pbs.org/wgbh. 2002.

19. Public Broadcasting System. Modern Meat: Introduction/Is your meat safe?/Industrial meat. *Frontline*. www.pbs.org/wgbh. April 18, 2002.

20. Public Broadcasting System. Modern Meat: Meat recalls. *Frontline*. www.pbs.org/wgbh.

21. Public Broadcasting System. Modern Meat: Supreme Beef vs. USDA. *Frontline*. www.pbs.org/wgbh. 2002.

22. Robert Wood Johnson Foundation. Public Health Leadership and Capacity: Ten years after the Jack-in-the-Box outbreak. www.rwjf.org/research. 2003.

23. Theno, David, PhD. Food Safety: Industry must raise the bar to ensure safer burgers. *News Release, Jack in the Box*. www.jackinthebox.com. August 1997.

24. U.S. Department of Agriculture. Color of cooked ground beef as it relates to doneness. *Technical Publications, Food Safety and Inspection Service*. Slightly Revised April 2003.

25. U.S. Department of Agriculture. Compliance guidelines for establishments on the FSIS microbiological testing program and other verification activities for *Escherichia coli* O157:H7. www.fsis.usda.gov. April 13, 2004.

26. U.S. Department of Agriculture. Evaluation Report – FSIS recall notification and industry guidance. *Evaluation and Analysis Division, Food Safety and Inspection Service*. September 2000.

27. U.S. Department of Agriculture. Fact Sheets: Foodborne Illness & Disease: Foodborne Illness: What consumers need to know. www.fsis.usda.gov.

28. U.S. Department of Agriculture. Fact Sheets: Meat Preparation: Beef…from farm to table. www.fisis.usda.gov.

29. U.S. Department of Agriculture. Fact Sheets: Production & Inspection: Accomplishments of the HACCP-based inspection models project/FSIS food recalls/FSIS import procedures for meat, poultry & egg products/Imported meat, poultry & egg products remain under USDA jurisdiction/Importing meat, poultry & egg products to the United States. *Food Safety and Inspection Service*. www.fsis.usda.gov.

30. U.S. Department of Agriculture. FSIS issues policy statement on beef and E. coli O157:H7; updated ground beef guidelines also available. *News and Information, Food Safety and Inspection Service*. January 19, 1999.

31. U.S. Department of Agriculture. FSIS sampling for ground beef shows E. Coli O157:H7 downward trend. source *News Release, Food Safety and Inspection Service* (Washington, D.C.). September 17, 2003.

32. U.S. Department of Agriculture. Guidance for beef grinders to better protect public health. *Food Safety and Inspection Service*. December 1998 (11 pages).

33. U.S. Department of Agriculture. Guidance for minimizing the risk of Escherichia coli O157:H7 in beef slaughter operations (Draft). *Food Safety and Inspection*. Revised December 1, 2000 (34 pages).

34. U.S. Department of Agriculture. New measures to address *E. coli* O157:H7 contamination (Backgrounder, Congressional and Public Affairs). *Food Safety and Inspection Service*. www.fsis.usda.gov/regulations_&_policies. September 2002.

35. U.S. Department of Agriculture. Questions and answers regarding directives 5000.2, 6420.2, and 10,010.1, Revision 1, and the compliance guidelines on *E. coli* O157:H7. www.fsis.usda.gov. May 17, 2004.

36. U.S. Department of Agriculture. Regulations & Policies: Acts & authorizing statutes. *Food Safety and Inspection Service*. www.fsis.usda.gov/regulations_&_policies.

37. U.S. Department of Agriculture. Revised directive for advanced meat recovery systems (Backgrounders/Key Facts). *Food Safety and Inspection Service*. www.fsis.usda.gov/OA/background. December 2002.

38. U.S. Department of Agriculture. Science: Microbiology: Raw ground beef – *E. Coli* testing results. *Food Safety and Inspection Service*. www.fsis.usda.gov/science.

39. U.S. Department of Agriculture. Update on the HAACP-based inspection models project – in-plant slaughter. (Backgrounders/Key Facts). *Food Safety and Inspection Service*. www.fsis.usda.gov/regulations_&_policies. March 2000.

40. U.S. Department of Agriculture. USDA rule on retained water in meat and poultry. *Backgrounders, Food Safety and Inspection Service*. www.fsis.usda.gov/OA/background. April 2001.

41. U.S. Department of Agriculture, Food Safety and Inspection Service. Beef products contaminated with *Escherichia coli* O157:H7. *Federal Register, Docket No. 97-068N, 9 CFR Chapter III (Rules and Regulations)*. January 19, 1999, Vol. 64, No. 11.

42. U.S. Department of Agriculture, Food Safety and Inspection Service. E. coli O157:H7 contamination of beef products. *Federal Register, Docket No. 00-022N, 9 CFR Part 417 (Rules and Regulations)*. October 7, 2002, Vol. 67, No. 194.

43. U.S. Department of Defense. Crisis communication strategies: Analysis: Case Study: Jack in the Box E. Coli crisis. DoD Joint Course in Communication, Class02-C, Team 1. www.ou.edu/deptcomm/dodjcc. .

44. Wotecki, Catherine. *E. coli* – An agent for change (speech). *U.S. Department of Agriculture, Food Safety and Inspection Service*. www.fsis.usda.gov/oa/speeches. September 25, 1997.

Vignette: Nutrition Labeling on Food Packaging

1. American Dietetic Association. Legislative Highlights: Final food labeling regulations. *Journal of the American Dietetic Association*. February 1993, Vol. 93, No. 2.

2. American Dietetic Association. Legislative Highlights: Health claims on food labels: An American Dietetic Association perspective (ADA timely statement). *Journal of the American Dietetic Association*. February 1988, Vol. 88, No. 2.

3. American Dietetic Association. President's Page: Health claims for foods: An impelling public policy issue for members. *ADA Reports.* April 1986, Vol. 86, No. 4:527-529.

4. Bren, Linda. New dietary guidelines give practical advice for healthier living. *FDA Consumer Magazine, U.S. Food and Drug Administration.* September-October 2000.

5. Center for Nutrition Policy and Promotion. The food guide pyramid update: Proposed food guide graphic and education materials. *Projects, CNPP.* www.usda.gov/cnpp.

6. Code of Federal Regulations. Title 21 – Food and Drugs, Chapter I (FDA), Part 101 (Food Labeling), Subpart F: Specific requirements for descriptive claims that are neither nutrient content claims nor health claims, Sec. 101.95: "Fresh," "freshly frozen," "fresh frozen," "frozen fresh." *Volume 2 (Government Printing Office).* Revised April 1, 2002.

7. Cooper, Richard M. Health claims on foods – reflections on the food/drug distinction and on the law of misbranding (Report of a Meeting). *American Journal of Clinical Nutrition.* October 1986, Vol. 44:560-566.

8. Dixon, Lori Beth, and Ernst, Nancy D. Choose a diet that is low in saturated fat and cholesterol and moderate in total fat: Subtle changes to a familiar message. *Supplement, Journal of Nutrition.* 2001.

9. Dow Jones Newswires. U.S. considers replacing food guide pyramid. *Wall Street Journal.* July 13, 2004.

10. Farley, Dixie. Look for "legit" health claims on foods. *FDA Consumer, U.S. Food and Drug Administration.*

11. Forbes, Allan L., MD. Dimensions of the issue of explicit health claims on food labels (Presidential Address). *American Journal of Clinical Nutrition.* April 1986, Vol. 43:629-635.

12. Formanek, Raymond, Jr. Proposed rules issued for bioengineered foods. *FDA Consumer, U.S. Food and Drug Administration.* March-April 2001.

13. Foulke, Judith E. Cooking up the new food label. *U.S. Food and Drug Administration.* www.fda.gov.

14. Geiger, Constance J., PhD, RD. Health claims: History, current regulatory status, and consumer research. *Journal of the American Dietetic Association.* November 1998, Vol. 98, No. 11:1312-1322.

15. Geiger, Constance J., PhD, RD, et al. Perspectives in Practice: Review of nutrition labeling formats. *Journal of the American Dietetic Association.* July 1991, Vol. 91, No. 7:808-815.

16. Golan, Elise, Kuchler, Fred, and Mitchell, Lorraine. Summary: Economics of food labeling (Agricultural Economic Report). *Economic Research Service, U.S. Department of Agriculture.* December 2000.

17. Kurtzweil, Paula. "Daily Values" encourage healthy diet. *U.S. Food and Drug Administration.* www.fda.gov/fdac.

18. Kurtzweil, Paula. Good reading for good eating. *U.S. Food and Drug Administration.* www.fda.gov/fdac.

19. Kurtzweil, Paula. "Nutrition Facts" to help consumers eat smart. *U.S. Food and Drug Administration.* www.fda.gov/fdac.

20. Kurtzweil, Paula. Nutritional info available for raw fruits, vegetables, fish. *U.S. Food and Drug Administration.* www.fda.gov/fdac.

21. Nestle, Marion. Dietary advice for the 1990s: The political history of the food guide pyramid. *Caduceus.* Winter 1993.

22. Nestle, Marion. Food lobbies, the food pyramid, and U.S. nutrition policy. International Journal of Health Services (Baywood Publishing Co., Inc.). 1993, Vol. 23, No. 3:483-496.

23. Pappas, Clement Dimitri. Maintaining a level playing field: The need for a uniform standard to evaluate health claims for foods and dietary supplements. *Food and Drug Law Journal.* 2000, Vol. 57: 25-41.

24. Saltos, Etta, PhD, RD. The food pyramid-food label connection. *FDA Consumer, U.S. Food and Drug Administration.* www.fda.gov/fdac.

25. Segal, Marian. Ingredient labeling: What's in a food? *U.S. Food and Drug Administration.* www.fda.gov/fdac.

26. Smyth, Stuart, and Phillips, Peter W.B. Labeling to manage marketing of GM foods. *Trends in Biotechnology* (Elsevier). September 2003, Vol. 21, No. 9:389-393.

27. Stehlin, Dori. A little "lite" reading. *U.S. Food and Drug Administration.* www.fda.gov/fdac/special/foodlabel/lite.html.

28. U.S. Department of Agriculture. Consumer Education and Information: Meat and poultry labeling terms. *Food Safety and Inspection Service.* www.fsis.usda.gov. Slightly revised August 2003.

29. U.S. Department of Agriculture. FOCUS ON: Food product dating. *Consumer Education and Information, Food Safety and Inspection Service.* Updated June 2001.

30. U.S. Department of Agriculture. Labeling and consumer protection: FSIS statement of interim policy on carbohydrate labeling statements. *Food Safety and Inspection Service.* www.fsis.usda.gov/OPPDE/larc. December 22, 2003.

31. U.S. Department of Agriculture. Labeling and Consumer Protection: Regulations for package dating. *Food Safety and Inspection Service.* www.fsis.usda.gov/OPPDE/larc/Policies/Dating.htm.

32. U.S. Department of Agriculture. Nutrition labeling proposed for raw meat and poultry products. *Backgrounders, Food Safety and Inspection Service.* January 2001.

33. U.S. Department of Agriculture. Revision of the food guidance system. *USDA Q&As.* July 12, 2004.

34. U.S. Department of Agriculture. Serving sizes in the food guide pyramid and on the nutrition facts label: What's different and why? *Nutrition Insights #22, USDA Center for Nutrition Policy and Promotion.* December 2000.

35. U.S. Department of Agriculture. The food guide pyramid. *Home and Garden Bulletin, Center for Nutrition Policy and Promotion.* 1992 (original version), No. 252.

36. U.S. Department of Agriculture. The food guide pyramid for young children. *Projects/Backgrounder/Center for Nutrition Policy and Promotion*. www.usda.gov/cnpp.

37. U.S. Department of Agriculture. USDA calls for public comment on revision of the food guidance system. *News Release* July 12, 2004, No. 0281.04.

38. U.S. Department of Agriculture. USDA's Food Guide: Background and development. *Human Nutrition Information Service*. September 1993, Misc. Publication No. 1514.

39. U.S. Department of Agriculture. USDA Food Safety and Inspection Service: Labeling of FSIS-regulated foods. *Food Safety and Inspection Service*.

40. U.S. Department of Agriculture. USDA unveils food guide pyramid for young children. *Press Release, Center for Nutrition Policy and Promotion*. March 25, 1999.

41. U.S. Department of Agriculture. Using the claim "certified organic by…" on meat and poultry product labeling. *Backgrounders, Food Safety and Inspection Service*. Updated March 2, 2000.

42. U.S. Department of Health and Human Services. Build a healthy base: Let the Pyramid guide your food choices. www.health.gov/dietaryguidelines.dga2000.

43. U.S. Department of Health and Human Services. Choose sensibly: Choose a diet that is low in saturated fat and cholesterol and moderate in total fat. www.health.gov/dietaryguidlines/dga2000.

44. U.S. Department of Health and Human Services. Dietary guidelines for Americans. www.health.gov/dietaryguidelines/dga2000.

45. U.S. Department of Health and Human Services. FDA announces proposal and draft guidance for food developed through biotechnology. *HHS News*. January 17, 2001.

46. U.S. Department of Health and Human Services. Guidance on labeling of foods that need refrigeration by consumers (Agency: Food and Drug Administration). *Federal Register*. February 24, 1997, Vol. 62, No. 36:8248-8252.

47. U.S. Department of Health and Human Services. The food label. *FDA Backgrounder, U.S. Food and Drug Administration*. July 9, 2003.

48. U.S. Food and Drug Administration. Claims that can be made for conventional foods and dietary supplements. *Office of Nutritional Products, Labeling, and Dietary Supplements, Center for Food Safety and Applied Nutrition*. September 2003.

49. U.S. Food and Drug Administration. Compliance policy guidance for FDA staff: Sec. 555.250 Statement of policy for labeling and preventing cross-contact of common food allergens. *Compliance Policy Guide*. www.fda.gov/ora/compliance_ref/cpg.

50. U.S. Food and Drug Administration. Consumer research on food labels. *CFSAN Consumer Studies Branch, Center for Food Safety and Applied Nutrition*. www.cfsan.fda.gov. Updated February 27, 2004.

51. U.S. Food and Drug Administration. Examples of revised nutrition facts panel listing trans fat. *Office of Nutritional Products, Labeling and Dietary Supplements, Center for Food Safety and Applied Nutrition*. www.cfsan.fda.gov. July 9, 2003.

52. U.S. Food and Drug Administration. Fact Sheet: Carbohydrates. www.fda.org/oc/initiatives/obesity. March 12, 2004.

53. U.S. Food and Drug Administration. FDA acts to provide better information to consumers on trans fats. *FDA Backgrounder*. www.fda.gov/oc/initiatives/transfat. July 9, 2003.

54. U.S. Food and Drug Administration. FDA to encourage science-based labeling and competition for healthier dietary choices. *FDA News*. July 10, 2003.

55. U.S. Food and Drug Administration. Guidance for Industry: Voluntary labeling indicating whether foods have or have not been developed using bioengineering (draft). *Center for Food Safety and Applied Nutrition*. January 2001.

56. U.S. Food and Drug Administration. Guidance on how to understand and use the nutrition facts panel on food labels. *FDA Center for Food Safety and Applied Nutrition*. www.cfsan.fda.gov.

57. U.S. Food and Drug Administration. Letter to food manufacturers about accurate serving size declaration on food products. *Office of Nutritional Products, Labeling and Dietary Supplements, Center for Food Safety and Applied Nutrition*. March 12, 2004.

58. U.S. Food and Drug Administration. Taking the guesswork out of good nutrition. *FDA Home Page*. www.fda.gov.

59. Zamiska, Nicholas. Food-pyramid frenzy. *Wall Street Journal*. July 29, 2004.

Looking Ahead: How to Ensure a Safe Food Supply

1. Abboud, Leila. Food industry wages fight against FDA import rules. *Wall Street Journal*. March 26, 2003.

2. Alvarez, Lizette. Consumers in Europe Resist Gene-Altered Foods. *New York Times*. February 11, 2003.

3. American Dietetic Association. Position of the American Dietetic Association: Biotechnology and the future of food. *ADA Reports, Journal of the American Dietetic Association*. February 1993, Vol. 93, No. 2: 190-192.

4. American Dietetic Association. Position of the American Dietetic Association: Food irradiation. *ADA Reports, Journal of the American Dietetic Association*. February 2000, Vol. 100, No. 2:246-253.

5. Associated Press. Irradiated Hamburgers to Appear on Future School Lunch Menus. May 29, 2003.

6. Associated Press. U.S. to Sue E.U. Over Ban on Modified Foods. *New York Times*. May 13, 2003.

7. Barboza, David and Day, Sherri. McDonald's Asks Meat Industry to Cut Use of Antibiotics. *New York Times*. June 20, 2003.

8. Becker, Elizabeth and Barboza, David. Battle Over Biotechnology Intensifies Trade War. *New York Times.* May 29, 2003.

9. Becker, Elizabeth. 3 Lawmakers on Meat Rules Tour a Model Plant. *New York Times.* August 1, 2003.

10. Becker, Elizabeth. Salmonella Survivor Endorses Push for Food Safety Agency. *New York Times.* February 12, 2003.

11. Bren, Linda. Genetic engineering: The future of foods? *FDA Consumer Magazine, U.S. Food and Drug Administration.* November-December 2003.

12. CDC. Frequently asked questions about food irradiation. *Division of Bacterial and Mycotic Diseases.* www.cdc.gov/ncidod/dbmd/diseaseinfo/foodirradiation.htm. Last reviewed September 29, 1999.

13. CDC. Overview of CDC food safety activities. *Food Safety Office.* www.cdc.gov/foodsafety.

14. Food Safety and Inspection Service. Emergency preparedness: Biosecurity & the food supply. *Fact Sheets.* www.fsis.usda.gov.

15. Food Safety and Inspection Service. Enhancing public health: Strategies for the future. *2003 FSIS Food Safety Vision.*

16. Food Safety and Inspection Service. Irradiation of raw meat and poultry, questions and answers. *Consumer Publications.* May 2000.

17. Food Safety and Inspection Service. Keeping food safe during an emergency. *USDA Consumer Alert.* September 17, 2003.

18. Helm, Ricki M., PhD. Food biotechnology: Is this good or bad? Implications to allergic diseases. *Annals of Allergy, Asthma, & Immunology.* June 2003, Vol. 90:90-98.

19. Henkel, John. Genetic engineering fast forwarding to future foods. *FDA Consumer Magazine, U.S. Food and Drug Administration.* April 1995 (revised February 1998).

20. Henney, Jane E., MD. Food safety and biotechnology: Are they related? (Remarks at Kansas State University by the Commissioner of Food and Drugs). *U.S. Food and Drug Administration.* March 10, 2000.

21. Humphrey, Christine M. The Food and Drug Administration's import alerts appear to be "misbranded." Food and Drug Law Journal. 2003, Vol. 58.

22. Leonhardt, David. Talks Collapse on U.S. Efforts to Open Europe to Biotech Food. *New York Times.* June 20, 2003.

23. Levy, Alan S., and Derby, Brenda M. Report on consumer focus groups on biotechnology. *FDA Center for Food Safety and Applied Nutrition.* 2000.

24. Lewis, Carol. A new kind of fish story: The coming of biotech animals. *FDA Consumer Magazine, U.S. Food and Drug Administration.* January-February 2001.

25. Public Broadcasting System. Modern Meat: Antibiotic debate overview/Opinions on antibiotics. *Frontline.* www.pbs.org/wgbh. 2002.

26. Public Health Reports. Science-based, unified approach needed to safeguard the nation's food supply. *News and Notes: Food Safety.* November/December 1998, Vol. 113.

27. Thompson, Larry. Are bioengineered foods safe? *FDA Consumer Magazine, U.S. Food and Drug Administration.* January-February 2000.

28. U.S. Department of Agriculture. Emergency incident response. *FSIS Directive* 6500.1. July 2, 2004.

29. U.S. Department of Agriculture. Experimental and sample products policy. *FSIS Directive* 7000.2. July 1, 2004.

30. U.S. Department of Agriculture. Fulfilling the vision: Initiatives in protecting public health. *Food Safety and Inspection Service.* July 2004.

31. U.S. Department of Agriculture. Homeland security threat condition response – monitoring and surveillance products in commerce. *FSIS Directive* 5420.3, Revision 1. July 2, 2004.

32. U.S. Department of Agriculture. USDA approves irradiation of meat to help improve food safety. *News Release* No. 0486.99. December 14, 1999.

33. U.S. Department of Agriculture. USDA/FDA education initiative: Evaluating the placement of food safety education in American schools (Executive Summary). *U.S. Food and Drug Administration.* May 11, 1998.

34. U.S. Department of Agriculture. USDA Homeland Security Efforts. May 2003.

35. U.S. Department of Health and Human Services. FDA to strengthen pre-market review of bioengineered foods. *HHS News,* No. POO-10. May 3, 2000.

36. U.S. Department of Health and Human Services. HHS creates food security research program, increases import exams more than five times to protect nation's food supply: Progress report details ongoing efforts to enhance the nation's food security. *News Release.* July 23, 2003.

37. U.S. Department of Health and Human Services. HHS issues new rules to enhance security in the U.S. food supply. *News Release.* October 9, 2003.

38. U.S. Food and Drug Administration. Agencies team up to protect food supply. *FDA Consumer Magazine.* March-April 2004.

39. U.S. Food and Drug Administration. CFSAN 3004 program priorities (Letter from center director). *Center for Food Safety and Applied Nutrition.* May 4, 2004.

40. U.S. Food and Drug Administration. Chapter 1: International inspection program, from Guide to International Inspections and Travel. www.fda.gov./ora/inspect_ref/giit.

41. U.S. Food and Drug Administration. Compliance policy guide. www.cfsan.fda.gov. Revised June 2004.

42. U.S. Food and Drug Administration. Fact sheet on FDA's new food bioterrorism regulation: Final rule: Administrative detention. *Protecting the Food Supply, Center for Food Safety and Applied Nutrition.* May 2004.

43. U.S. Food and Drug Administration. Fact sheet on FDA's new food bioterrorism regulation: Interim final rule – prior notice of imported food shipments. *Protecting the Food Supply, Center for Food Safety and Applied Nutrition.* October 2003.

44. U.S. Food and Drug Administration. FDA and CBP announce their transitional compliance policy on food imports under the Bioterrorism Act. *FDA News,* No. P03-103. December 11, 2003.

45. U.S. Food and Drug Administration. FDA and CBP bolster safeguards on imported food. *FDA News.* December 3, 2003.

46. U.S. Food and Drug Administration. FDA finalizes rule on administrative detention of suspect food. *FDA News.* May 27, 2004.

47. U.S. Food and Drug Administration. Food irradiation: A safe measure. *FDA Consumer Magazine.* May-June 1998.

48. U.S. Food and Drug Administration. Food safety and security constituent update. *Center for Food Safety and Applied Nutrition.* June 25, 2004.

49. U.S. Food and Drug Administration. Food safety initiative. *Center for Veterinary Medicine.* www.fda.gov/cvm/fsi.

50. U.S. Food and Drug Administration. Food safety progress report, Fiscal Year 2000. www.cfsan.fda.gov. August, 2001.

51. U.S. Food and Drug Administration. Guide to inspections of manufacturers of miscellaneous food products – Volumes I and II. www.fda.gov/ora.

52. U.S. Food and Drug Administration. Guide to international inspections and travel (Contents). www.fda.gov/ora/inspect_ref/giit.

53. U.S. Food and Drug Administration. Healthy People 2010 focus area data progress review: Focus area 10: Food safety. *FDA/FSIS/CDC* (jointly). www.cfsan.fda.gov. May 11, 2004.

54. U.S. Food and Drug Administration. Healthy People 2010 food safety data progress review: Food safety education examples. *FDA/FSIS/CDC* (jointly). www.cfsan.fda.gov. May 11, 2004.

55. U.S. Food and Drug Administration. Import program system information. www.fda.gov/ora/import. Last update December 17, 2003.

56. U.S. Food and Drug Administration. Introduction to FDA's Import Refusal Report (IRR). www.fda.gov/ora/oasis. Updated February 21, 2003.

57. U.S. Food and Drug Administration. National food safety programs. *FDA/USDA/EPA/CDC* (jointly) www.foodsafety.gov. Updated June 24, 2005.

58. U.S. Food and Drug Administration. Prior notice of imported foods (Compliance summary information). *Center for Food Safety and Applied Nutrition.* www.cfsan.fda.gov. Updated May 2004.

59. U.S. Food and Drug Administration. Prior notice of imported food questions and answers (Edition 2). *Guidance for Industry.* www.cfsan.fda.gov. May 2004.

60. U.S. Food and Drug Administration. Progress report to Secretary Tommy G. Thompson: Ensuring the safety and security of the nation's food supply. *Center for Food Safety and Applied Nutrition.* July 23, 2003.

61. U.S. Food and Drug Administration. Regulatory issues in agricultural biotechnology. *FDA Veterinarian Newsletter.* January/February 1998, Vol. XIII, No. 1.

62. U.S. Food and Drug Administration. Testing for rapid detection of adulteration of food. *Report to Congress.* www.fda.gov/oc/bioterrorisim. October 2003.

Chapter 8. *Advances in Maternal and Child Health*

Looking Back

1. Birth defects rising in the U.S.: Environmental toxicity suspected. http://healthandenergy.com/birth_defects.htm. November 17, 1999.

2. Brody, Jane E. Experts strive to make more pregnancies full term. *New York Times.* April 8, 2003.

3. Brody, Jane E. Premature births rise sharply, confounding obstetricians. *New York Times.* April 8, 2003.

4. California Birth Defects Monitoring Program. www.cbdmp.org/spd_history.htm.

5. CDC. Achievements in Public Health, 1900-1999: Family planning (reported by Division of Reproductive Health, National Center for Chronic Disease Prevention and Health Promotion). *MMWR.* December 03, 1999, Vol. 48, No. 47:1073-1080.

6. CDC. Achievements in public health, 1900-1999: Healthier mothers and babies. *MMWR.* October 1, 1999, Vol. 48, No. 38:849-858.

7. CDC. Infant and maternal mortality in the United States, 1900-99. *Population and Development Review.* December 1999, Vol. 25, No. 4.

8. CDC. *MMWR.* September 4, 1998, Vol. 47, No. 34:705-7.

9. CDC. Trends and patterns of birth defects and genetic diseases with associated mortality in the United States, 1979-1992: An analysis of multiple-cause mortality data. *Genetic Epidemiology.* 1997;14: 493-505.

10. DeLee, J.B. The prophylactic forceps operation. *American Journal of Obstetrics Gynecology*. 1920-21; 1:34-35, 77-84.

11. Harris, John, MD, MPH. Transcript of testimony presented by director, California Birth Defects Monitoring Program, on behalf of March of Dimes Birth Defects Foundation. Before the Senate Health, Education, Labor and Pensions Committee Subcommittee on Public Health. March 6, 2002.

12. Johnson, John W. C. The Millennial Mark, from Transaction of the Sixty-Third Annual Meeting of the South Atlantic Association of Obstetricians and Gynecologists. *American Journal of Obstetrics and Gynecology*. 2001, Vol. 185:261-4.

13. March of Dimes. Maternal, infant, and child health in the United States, 2001. *Perinatal Data Center*. February 2002, Vol. 9:1131-98.

14. Meckel, Richard A. Save the babies: American public health reform and the prevention of infant mortality, 1850-1929. *Johns Hopkins University Press*. April 1, 1990.

15. Medical and nursing services for the maternal cases of the National Health Survey. *Public Health Reports*. 1941;56:855-856.

16. Mekdeci, Betty, and Schettler, Ted, MD, MPH. Birth defects and the environment. www.protectingourhealth.org/newscience/birthdefects.

17. National Center for Health Statistics. Report of final natality statistics, 1996. U.S. Department of Health and Human Services, Public Health Service, CDC. DHHS publication no. (PHS) 98-1120. 1998, Vol. 46, No. 11.

18. Number of low birth weight infants born in America rose between 1990 and 2000. *Medical Study News*. www.nyam.org. October 5, 2004.

19. Shaw Crouse, Janice, PhD, and Vineyard, Angie. Birthing babies: Maternal mortality rates plunge over 20th century. Beverly La Haye Institute. July-August 2002, *Data Digest*. Vol. 3, No 4.

20. TEF/Vater International. www.tefvater.org/cardiac.html.

21. Whitridge, Williams J. A criticism of certain tendencies in American obstetrics. *New York State Journal of Medicine*. 1992;22:493-9

Case Study: Folic Acid

1. Botto, Lorenzo, MD, *Medical Progress*. Vol. 341, No. 20:1509-1519.

2. D'Oria, Robyn. Folic acid prevents birth defects and major diseases. The Medical Center at Princeton. www.pacpubserver.com/new/health/f-h/hm012300.html. January 23, 2000.

3. Einarson, A., Parshuram, C., Koren, G. Periconceptional use of folic acid to reduce the rates of neural tube defects: Is it working? *Reproductive Toxicology*. 2000, Vol. 14:291-292.

4. March of Dimes. Folic acid vitamin use by women reaches all-time high, March of Dimes survey finds. *Press Release*. www.marchofdimes.com.

5. Wald, Nicholas J. Folic acid and the prevention of neural-tube defects. *New England Journal of Medicine*. January 8, 2004, Vol. 350, No. 2.

6. Werler, Martha M., ScD, Louik, Carol, ScD, and Mitchell, Allen, MD. Achieving a public health recommendation for preventing neural tube defects with folic acid. *American Journal of Public Health*. November 1999, Vol. 89, No. 11:1637-1639.

Vignette: Amniocentesis

1. Ethical Aspects of termination of pregnancy following prenatal diagnosis. *International Journal of Gynecological Obstetrics*. 1992.

2. Fuchs, F. and Riis, P. Antenatal sex determination. *Nature* (London). 1956, Vol. 177:330.

3. Harris, Ryan A., Washington, A. Eugene, Nease, Jr., Robert F., Kupperman, Miriam. Cost utility of prenatal diagnosis and the risk-based threshold. *The Lancet*. www.thelancet.com. January 24, 2004, Vol. 363.

4. Lesser, Yael, PhD. Elective amniocentesis in low-risk pregnancies: Decision making in the era of information and uncertainty. Bar Ilan University.

5. Nadler, H.L., and Gerbie, A.B. Role of amniocentesis in the intra-uterine diagnosis of genetic defects. *New England Journal of Medicine*. 1970, Vol. 282:596.

6. Woo, Joseph. A short history of amniocentesis, fetoscopy and chorionic villus sampling. www.ob-ultrasound.net/amniocentesis.html.

Looking Ahead: Genetic Screening

1. American Academy of Pediatrics. Newborn Screening Task Force: Serving the family from birth to medical home; Newborn screening: a blueprint for the future; A call for a national agenda on state newborn screening programs. *Pediatrics*. 2000;106:389-427.

2. Angier, Natalie. Not just genes: Moving beyond nature vs. nurture. *New York Times*. February 25, 2003.

3. Brody, Jane E. Genes may draw your road map, but you still chart your course. *New York Times*. February 25, 2003.

4. Juengst, Eric T., PhD. What should we mean by "prevention" in public health genetics? From the 1st Annual Conference on Genetics and Public Health. May 1998.

5. Khoury, Muin J., MD, PhD. Challenges and opportunities: A Framework for genetics and public health. From the 1st Annual Conference on Genetics and Public Health. May 1998.

6. Kolata, Gina. Genetic revolution: How much, how fast? *New York Times.* February 25, 2003.

7. Kolata, Gina. Using genetic tests, Ashkenazi Jews vanquish a disease. *New York Times.* February 18, 2003.

8. Murray, Robert F., MD. Genetic screening in the genome era: A minority perspective. From the 1st Annual Conference on Genetics and Public Health. May 1998.

Chapter 9. *Oral Health*

Looking Back

1. Academy of General Dentistry. A Millenium of Dentistry – A look into the past, present and future of dentistry. *Consumer Information/Oral Health Topics/History.*

2. Allukian, Myron, Jr., DDS, MPH. From Paul Revere to Fluoridation and AIDS: A brief history of dental public health programs in boston and massachusetts. *Journal of the Massachusetts Dental Society.* Vol. 49, No. 1, Spring 2000.

3. Angier, Natalie. Roots and all: A history of teeth. *New York Times.* August 5, 2003.

4. BDA Museum. BDA Museum Dental History Gallery. www.bda-dentistry.org.uk.

5. Bellis, Mary. History of Dentistry Instruments. National Academy for State Health Policy. November 2002.

6. Bellis, Mary. History of Dentistry and Dental Care. *What You Need to Know About Inventors.* http://inventors.about.com/library/inventors/bldental.htm.

7. California Dental Association. History of Dentistry. *California Dental Association Online.* Articles on Dental Health.

8. Dougherty, Matthew. A Biochemist Who Led Dental Education: William Gies' 1926 report on dental education is still relevant today. *Columbia University Health Sciences InVivo,* Vol. 2, No. 6, March 26, 2003.

9. Field, Marilyn J., Ph.D., Editor. Dental Education at the Crossroads: Challenges and Change. Institute of Medicine. *National Academy Press,* Washington, D.C. 1995.

10. History of Dentistry. www.sheridanc.on.ca/academic/computing/comp4064/projects/buchalski/history.

11. Hyson, John M., Jr., DDS, MS, MA. Women Dentists: The Origins. *Journal of the California Dental Association.* 2002.

12. Ismail, Amid I., BDS, MPH, DrPH, Hasson, Hana, DDS, MS, Sohn, Woosung, DDS, PhD, DrPH. Dental Caries in the Second Millenium. *NIH Consensus Development Conference on Dental Caries Diagnosis and Management.* March 26-28, 2001.

13. Lakatos, Monica J., D.D.S. The History of Dentistry. *Northshore Dental Associates,* North Muskegon, Michigan.

14. Lucretia Vaile Museum: Tools of the Trade. The History of Dentistry. www.ci.palmer-lake.co.us/plhs/dentaltools.html.

15. Massachusetts General Hospital. Oral & Maxillofacial Surgery. www.mgh.harvard.edu/oralsurgery/history.htm.

16. Maxillofacial Center. Thomas Emerson Bond, Jr., A.M., M.D. www.maxillofacialcenter.com/BondBook/book/main.html.

17. National Institutes of Health. NIDR Turns 50, Gets New Name. *Press Release, National Institute of Dental Research.* October 22, 1998.

18. PDA International Hall of Fame of Dentistry. Dr. Chapin A. Harris. www.fauchard.org/awards/fame08.htm.

19. Shayne's Dental Site. History of Dentistry. www.dental-site.itgo.com/ancientpeople.htm.

20. The History of Dentistry. www.drteladent.com.

21. Today in Science History. Harvard School of Dental Medicine. www.todayinsci.com.

22. University of Maryland. 2002-2003 Facts & Figures, Baltimore College of Dental Surgery, Dental School. www.umaryland.edu.

23. University of Maryland. Dental School and Dental Hygiene Program. *Student Answer Book.* www.umaryland.edu/student/sab/schools_dental.html.

24. University of Michgan. School of Dentistry. *Dean's Message.* www.dent.umich.edu/about

25. University of Rochester Medical Center. History of the Eastman Dental Center. Web site of *the University of Rochester.*

26. University of Western Ontario. History of Dentistry. *Division of Community Dentistry.* April 2001.

27. U.S. Public Health Service. Oral Health in America: A Report of the Surgeon General. www.nidr.nih.gov/sgr/sgrohweb/home/htm. July 2000.

Case Study: Fluoridation

1. American Academy of Family Physicians. Fluoridation of Public Water Supplies. www.aafp.org/x1585.xml. 2003.

2. American Dental Association. Fluoride and Fluoridation. www.ada.org/public/topics/fluoride/facts-intro.html.

3. American Dental Association. Status of Community: U.S. communities recently voting to adopt fluorida-tion. www.ada.org/goto/fluoride. 2005.

4. Association of State and Territorial Health Officials. Community Water Fluoridation: A State Best Practice in Dental Caries Prevention. January 2003.

5. CDC. Frequently Asked Questions, Water Fluoridation. *Resource Library, National Center for Chronic Disease Prevention and Health Promotion.* March 2002.

6. CDC. Public Health Focus: Fluoridation of Community Water Systems. *MMWR Weekly.* May 29, 1992.

7. CDC. Achievements in Public Health, 1900-1999: Fluoridation of Drinking Water to Prevent Dental Caries. *MMWR Weekly.* October 22, 1999.

8. CDC. Fluoridation Status: Percentage of U.S. population on public water supply systems receiving fluoridated water. *National Oral Health Surveillance System.* http://www2.cdc.gov/nohss/FluoridationV.asp. Last reviewed October 25, 2004.

9. Dyck, Bonnie C., RDH, MPH. Community Water Fluoridation: From the Past Toward the Year 2000. *P&G Dental ResourceNet Archives.*

10. Easley, Dr. Michael W. Fluoridation: A Triumph of Science Over Propaganda. American College of Science and Health, *Priorities for Health.* Volume 8, Number 4, 1996.

11. Easley, Michael W., D.D.S. M.P.H. A Brief History of Community Water Fluoridation in America. State University of New York at Buffalo. 1999.

12. FluorideWorks! Q&A. www.fluorideworks.org/qa.htm.

13. National Institute of Dental and Craniofacial Research. The Story of Fluoridation. www.nidcr.nih.gov/health/fluorideStory.asp.

14. South Africa Department of Health. Water Fluoridation: A manual for water plant operators (Chapter One: Fluoridation and Public Health). Pp. 3-16. www.doh.gov.za.

15. Texas Health Steps (EPSDT-Medicaid). Water Fluoridation Costs in Texas. www.tdh.state.tx.us/dental/dental-txt/flstudy.htm. May 2000.

16. University of Toronto. Directory Record: William Lorne Hutton. www.fis.utoronto.ca/hilscan.

17. World Health Organization. Fluoride in Drinking Water. *Environmental Health Information from* www.who.int.

Vignette: Dental Sealants

1. El-Mowafy, Omar, BDS, PhD, FADM. What if Michael Buonocore Had Been Unsuccessful in His Mission? *Journal of the Canadian Dental Association.* Vol. 69, No. 3, March 2003.

2. Kugel, Gerard, D.M.D., M.S., Ferrari, Marco, M.D., D.D.S., Ph.D. The Science of Bonding: From First to Sixth Generation. *JADA,* Vol. 131, June 2000.

3. P&G DentalResource Net. Pit and Fissure Sealants: The Added Link in Preventive Dentistry.

Looking Ahead: Oral Diseases, Still a Neglected Epidemic

1. Allukian, Myron, Jr., DDS, MPH. The Neglected Epidemic and the Surgeon General's Report: A Call to Action for Better Oral Health. *American Journal of Public Health.* June 2000, Vol. 90, No. 6.

2. Allukian, Myron, Jr., DDS, MPH. *Oral Diseases: The Neglected Epidemic. Principles of Public Health Practice,* Second Edition (Scutchfield, F.D. and Keck, C.W., editors). Pp. 387-408. 2003.

3. American Academy of Pediatric Dentistry, et al. Oral health – integration and collaboration: Testimony for the 2005 Global Health Summit. Philadelphia, Pennsylvania. June 5, 2005.

4. Downs, Martin F. Obese young adults more likely to have gum disease. *Reuters Health/Journal of Periodontology.* June 5, 2003, Vol. 74:610-615.

5. Garrett, Michael, DDS. Role of Dental Public Health Professionals in Community Alliances.

6. Gilbert, Susan. Oral hygiene may help more than teeth and gums. *New York Times.* August 5, 2003.

7. Lewin, Tamar. Universities Learn Value of Neighborliness. *New York Times.* March 12, 2003.

8. McCook, Alison. Experts say babies need dental check at 6 months. *Reuters Health/Pediatrics.* 2003, Vol. 111:1113-1116.

9. National Institute of Dental and Craniofacial Research. Draft Outline – National Oral Health "Call to Action." www.nidcr.nih.gov/scripts.

10. Shulman, Shanna, Kell, Megan, Rosenbach, Margo. SCHIP takes a bite out of the dental access gap for low-income children, Final Report. Centers for Medicare & Medicaid Services (CMS), U.S. Department of Health and Human Services. *Mathematica Policy Research, Inc.* November 16, 2004.

Chapter 10. *Addiction*

Looking Back

1. Amos, Amanda and Haglund, Margaretha. From social taboo to "torch of freedom": The marketing of cigarettes to women. *Tobacco Control.* 2000;9:3-8.

2. Archer, Loran, PhD, Grant, Bridget F., PhD, and Dawson, Deborah A., PhD. What if Americans drank less? The potential effect on the prevalence of alcohol abuse and dependence. *American Journal of Public Health.* January 1995, Vol. 85, No. 1:61-66.

3. Associated Press. National Drug Use Survey Finds Treatment is Rare. *Wall Street Journal Online.* September 5, 2003.

4. Benson, Etienne. A new treatment for addiction. *Monitor on Psychology/APA Online.* Vol. 34, No. 6, June 2003.

5. Bergner, Lawrence, MD, MPH. Cigarettes and the Surgeon General's Report: Letter to the Editor with response from Mark Parascandola, PhD. *American Journal of Public Health.* September 2001, Vol. 91, No. 9:1345.

6. Bondy, Susan, PhD. Alcohol availability and alcoholism: Q&A response to Robert J. Petersen, MD. *JAMA.* December 20, 1995. Vol. 274, No. 23:1832.

7. California Narcotic Officers' Association. Alcohol – A potent drug. *Narcotic Educational Foundation of America.* www.cnoa.org.

8. Carpenter, Siri. Cognition is central to drug addiction. *Monitor on Psychology.* Vol. 32, No. 5, June 2001.

9. CDC. Women and smoking: A Report of the Surgeon General 2001. *National Center for Chronic Disease Prevention and Health Promotion/Tobacco Information and Prevention Source (TIPS).*

10. CDC. Chronology of significant developments related to smoking and health, 1964-2002. *National Center for Chronic Disease Prevention and Health Promotion/TIPS.* www.cdc.gov/tobacco/overview/chron96.htm. Last reviewed December 16, 2003.

11. CDC. Selected actions of the U.S. government regarding regulation of tobacco sales, marketing, and use. *National Center for Chronic Disease Prevention and Health Promotion/TIPS.* www.cdc.gov/tobacco/overview/regulate.htm. Last reviewed March 31, 2003.

12. CDC. Timeline of Tobacco Addiction Milestones by Topic, 1964-2202.

13. CDC. Surgeon General's Reports. *National Center for Chronic Disease Prevention and Health Promotion/TIPS.* www.cdc.gov./tobacco/sgr/index.htm.

14. CDC. Organizations. *National Center for Chronic Disease Prevention and Health Promotion/Taking Action Against Secondhand Smoke.* www.cdc.gov/tobacco/ETS_Toolkit/PublicPlaces/organizations.htm.

15. Courtwright, David T. The hidden epidemic: Opiate addiction and cocaine use in the South, 1860-1920. *Journal of Southern History.* Vol. XLIX, No. 1:57-72, February 1983.

16. Dunlap, Eloise, PhD, and Johnson, Bruce D., PhD. The setting for the Crack Era: Macro forces, micro consequences (1960-1992). *Journal of Psychoactive Drugs.* Vol. 24(4):307-321, Oct-Dec 1992.

17. Ernster, Virginia L., PhD. Mixed messages for women: A social history of cigarette smoking and advertising. *New York State Journal of Medicine.* July 1985.

18. Escamilla, Gina, BA, Cradock, Angie L., MS, and Kawachi, Ichiro, MD, PhD. Women and smoking in Hollywood movies: A content analysis. *American Journal of Public Health.* March 2000, Vol. 90, No. 3:412-414.

19. Fee, Elizabeth et al. The smoke nuisance. *American Journal of Public Health.* June 2002, Vol. 92, No. 6:931.

20. Foster, Susan E., MSW, et al. Alcohol consumption and expenditures for underage drinking and adult excessive drinking. *JAMA.* February 26, 2003, Vol. 289, No. 8:989-995.

21. Hamid, Ansley, PhD. The developmental cycle of a drug epidemic: The cocaine smoking epidemic of 1981-1991. *Journal of Psychoactive Drugs.* Vol. 24(4):337-348, Oct-Dec 1992.

22. Hanson, Glen R., PhD, DDS, and Li, Ting-Kai, MD. Public health implications of excessive alcohol consumption. *JAMA.* February 26, 2003, Vol. 289, No. 8:1031-1032.

23. Hassmiller, Kristen M., MHSA, et al. Nondaily smokers: Who are they? *American Journal of Public Health.* August 2003, Vol. 93, No. 8:1321-1327.

24. Helmuth, Laura. Beyond the Pleasure Principle. *Science.* Vol. 294, November 2, 2001.

25. In the know ZONE. Addiction/Definition of Addiction/Mechanisms of Addiction/Definition of Addiction. www.intheknowzone.com/tobacco/addiction.htm.

26. JustFacts.org. General alcohol info. www.justfacts.org/jf/alcohol/general.asp.

27. JustFacts.org. Alcoholism. www.justfacts.org/jf/alcohol/alcoholism.asp.

28. JustFacts.org. Binge drinking. www.justfacts.org/jf/alcohol/binge.asp.

29. Le, A.D. et al. Nicotine increase alcohol self-administration and reinstates alcohol seeking in rats. *Psychopharmacology,* 168:216-221, 2003.

30. Leshner, Alan I., PhD. What does it mean that addiction is a brain disease? *Monitor on Psychology.* Vol. 32, No. 5, June 2001.

31. MADD Online. Researchers identify alcohol-related genes. www.madd.org/stats.

32. McGrady, Gene A., MD, MPH, and Pederson, Linda L., PhD. Do sex and ethnic differences in smoking initiation mask similarities in cessation behavior? *American Journal of Public Health.* June 2002, Vol. 92, No. 6:961-965.

33. Midanik, Lorraine T., PhD, and Greenfield, Thomas K., PhD. Trends in social consequences and dependence symptoms in the United States: The National Alcohol Surveys, 1984-1995. *American Journal of Public Health.* January 2000, Vol. 90, No. 1:53-56.

34. Musto, David F. Opium, cocaine and marijuana in American history. *Scientific American.* July 1991.

35. National Institute of Drug Abuse. Cigarettes and other nicotine products. *NIDA InfoFacts.* www.drugabuse.gov/Infofax/tobacco.html.

36. National Institute of Drug Abuse. Nicotine Addiction. *NIDA Research Report Series (DHHS and NIH).* July 1998.

37. National Institute of Drug Abuse. Crack and cocaine. *NIDA InfoFacts.* www.nida.nih.gov/Infofax/cocaine.html.

38. Nelson, David E., MD, MPH, et al. State trends in health risk factors and receipt of clinical preventive services among U.S. adults during the 1990s. *JAMA.* May 22-29, 2002, Vol 287, No. 20:2659-2667.

39. NHTSA. Alcohol: How much is too much? www.nhtsa.dot.gov/people/injury/alcohol/alcohol_screening/Brochure.html. July 2002.

40. Nicolaides, Betty M. The state's "sharp line between the sexes": Women, alcohol and the law in the United States, 1850-1980. *Addiction.* 1996; 91 (8):1211-1229.

41. O'Connor, Anahad. New ways to loosen addiction's grip. *New York Times.* August 3, 2004.

42. Parascandola, Mark, PhD. Cigarettes and the U.S. Public Health Service in the 1950s. *American Journal of Public Health.* February 2001, Vol. 91, No. 2:196-205.

43. Picciotto, Marina R. and Corrigall, William A. Neuronal systems underlying behaviors related to nicotine addiction: Neural circuits and molecular genetics. *Journal of Neuroscience.* May 1, 2002, 22(9):3338-3341.

44. SmokeHelp.org. Deadly smoke: Major toxic agents in cigarette smoke. From *"A Report of the Surgeon General, 1989."* www.smokehelp.org/html/smoke.html.

45. White, William A. Psychiatric Symptoms of Opium and Cocaine Use (Historical Note). *Journal of Nervous and Mental Disease.* Vol. 190, No. 2:107, February 2002.

Case Study: Tobacco

1. Action on Smoking and Health. Big Tobacco and Women: What the tobacco industry's confidential files reveal. *Cancer Research Campaign.* November 22, 1998. www.ash.org.uk.

2. American Cancer Society. Anti-smoking efforts reach 40-year milestone. *ACS News Center.* January 11, 2004. www.cancer.org

3. American Journal of Public Health. Entire issue devoted to tobacco and smoking. *APHA.* February 2004.

4. Associated Press. Third-world smoking deaths reach par with rich nations. *Wall Street Journal Online.* September 11, 2003.

5. American Nonsmokers' Rights Foundation. Ordinance Counts Summary: Municipalities with 100% smoke-free workplace and/or restaurant ordinances//Municipalities with 100% smoke-free ordinances//Municipalities with 100% smoke-free freestanding bar ordinances//Municipalities with 100% smoke-free ordinances in all workplaces, restaurants, and bars//Smoking law status in major U.S. travel destinations//Number of ordinances with 100% smoke-free workplaces, restaurants, and bars: Enactment by year. www.no-smoke.org. January 7, 2004.

6. American Psychological Association. Testimony on tobacco policy by Jack E. Henningfield, PhD. *APA Online/Public Policy Office.* June 3, 2003.

7. Barbeau, Elizabeth M., ScD, MPH, et al. Coverage of smoking-cessation treatment by union health and welfare funds. *American Journal of Public Health.* September 2001, Vol. 91, No. 9:1412-1415.

8. Bayer, Ronald, PhD, Gostin, Lawrence O., JD, LLD, Javitt, Gail H., JD, MPH, and Brandt, Allan, PhD. Tobacco advertising in the United States: A proposal for a constitutionally acceptable form of regulation. *JAMA.* June 12, 2002, Vol. 287, No. 22:2990-2995.

9. Brooks, Daniel R., MPH, and Mucci, Lorelei A., MPH. Support for smoke-free restaurants among Massachusetts adults, 1992-1999. *American Journal of Public Health.* February 2001, Vol. 91, No. 2:300-303.

10. Bryan-Jones, Katherine and Bero, Lisa A., PhD. Tobacco industry efforts to defeat Occupational Safety and Health Administration Indoor Air Quality Rule. *American Journal of Public Health.* April 2003, Vol. 93, No. 4:585-592.

11. Business Wire. Nicotine-free cigarettes show promise in new quit-smoking study: One out of three smokers quit using Quest 3. *Business Wire/Gale Group.* October 6, 2003.

12. CDC. Tobacco use in the United States. *National Center for Chronic Disease Prevention and Health Promotion/TIPS.* www.cdc.gov/tobacco/overview/tobus.us.htm.

13. CDC. Annual deaths attributable to cigarette smoking – United States, 1995-1999. *National Center for Chronic Disease Prevention and Health Promotion/TIPS.* www.cdc.gov/tobacco/overview/attrdths.htm.

14. CDC. Cigarette smoking-attributable morbidity – United States, 2000. *MMWR Highlights.* September 5, 2003/Vol. 52/No. 35.

15. CDC. Annual smoking-attributable mortality, years of potential life lost, and economic costs – United States, 1995-1999. *MMWR Highlights.* April 12, 2002, Vol. 51, No. 14.

16. CDC. Office of Smoking and Health (OSH) Summary for 2002. *National Center for Chronic Disease Prevention and Health Promotion/TIPS.* Last reviewed April 11, 2003.

17. CDC. Cigarette smoking among adults – United States, 2001. *MMWR Highlights.* October 10, 2003, Vol. 52, No. 40.

18. CDC. 40th Anniversary of the First Surgeon General's Report on Smoking and Health/Prevalence of cigarette use among 14 racial/ethnic populations – United States, 1999-2001. *MMWR.* January 30, 2004, Vol. 53, No. 3.

19. CDC. State-specific prevalence of current cigarette smoking among adults – United States, 2002. *MMWR Highlights.* January 9, 2004/Vol. 52/No. 53.

20. CDC. Trends in current cigarette smoking by grade in school – United States, 1975-2001. *National Center for Chronic Disease Prevention and Health Promotion/Tobacco Information and Prevention Source (TIPS).* www.cdc.gov/tobacco/research_data/youth/smkne.htm.

21. CDC. Tobacco use among middle and high school students – United States, 2002 (MMWR Highlights). *National Center for Chronic Disease Prevention and Health Promotion/Tobacco Information and Prevention Source (TIPS).* www.cdc.gov/tobacco/reserach_data/youth/mmwr5245_highlights.htm.

22. CDC. Preventing chronic diseases: Investing wisely in health/Preventing tobacco use. *CDC Chronic Disease Prevention.* Revised April 2003.

23. CDC. Targeting tobacco use: The nation's leading cause of death 2003. *CDC At a Glance.* Revised June 2003.

24. CDC. Nebraska/Implementing a comprehensive tobacco control program to reduce tobacco use. *Tobacco Free Nebraska Program.* www.cdc.gov/tobacco/index.htm.

25. CDC. Oregon/Reaching target groups with high rates of tobacco use through comprehensive tobacco control: A policy-based approach. *Oregon Tobacco Prevention and Education program.* www.cdc.gov/tobacco/index.htm.

26. CDC. Washington/Identifying and eliminating disparities in tobacco use through a cross-cultural workshop. *Washington State Department of Health.* www.cdc.gov/tobacco/index.htm.

27. CDC. Sports initiatives – tobacco-free sports. *National Center for Chronic Disease Prevention and Health Promotion/TIPS.* www.cdc.gov/tobacco/sports_initiatives_splash.htm. Last reviewed October 23, 2003.

28. CDC. Campaigns & Events. *National Center for Chronic Disease Prevention and Health Promotion/TIPS.* www.cdc.gov/tobacco/campaigns_events.htm. Last reviewed September 23, 2003.

29. CDC. 2004 Tobacco Control Media Event Calendar. *National Center for Chronic Disease Prevention and Health Promotion/TIPS.* www.cdc.gov/tobacco/calendar/calendar.htm. Last reviewed January 14, 2004.

30. CDC. January 11, 2004, marks the 40th anniversary of the inaugural Surgeon General's Report on Smoking and Health. *National Center for Chronic Disease Prevention and Health Promotion/TIPS.* www.cdc.gov/tobacco/overview/anniversary.htm. Page last reviewed January 29, 2004.

31. CDC. Prevalence of current cigarette smoking among adults and changes in prevalence of current and some day smoking – United States, 1996-2001. *MMWR.* August 11, 2003, Vol. 52, No.14:303-307.

32. CDC. New guidelines challeng all clinicians to help smokers quit. *National Center for Chronic Disease Prevention and Health Promotion/TIPS.* June 27, 2000.

33. CDC. State Medicaid coverage for tobacco-dependence treatments – United States, 1994-2002. *MMWR Highlights.* January 30, 2004, Vol. 53, No. 3.

34. CDC. Point-of-purchase tobacco environments and variation by store type – United States, 1999. *MMWR Highlights* March 8, 2002, Vol. 51, No. 9.

35. CDC. Domestic cigarette advertising and promotional expenses – United States, 1963-1994. *National Center for Chronic Disease Prevention and Health Promotion/TIPS.* Last reviewed March 25, 2003.

36. CDC. An online tool kit: What is secondhand smoke? *National Center for Chronic Disease Prevention and Health Promotion/Taking Action Against Secondhand Smoke.* www.cdc.gov/tobacco/ETS_Toolkit/index.htm.

37. Fagan, Pebbles, PhD, MPH, et al. Eliminating tobacco-related health disparities: Directions for future research. *American Journal of Public Health.* February 2004, Vol. 94, No. 2:211-217.

38. Federal Trade Commission. Cigarette report for 1999. www.ftc.gov/opa/2002/03/cigarette.htm. March 13, 2001.

39. Federal Trade Commission. Report to Congress for 1998 pursuant to the Federal Cigarette Labeling and Advertising Act. www.ftc.gov/opa/2000/06/cig98.htm. June 27, 2000.

40. Federal Trade Commission. Report to Congress for 1997 pursuant to the Federal Cigarette Labeling and Advertising Act. www.ftc.gov/opa/1999/07/cig-97.htm. July 28, 1999.

41. Federal Trade Commission. FTC Report to Congress shows increases in smokeless tobacco revenues and advertising and promotional expenditures. *Press Release.* August 12, 2003.

42. Fichtenberg, Caroline M., MS, and Glantz, Stanton A., PhD. Association of the California tobacco control program with declines in cigarette consumption and mortality from heart disease. *New England Journal of Medicine.* December 14, 2000, Vol. 343, No. 24:1772-1777.

43. Fiore, Michael C., MD, MPH, et al. Preventing 3 million premature deaths and helping 5 million smokers quit: A National action plan for tobacco cessation. *American Journal of Public Health.* February 2004, Vol. 94, No. 2:205-210.

44. Folsom, Aaron R., MD, MPH, and Watson, Robert L., DVM, PhD, MPH. Estimating the numbers of smoking-related deaths. *JAMA.* November 8, 2000, Vol. 284, No. 18:2319-2321.

45. Givel, Michael, PhD, and Glantz, Stanton A., PhD. The "Global Settlement" with the tobacco industry: 6 years later. *American Journal of Public Health.* February 2004, Vol. 94, No. 2:218-224.

46. Glantz, Stanton A., PhD. An evaluation of: The impact of nonsmoking ordinances on restaurant financial performance, Deloitte & Touche LLP, Washington, D.C. *University of California, San Francisco.* October 2003.

47. Gross, Cary P., MD, et al. State expenditures for tobacco-control programs and the tobacco settlement. *New England Journal of Medicine.* October 3, 2002, Vol. 347, No. 14:1080-1086.

48. Healthy People 2010. Tobacco Use. www.healthypeople.gov.

49. Hoag, Christina. Anti-smoking push loses most of budget. *Miami Herald.* May 29, 2003.

50. Houston, Thomas, MD, and Kaufman, Nancy J., RN, MS. Tobacco control in the 21st century: Searching for answers in a sea of change. *JAMA.* August 9, 2000, Vol. 284, No. 6:752-753.

51. Kahn, Robert S., MD, MPH, Certain, Laura, BA, and Whitaker, Robert C., MD, MPH. A re-examination of smoking before, during, and after pregnancy. *American Journal of Public Health.* November 2002, Vol. 92, No. 11:1801-1808.

52. Kaufman, Marc. Surgeon General Favors Tobacco Ban. *Washington Post.* June 4, 2003.

53. Lasser, Karen, MD, et al. Smoking and mental illness: A population-based prevalence study. *JAMA.* November 22/29, 2000, Vol. 284, No. 20:2606-2610.

54. Magzamen, Sheryl, MPH, and Glantz, Stanton A., PhD. The new battleground: California's experience with smoke-free bars. *American Journal of Public Health.* February 2001, Vol. 91, No. 2:245-252.

55. Morrison, Alan B., BA, LLB. Counteracting cigarette advertising. *JAMA.* June 12, 2001, Vol. 287, No. 22.

56. New York State Department of Health. Cigarette use by youth in New York State. *Fact Sheet.* Revised October 2003. www.health.state.ny.us/nysdoh/tobacco/reports/trends/youth_cigarette_use.htm.

57. New York State Department of Health. Trends in cigarette use by youth in New York State: Youth tobacco survey 2000-2202. Revised October 2003. www.health.state.ny.us/nysdoh/tobacco/reports/trends/youth_tobacco_survey_2000-2002.htm.

58. New York State Department of Health. New York anti-smoking campaign recognized as one of the largest in the nation. *DOH News From the Commissioner.* February 16, 2001.

59. New York State Department of Health. Cigarette smoking among adults – New York State 2000. *Tobacco.* April 2003.

60. New York State Department of Health. Smokers quitline makes dramatic strides in the fight against smoking in New York State. *DOH News From the Commissioner.* April 2001.

61. New York State Department of Health. Secondhand smoke – it takes your breath away. *Info for Consumers.* www.health.state.ny.us/nysdoh/smoking/second/second.htm.

62. New York State Department of Health. A Guide to the New York State Clean Indoor Air Act//Regulation of smoking in public and work places: Effective July 24, 2003. *Clean Indoor Air Act.* www.health.state.ny.us/nysdoh/clean_indoor_air_act/general.htm.

63. New York State Department of Health. State Health Department announces new toll-free info line and Web site information for tomorrow's implementation of the Clean Indoor Air Act. *DOH News From the Commissioner.* July 2003.

64. Parker-Pope, Tara. Getting "Smober": Smokers Seeking to Quit Find Some Help on the Web. *Wall Street Journal Online.* April 22, 2003.

65. Pickett, Kate E., PhD, et al. Coverage of tobacco dependence treatments for pregnant smokers in Health Maintenance Organizations. *American Journal of Public Health.* September 2001, Vol. 91, No. 9:1393-1394.

66. PR Newswire. American Cancer Society reminds women who smoke – Lung cancer more deadly than breast cancer, as part of its women's health celebrations during Breast Cancer Awareness Month. *PR Newswire Association, Inc./Gale Group.* October 6, 2003.

67. PR Newswire. Smokers with breast cancer twice as likely to die than nonsmokers. *PR Newswire Association, Inc./Gale Group.* October 20, 2003.

68. PR Newswire. Lung cancer screening motivates smokers to quit. *PR Newswire Association, Inc./Gale Group.* October 31, 2003.

69. PR Newswire. More than 6,000 Pennsylvania residents use effective stop-smoking program in first year of operation; American Cancer Society's Great American Smokeout November 20. *PR Newswire Association, Inc./Gale Group.* November 12, 2003.

70. PR Newswire. More smokers quit with help from Wisconsin quit line; $7 million saved in healthcare costs. *PR Newswire Association, Inc./Gale Group.* October 14, 2003.

71. PR Newswire. NYC firefighters and EMS workers go tobacco-free; Fire Department New York tobacco-cessation program shows 40 percent quit rate at 6 months. *PR Newswire Association, Inc./Gale Group.* October 29, 2003.

72. PR Newswire. Nation's leading smoking-cessation provider become independent; expansion of infrastructure and service will meet growing demand. *PR Newswire Association, Inc./Gale Group.* November 12, 2003.

73. PR Newswire. Statewide ads to promote Quitplan stop-smoking programs; ads show smokers a better way to quit than by themselves. *PR Newswire Association, Inc./Gale Group.* November 10, 2003.

74. Rohrbach, Louise Ann, PhD, MPH, et al. Independent evaluation of the California Tobacco Control Program: Relationships between program exposure and outcomes, 1996-1998. *American Journal of Public Health.* June 2002, Vol. 92, No. 6:975-983.

75. Schroeder, Steven A., MD. Tobacco control in the wake of the 1998 Master Settlement Agreement. *New England Journal of Medicine.* January 15, 2004, 350;3:293-301.

76. Skeer, Margie, MSW, MPH et al. Town-level characteristics and smoking-policy adoption in Massachusetts: Are local restaurant smoking regulations fostering disparities in health protection? *American Journal of Public Health.* February 2004, Vol. 94, No. 2:286-292.

77. Sturm, Roland. The effects of obesity, smoking, and drinking on medical problems and costs. *Health Affairs.* March/April 2002.

78. Tang, Hao, MD, PhD, et al. Changes in attitudes and patronage behaviors in response to a smoke-free bar law. *American Journal of Public Health.* April 2003, Vol. 93, No. 4:611-617.

79. Taylor, Donald H., Jr., PhD, et al. Benefits of smoking cessation for longevity. *American Journal of Public Health*. June 2002, Vol. 92, No. 6:990-996.

80. Tsoukalas, Theodore, PhD, and Glantz, Stanton A., PhD. The Duluth Clean Indoor Air Ordinance: Problems and success in fighting the tobacco industry at the local level in the 21st century. *American Journal of Public Health*. August 2003, Vol. 93, No. 8:1214-1221.

81. U.S. Department of Health and Human Services. *Reducing Tobacco Use: A Report of the Surgeon General*. Atlanta, Georgia: U.S. Department of Health and Human Services, Centers for Disease Control and Prevention, National Center for Chronic Disease Prevention and Health Promotion, Office on Smoking and Health, 2000.

82. U.S. Environmental Protection Agency. Health Effects. *Smoke-free homes*. www.epa.gov/smokefree/healthrisks.html.

83. U.S. Environmental Protection Agency. Fact Sheet: Respiratory health effects of passive smoking. *Indoor Air – Secondhand Smoke*. www.epa.gov/iaq/pubs/etsfs.html.

84. U.S. Environmental Protection Agency. Setting the record straight: Secondhand smoke is a preventable health risk. *Indoor Air – Secondhand Smoke*. www.epa.gov/iaq/pubs/strsfs.html.

85. U.S. Environmental Protection Agency. What you can do about secondhand smoke as parents, decision-makers, and building occupants. *Indoor Air – Secondhand Smoke*. www.epa.gov/iaq/pubs/etsbro.html.

86. U.S. Public Health Service. Treating Tobacco Use and Dependence – Clinician's Packet/A How-To Guide for Implementing the Public Health Service Clinical Practice Guideline. www.surgeongeneral.gov/tobacco/clinpack.html. March 2003.

87. U.S. Public Health Service. Achievements in Tobacco-Cessation Case Studies. www.surgeongenerl.gov/tobacco/smcasest.htm.

88. Wakschlag, Lauren S., PhD, et al. Maternal smoking during pregnancy and severe antisocial behavior in off-spring: A review. *American Journal of Public Health*. June 2002, Vol. 92, No. 6:966-974.

Vignette: Mothers Against Drunk Driving (MADD)

1. Amednews.com. NBC's liquor advertisements: A network drunk on greed (editorial). www.ama-assn.org/amednews. January 28, 2002.

2. Amednews.com. A win for health and safety: NBC wisely puts the lid back on hard liquor ads (editorial). www.ama-assn.org/amednews. April 15, 2002.

3. Aversa, Jeannine. Alcohol ads touting health benefits must also warn of risks, government says. *Detroit News*. March 1, 2003.

4. Insurance Institute for Highway Safety. Q&A: Alchohol: General/Administrative License Suspension/Deterrence & Enforcement www.highwaysafety.org/safety_facts/qanda/alcohol_general.htm, etc. As of June 2003.

5. JustFacts.org. Drinking & Driving. www.justfacts.org/jf/alcohol/laws.asp Lord, Janice. Really MADD: Looking Back at 20 years. *Driven magazine*. Spring 2000. www.madd.org/aboutus

6. Leads from the Morbidity and Mortality Weekly Report, CDC. Safety-belt use among drivers involved in alcohol-related fatal motor-vehicle crashes – United States, 1982-1989. *JAMA*. July 10, 1991, Vol 266, No. 2.

7. MADD. About Us/MADD timeline/MADD milestones 1980-2003. www.madd.org.

8. MADD. What is MADD's position on liquor advertising on television? www.madd.org/aboutus.

9. MADD. Who founded MADD? www.madd.org/aboutus.

10. MADD. Kentucky bus crash: A legacy of hope. *Driven*. Spring 1998. www.madd.org/aboutus.

11. MADD. Stats & Resources/Statistics/General Statistics/Did you know. www.madd.org/stats.

12. MADD. BAC and impairment/Number of drinks and BAC in two hours of drinking/Relative fatality risk for drivers in single-vehicle crashes by BAC/Drunk driving in the United States. www.madd.org/stats.

13. MADD. NADS awarded $2.9 million for alcohol and driver performance research. *Press Release*. December 31, 2002.

14. NHTSA. The economic impact of motor vehicle crashes 2000. www.nhtsa.dot.gov/people/economic/EconImpact2000/summary.htm.

15. NHTSA. 2001 National Survey of Drinking and Driving, Volume 1, Summary Report. *U.S. Department of Transportation*. Report No. DOT HS 809 549. June 2003.

16. NHTSA. Alcohol and Highway Safety 2001: A review of the state of knowledge; Executive Summary. *U.S. Department of Transportation*.

17. NHTSA. Open Container Laws. Traffic Safety Facts: Laws. *U.S. Department of Transportation*. Volume 1, Number 1, May 2003.

18. NHTSA. Impaired driving in the United States. *U.S. Department of Transportation*. www.nhtsa.dot.gov/people/injury/alcohol/impaired_driving_pg2/US.htm.

19. NHTSA. USDOT releases 2002 highway fatality statistics. *U.S. Department of Transportation Press Release* (NHTSA 32-03). July 17, 2003.

20. NHTSA/NCSA. Traffic Safety Facts 2002: Overview/Older Population/Alcohol. *National Center for Statistics & Analysis*. DOT HS 809 612/611/606.

21. NHTSA/NIAAA. Sentencing and dispositions of youth DUI and other alcohol offenses: A guide for judges and prosecutors; III. The Laws. www.nhtsa.dot.gov/people/injury/alcohol/youthdui/section3.html.

22. Wald, Matthew L. Senate version of bill pushes states to adopt stiff drunken driving penalties. *New York Times.* June 17, 2005.

Looking Ahead: Fighting Addiction in Young Women

1. Alcohol Policies Project. CSPI backs FTC actions on alcohol ads. *Center for Science in the Public Interest Press Release.* August 7, 1998.

2. Barrett, Devlin. Study: Girls more easily addicted to drugs. *Associated Press.* February 5, 2003.

3. Biener, Lois, PhD, and Albers, Alison B., PhD. Young adults: Vulnerable new targets of tobacco marketing. *American Journal of Public Health.* February 2004, Vol. 94, No. 2:326-330.

4. Business Wire. Baseball's "Mr. October" Reggie Jackson returns to the World Series to turn kids into C.H.A.M.P.S.S. *Business Wire/Gale Group.* October 22, 2003.

5. CNN. Report: Philip Morris polled teens on smoking. www.cnn.com/HEALTH/9612/15/youth.smoking/index.html. December 15, 1996.

6. Curie, Charles G., M.A., A.C.S.W. and Clark, H. Westley, M.D., J.D., M.P.H. "Dear Physician" letter concerning opioid addiction treatment. *Substance Abuse and Mental Health Services Administration, U.S. Department of Health and Human Services.* Received February 10, 2003.

7. CASA. 2001 Annual Report: A drug-free future begins here. *The National Center on Addiction and Substance Abuse at Columbia University.*

8. CASA. Big differences in why girls vs boys use cigarettes, alcohol and drugs; consequences swifter and harsher for girls – CASA's new report call for nationwide overhaul in prevention and treatment programs. *Press Release, The National Center on Addiction and Substance Abuse at Columbia University.* February 5, 2003.

9. CASA. CASAInside. *The National Center on Addiction and Substance Abuse at Columbia University* Spring, 2002.

10. CASA. The Formative Years: Pathways to substance abuse among girls and young women aged 8-22 (with accompanying statement by Joseph A. Califano, Jr., chairman and president). *The National Center on Addiction and Substance Abuse at Columbia University.* February 2003.

11. CASA. Warning signs and times of increased risk for substance abuse among girls and young women.

12. CDC. Minnesota: Reducing tobacco use among teenagers through a comprehensive tobacco-control program. *Minnesota Department of Health.* www.cdc.gov/tobacco/index.htm.

13. Center on Alcohol Marketing and Youth. Raised on radio: Underage youth more likely to hear alcohol ads on radio than adults. *Press Release.* January 22, 2004.

14. Ellickson, Phyllis L., PhD, et al. From adolescence to young adulthood: Racial/ethnic disparities in smoking. *American Journal of Public Health.* February 2004, Vol. 94, No. 2:293-299.

15. Elliott, Victoria Stagg. AMA wants to ban booze ads aimed at teens. *Amednews.com.* January 13, 2003.

16. Federal Trade Commission. FTC report cites improvements in alcohol industry self-regulation. *Press Release.* September 9, 2003.

17. Hays, Constance L. Philip Morris assembles $100 million anti-smoking program aimed at teens. *New York Times.* December 3, 1998.

18. Healthy People 2010. Tobacco use objective 7-2. "Increase the proportion of middle, junior high, and senior high schools that provide…." www.healthypeople.gov/document/html/objectives/07-02.htm.

19. Helfand, William H., Lazarus, Jan, and Theerman, Paul. The "truth" tobacco memorial. *American Journal of Public Health.* February 2001, Vol. 91, No. 2:195.

20. Hingson, Ralph W., Sc.D. et al. Magnitude of alcohol-related mortality and morbidity among U.S. college students aged 18-24. *Journal of Studies on Alcohol.* March 2002.

21. Kiefe, Catarina I., PhD, MD. et al. Ten-year changes in smoking among young adults: Are racial differences explained by socioeconomic factors in the CARDIA study? *American Journal of Public Health.* February 2001, Vol. 91, No. 2:213-218.

22. Landers, Peter. Why treating addicts is tough play for drug firms. *Wall Street Journal Online.* April 28, 2003.

23. Landman, Anne, BA, Ling, Pamela M., MD, MPH, and Glantz, Stanton A., PhD. Tobacco industry youth-smoking prevention programs: Protecting the industry and hurting tobacco control. *Forum on Youth Smoking/American Journal of Public Health.* June 2002, Vol. 92, No. 6:917-930.

24. Levy, David T., PhD, Cummings, K. Michael, PhD, and Hyland, Andrew, PhD. A simulation of the effects of youth initiation policies on overall cigarette use. *American Journal of Public Health.* August 2000, Vol. 90, No. 8:1311-1314.

25. MADD. CASA Report on underage drinking. www.madd.org/stats.

26. MADD Online. Why 21? www.madd.org/stats.

27. MADD Online. Age of first use of alcohol. www.madd.org/stats.

28. MADD Online. Youth statistics. www.madd.org/stats.

29. Marcus, Adam. Magazines shower teens with alcohol ads. *ABC News/HealthScoutNews.* May 14, 2003.

30. McGough, Robert. The growing brain may make teens more prone to addiction. *Wall Street Journal Online.* June 19, 2003.

31. Miller, Ted R., Ph.D. The Limiting Factor: economic costs of underage drinking. *Driven.* Fall 1999. www.madd.org/stats.

32. Mowery, Paul D., MA, et al. Progression to established smoking among U.S. youths. *American Journal of Public Health.* February 2004, Vol. 94, No. 2:331-337.

33. Nagourney, Eric. Perceptions: When Ads Work Too Well. *New York Times.* July 22, 2003.

34. Niederdeppe, Jeff, MA, Farrelly, Matthew C., PhD, and Haviland, M. Lyndon, DrPH. Confirming "truth": More evidence of a successful tobacco countermarketing campaign in Florida. *American Journal of Public Health.* February 2004, Vol. 94, No. 2:255-256.

35. New York State Department of Health. State awards $4.4 million in youth-empowerment grants. *DOH News From the Commissioner.* April 17, 2001.

36. New York State Department of Health. A Guide for Tobacco Merchants: Retail tobacco dealers and New York's youth access tobacco control laws. *Info for Consumers.* www.health.state.ny.us/nysdoh/smoking/tobguide.htm. Effective October 21, 2002.

37. New York State Department of Health. A Guide for Tobacco Merchants: Vending machines and New York's youth access tobacco control laws. *Info for Consumers.* www.health.state.ny.us/nysdoh/smoking/vendmach.htm. Effective October 21, 2002.

38. New York State Department of Health. State Health Department issues enforcement actions against tobacco vendors selling to minors. *DOH News From the Commissioner.* March 2, 2001.

39. NHTSA. Alcohol beverage control enforcement: Legal research report. *Pacific Institute for Research and Evaluation.* April 2003.

40. PR Newswire. Tobacco use common in schools demonstrating poor academic performance; Tobacco experimentation more prevalent in asthmatic children than nonasthmatics. *Tobacco Dependence Category Overview, Gale Group.* November 2003.

41. PR Newswire. Missouri receives "F" for failing to meet nation's goals to reduce smoking among women and girls. *PR Newswire Association, Inc./Gale Group.* October 6, 2003.

42. Reuters Health. More alcohol ads in magazines with teen readers. http://myhealth.memorialmedical.com/HealthNews/reuters. May 13, 2003.

43. Schwartzwelder, Scott, PhD. Brain 101. *Driven.* Fall 1998. www.madd.org/stats.

44. ScienCentralNews. Alcohol and Ads. *ScienCentral, Inc.* February 5, 2004. www.sciencentral.com.

45. Sly, David F., PhD, Hopkins, Richard S., MD, MSPH, Trapido, Edward, ScD, and Ray, Sarah, MA. Influence of a counteradvertising media campaign on initiation of smoking: The Florida "truth" campaign. *American Journal of Public Health.* February 2001, Vol. 91, No. 2:233-238.

46. Tapert, Susan F., PhD et al. Neural responses to alcohol stimuli in adolescents with alcohol-use disorder. *Archives of General Psychiatry.* Vol. 60, No. 7, July 2003.

47. Teinowitz, Ira. Alcohol marketers change ad guidelines: To buy ads in media reaching a 70% adult audience. *AdAge.com.* September 9, 2003.

48. Thomas, Karen. Report: Teen girls big alcohol consumers. *USA Today.* February 27, 2002.

49. Toomey, Traci L., Ph.D. and Wagenaar, Alexander C., Ph.D. Environmental policies to reduce college drinking: Options and research findings. *Journal of Studies on Alcohol.* Supplement No. 14:193-205, 2002.

Chapter 11. *U.S. Public Health Infrastructure*

Looking Back

1. CDC Office of the Director, Epidemiology Program Office. Achievements in Public Health, 1900-1999: Changes in the Public Health System. *JAMA* (2000;283:735-738) and *MMWR* (1999;48:1141-1147).

2. Grant-Makers Health. Strengthening the public health system for a healthier future. Issue brief No.17 February 2003. www.gih.org.

3. Kinney, Eleanor D. The Evolution of Public Health Regulation. http://academic.udayton.edu/health/syllabi/Bioterrorism/4PHealthLaw/PHLaw00k.htm.

4. Klaucke DN, Buehler JW, Thacker SB, et al. Guidelines for evaluating surveillance systems. *MMWR.* 1988; 37(s-5):1-18.

5. U.S. Department of Health and Human Services, Centers for Disease Control and Prevention. Public Health's Infrastructure: A Status Report Prepared for the Appropriations Committee of the United States Senate. www.phppo.cdc.gov/documents/phireport2_16.pdf.

6. U.S. Public Health Service. A Proud Past, a Healthy Future. www.osophs.dhhs.gov/phs200.

Case Study: The Creation of CDC

1. CDC Office of the Director. Futures Initiative: Creating the future of CDC in the 21st century. www.cdc.gov/futures/od_options/od_faq.htm. *MMWR.* 1996;45:526-528.

2. Etheridge, Elizabeth W., Ph.D. From her book, Sentinel for Health: A History of the Centers for Disease Control. University of California Press (Berkeley, Calif.). 1992.

3. Gerberding, Julie L., MD, MPH. CDC's Role in Promoting Healthy Lifestyles. Testimony of the CDC Director Before the U.S. Senate Committee on Appropriations, Subcommittee on Labor, HHS, Education and Related Agencies. February 17, 2003.

4. www.uic.edu/sph/prepare/courses/ph410/resources/cdchistory.htm.

Vignette: The Surgeon General Report of 1964

1. CDC. 40th Anniversary of the First Surgeon General's Report on Smoking and Health. *MMWR*. 2004; 53:49.
2. CDC. History of the 1964 Surgeon General's Report on Smoking and Health. http://www.cdc.gov/tobacco/30yrsgen.htm.
3. CDC. January 11, 2004, Marks the 40th Anniversary of the Inaugural Surgeon General's Report on Smoking and Health. *Press Release.*
4. Fee, Elizabeth and Brown, Theodore M. The Unfulfilled Promise of Public Health: Déjà Vu All Over Again. *Health Affairs*. November-December 2002, Vol. 21, No. 6:32-34.
5. McMillen, Robert C., PhD, et al. Smoking in America: 35 Years after the Surgeon General's Report: A Report on the 2000 National Social Climate Survey. *Tobacco Control. Surveys and Program Evaluations* (Paper NSC1). http://repositories.cdlib.org/tc/surveys/NSC1. November 1, 2000.
6. U.S. Department of Health and Human Services. Luther Leonidas Terry (1961-1965). www.surgeongeneral.gov/library/history/bioterry.htm.
7. U.S. National Library of Medicine. http://profiles.nlm.nih.gov/NN/Views/Exhibit/narrative/system.html
8. U.S. National Library of Medicine. Changing Conceptions of Public Health. http://profiles.nlm.nih.gov/NN/Views/Exhibit/narrative/conceptn.html.
9. U.S. National Library of Medicine. The 1964 Report on Smoking and Health. http://profiles.nlm.nih.gov/NN/Views/Exhibit/narrative/smoking.html.

Looking Ahead: Public Health - A 21st Century Perspective

1. Altman, Lawrence K., MD. A public health quandary: When should the public be told? *New York Times*. February 15, 2005.
2. Altman, Lawrence K., MD. Rising from the ranks to lead the WHO *New York Times*. July 22, 2003.
3. Barclay, Laurie, MD. Vision to restore the American health system: A newsmaker interview with Floyd E. Bloom, MD. *Medscape Medical News*. February 14, 2003.
4. Boufford, Jo Ivey, and Lee, Phillip R. Health Policies for the 21st Century: Challenges and Recommendations for the U.S. Department of Health and Human Services September 2001. www.milbank.org/010910healthpolicies.html.
5. CDC & Health Resources and Services Administration. www.cdc.gov/programs/bt01.htm.
6. CDC. Anthrax: What You Need To Know. Emergency Preparedness and Control. www.bt.cdc.gov/agent/anthrax/needtoknow.asp.
7. CDC. Programs in Brief. www.cdc.gov/programs/chronic.htm.
8. CDC. Youth Media Campaign. www.cdc.gov/youthcampaign/index.htm.
9. Center for Nonproliferation Studies at the Monterey Institute of International Studies. Glossary. www.nti.org/e_research/e6_glossary.html
10. Chang M, Glynn MK, Groseclose SL. Endemic, notifiable bioterrorism-related diseases, United States, 1992-1999. *Emerging Infectious Diseases*. May 2003.
11. Fauci, Anthony S. Infectious Diseases: Considerations for the 21st Century. National Institute of Allergy and Infectious Diseases, National Institutes of Health (Bethesda, MD).
12. Grady, Denise, and Altman, Lawrence K. Experts see gains and gaps in planning for terror attack. *New York Times*. March 25, 2003.
13. Grady, Denise. Learning the science of leading. *New York Times*. July 15, 2003.
14. Harrell, James A., Baker, Edward L., MD, MPH, and the Essential Services Work Group. The Essential Services of Public Health. American Public Health Association. www.apha.org/ppp/science/10ES.htm.
15. Herper, Matthew. Bush aims biotech at bioterror. *Forbes*. January 29, 2003.
16. Orleans, C. Tracy, PhD. *Press Release,* American Journal of Health Promotion. December 20, 1999.
17. Public Health Functions Steering Committee. Public Health in America. Fall 1994. www.health.gov/phfunctions/public.htm. January 1, 2000.
18. Titmuss, Richard M. *Social Policy: An Introduction*. Pantheon Books (New York). 1974.